AUTISM SPECTRUM DISORDER IN THE FIRST YEARS OF LIFE

Also Available

Asperger Syndrome, Second Edition
*Edited by James C. McPartland, Ami Klin,
and Fred R. Volkmar*

Autism Spectrum Disorder in the First Years of Life

Research, Assessment, and Treatment

Edited by
Katarzyna Chawarska
Fred R. Volkmar

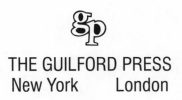

THE GUILFORD PRESS
New York   London

The authors have checked with sources believed to be reliable in their efforts
to provide information that is complete and generally in accord with the
standards of practice that are accepted at the time of publication. However,
in view of the possibility of human error or changes in behavioral, mental
health, or medical sciences, neither the authors, nor the editors and publisher,
nor any other party who has been involved in the preparation or publication
of this work warrants that the information contained herein is in every
respect accurate or complete, and they are not responsible for any errors or
omissions or the results obtained from the use of such information. Readers
are encouraged to confirm the information contained in this book with other
sources.

Library of Congress Cataloging-in-Publication Data

Names: Chawarska, Katarzyna, editor. | Volkmar, Fred R., editor.
Title: Autism spectrum disorder in the first years of life : research,
    assessment, and treatment / edited by Katarzyna Chawarska and Fred R.
    Volkmar.
Description: New York : The Guilford Press, [2020] | Includes
    bibliographical references and index. |
Identifiers: LCCN 2020012272 | ISBN 9781462543236 (hardcover)
Subjects: LCSH: Autism spectrum disorders in children.
Classification: LCC RJ506.A9 A923744 2020 | DDC 618.92/85882—dc23
LC record available at https://lccn.loc.gov/2020012272

About the Editors

Katarzyna Chawarska, PhD, is Emily Fraser Beede Professor of Child Psychiatry in the Child Study Center at Yale University School of Medicine. She is Director of the Social and Affective Neuroscience of Autism Program and the Infant and Toddler Developmental Disabilities Clinic. Dr. Chawarska is a leading expert on identifying early prognostic markers and novel treatment targets in autism spectrum disorder (ASD). Her recent work focuses on improving understanding of attentional and affective processes involved in development of core and comorbid features in ASD, as well as investigating the links between development of brain connectivity during prenatal and early neonatal periods and later outcomes in infants at risk for ASD.

Fred R. Volkmar, MD, is Goodwin Endowed Chair of Special Education (part time) at Southern Connecticut State University and Irving B. Harris Professor of Child Psychiatry, Pediatrics, and Psychology (part time) in the Child Study Center at Yale University School of Medicine. He has served as Director of the Child Study Center as well as Chief of Child Psychiatry at Yale–New Haven Hospital. Dr. Volkmar was the primary author of the American Psychiatric Association's DSM-IV autism and pervasive developmental disorders section. He has published several hundred scientific papers and chapters as well as a number of books, including *Asperger Syndrome, Second Edition; Healthcare for Children on the Autism Spectrum; Handbook of Autism and Pervasive Developmental Disorders, Fourth Edition; Encyclopedia of Autism*; and, most recently, *Autism and Pervasive Developmental Disorders, Third Edition*. He serves as Editor of the *Journal of Autism and Developmental Disorders*.

Contributors

Amina Abubakar, PhD, KEMRI–Wellcome Trust Research Programme, Kilifi, Kenya, and Institute for Human Development, Aga Khan University, Nairobi, Kenya

Adham Atyabi, PhD, Department of Computer Science, University of Colorado, Colorado Springs, Colorado, and Center for Child Health, Behavior, and Development, Seattle Children's Research Institute, Seattle, Washington

Jessica Bradshaw, PhD, Department of Psychology, University of South Carolina, Columbia, South Carolina

Ludivine Brunissen, BS, Yale Child Study Center, Yale School of Medicine, New Haven, Connecticut

Emily Campi, BS, University of Southern California Mrs. T. H. Chan Division of Occupational Science and Occupational Therapy, Los Angeles, California

Katarzyna Chawarska, PhD, Yale Child Study Center, Yale School of Medicine, New Haven, Connecticut

Petrus J. de Vries, PhD, Division of Child and Adolescent Psychiatry, University of Cape Town, Cape Town, South Africa

Kelsey Jackson Dommer, MS, Center for Child Health, Behavior, and Development, Seattle Children's Research Institute, Seattle, Washington

Jed T. Elison, PhD, Institute of Child Development, University of Minnesota, Minneapolis, Minnesota

Joseph K. Gona, PhD, Neuroscience Unit, KEMRI–Wellcome Trust Research Programme, Kilifi, Kenya

Jonathan Green, MD, Manchester Academic Health Sciences Centre, University of Manchester, and Royal Manchester Children's Hospital, Manchester, United Kingdom

Rebecca Grzadzinski, PhD, Carolina Institute for Developmental Disabilities, University of North Carolina at Chapel Hill, Chapel Hill, North Carolina

Connie Kasari, PhD, Department of Human Development and Psychology, Graduate School of Education and Information Studies, University of California, Los Angeles, Los Angeles, California

Julie A. Kientz, PhD, Department of Human Centered Design and Engineering, University of Washington, Seattle, Washington

Catherine Lord, PhD, David Geffen School of Medicine, University of California, Los Angeles, and Semel Institute of Neuroscience and Human Behavior, Los Angeles, California

Megan Lyons, MS, Yale Child Study Center, Yale School of Medicine, New Haven, Connecticut

Suzanne L. Macari, PhD, Yale Child Study Center, Yale School of Medicine, New Haven, Connecticut

Marilena Mademtzi, PhD, Yale Child Study Center, Yale School of Medicine, New Haven, Connecticut

Rachel Mapenzi, Neuroscience Unit, KEMRI–Wellcome Trust Research Programme, Kilifi, Kenya

Meghan Miller, PhD, MIND Institute, University of California, Davis, Sacramento, California

Charles R. Newton, MD, Neuroscience Unit, KEMRI–Wellcome Trust Research Programme, Kilifi, Kenya

Roald A. Øien, PhD, UiT–The Arctic University of Norway, Tromso, Norway

Sally Ozonoff, PhD, MIND Institute, University of California, Davis, Sacramento, California

Joseph Piven, MD, Carolina Institute for Developmental Disabilities, University of North Carolina at Chapel Hill, Chapel Hill, North Carolina

Maria Pizzano, PhD, Center for Autism Research and Treatment, University of California, Los Angeles, Los Angeles, California

Kelly K. Powell, PhD, Yale Child Study Center, Yale School of Medicine, New Haven, Connecticut

Kenneth Rimba, BA, Neuroscience Unit, KEMRI–Wellcome Trust Research Programme, Kilifi, Kenya

Kavita Ruparelia, BA, Department of Pediatrics and Child Health, Muhimbili University of Health and Allied Sciences, Dar es Salaam, United Republic of Tanzania

Celine A. Saulnier, PhD, Neurodevelopmental Assessment and Consulting Services, Decatur, Georgia

Frederick Shic, PhD, Department of Pediatrics, University of Washington, Seattle, Washington, and Center for Child Health, Behavior, and Development, Seattle Children's Research Institute, Seattle, Washington

Andy Shih, PhD, Autism Speaks, New York, New York

Robin Sifre, MA, Institute of Child Development, University of Minnesota, Minneapolis, Minnesota

Fons J. R. van de Vijver, PhD, Department of Culture Studies, Tilburg University, Tilburg, The Netherlands

Angelina Vernetti, PhD, Yale Child Study Center, Yale School of Medicine, New Haven, Connecticut

Fred R. Volkmar MD, Yale Child Study Center, Yale School of Medicine, and Department of Special Education, Southern Connecticut State University, New Haven, Connecticut

Lisa Wiesner, MD, Department of Pediatrics, Yale School of Medicine, New Haven, Connecticut

Contents

Introduction

Katarzyna Chawarska and Fred R. Volkmar

In the more than three-quarters of a century since Leo Kanner's (1943) classic description of autism, tremendous advances in our understanding of the development of this spectrum disorder have been made. Despite a slow initial progress, the 1970s marked the emergence of key findings on the validity of autism as a condition (Kolvin, 1971; Rutter, 1972), its strong neurobiological (Ritvo, 1977; Volkmar & Nelson, 1990) and genetic (Folstein & Rutter, 1977) origins, and the importance of structured interventions for teaching (Bartak & Rutter, 1973). As a result of these findings, autism was officially recognized in the American Psychiatric Association's (1980) landmark third edition of the *Diagnostic and Statistical Manual of Mental Disorders* (DSM-III). As noted in subsequent chapters, this diagnostic classification has been "tweaked" in numerous ways over time, raising some important conceptual issues and challenges for early diagnosis. However, the importance of autism's official recognition cannot be overemphasized. Between 1943 and 1979, the rate of publication of empirical research on autism gradually rose, but after the publication of DSM-III in 1980, it exploded. A considerable body of work now exists on the development of autism, its neurological basis, and approaches to treatment (Volkmar, 2019).

However, this work remains spotty in its coverage with, until relatively recently, comparatively less focus on autism as it first develops in the early stages of life. Fortunately, this has now changed dramatically thanks to advances in early screening and diagnosis as well as methods for studying the social and communication development of young and disabled children. Developing early screening and surveillance tools as well as improving the precision of early diagnostic instruments has enabled clinicians to identify autism cases as early as in the second year of life, facilitating implementation of early intervention as well as research into early expression of the syndrome. Prospective studies of younger siblings of children with autism spectrum disorder (ASD), some of which begin during pregnancy, provide an unprecedented opportunity to study the emergence of autism *in statu nascendi,* from its prodromal into the early syndromal stage, with the hope of identifying very early prognostic markers as well as risk and protective factors. Jointly, the development of early screening tools and prospective sibling studies may help identify the tools needed to address heterogeneity in syndrome expression, to discover novel treatment targets, and to develop more targeted and individualized interventions specific to the early developmental epoch marked by high brain plasticity. Novel experimental methods relying on eye tracking, physiology, and brain imaging have proved to be helpful in intensifying the early markers of ASD and for tracking the development of ASD over time.

Presently, many research groups around the world are concerned with these questions, and their efforts are reflected in this volume. Indeed, these last few years have witnessed a true explosion of work focused on understanding the mechanisms contributing to the development of autism, improving early detection, and testing new interventions for young children with the disorder. The chapters in this volume provide a state-of-the-art view on current research into the mechanisms, new approaches to diagnosis, and assessment and treatment of autism. The latter theme is particularly important, given the significant impact that early detection and intervention have on improving later outcomes (Magiati & Howlin, 2019).

In Chapter 1, Volkmar and Øien review current and recurring challenges in the early screening and diagnosis of autism. The impact of DSM-5 (American Psychiatric Association, 2013) on early diagnosis remains unclear but is a source of concern, particularly for the most cognitively able young children (Barton, Robins, Jashar, Brennan, & Fein, 2013). As the authors discuss, the move to a diagnosis of "autism spectrum disorder" has paradoxically led to a swing back to a narrower concept that is more consistent with the prototypical cases described by Kanner (1943). They also highlight some of the challenges that other factors, such as gender and culture, pose for early diagnosis.

In Chapter 2, Campi, Lord, and Grzadzinski then provide a thoughtful and comprehensive summary of current approaches to screening, its uses, and its limitations. They note the importance of screening but also the complex nature of early symptoms and the many challenges faced in implementing effective screening instruments. Indeed, these challenges have led some groups, notably the U.S. Preventive Services Task Force, to raise concerns about current support for early universal screening in cases where no parental concern exists (Siu & the U.S. Preventive Services Task Force, 2016, p. 691), since children with ASD are typically identified by family members or primary care physicians, not through screening processes. The Task Force recommendation highlights important gaps in the current literature on the long-term evidence for early intervention outcomes and the critical need for well-designed studies on the direct impact of early universal screening on later outcomes. Campi and her colleagues provide a nuanced description of the rationale for early screening and the mounting evidence for its benefits, including lowering the average age at first diagnosis and the rate of cases missed by parents and pediatricians, identifying non-ASD neurodevelopmental disorders, and facilitating referral to evaluation and services for young children at risk for ASD. The authors stress the role of accessible and inclusive screening procedures in decreasing the disparity in age of first diagnosis among minority, undereducated, and low-socioeconomic-status families. They warn against a shift in research toward the utility of screening and the long-term outcomes of early diagnosis, which are difficult to quantify, at the expense of research on early markers and novel treatments and interventions. The authors emphasize the need for longitudinal research, from initial screening into adulthood, as well as research into the implementation and feasibility of screening procedures.

In Chapter 3, Macari and her colleagues review progress in aspects of psychological assessment of young children at risk for ASD. They highlight the move to look past what are usually regarded as core features of the syndrome to more general psychological development, including areas such as attachment, temperament, and emotional expressivity. Other areas where important progress has been made include aspects of communication, adaptive skills, and potential predictors of later psychiatric comorbidities.

In Chapter 4 on early interventions, Pizzano and Kasari review evidence for the benefits of early interventions aimed at young children with ASD, in addition to targets for future improvements in current intervention models and research designs. Their chapter summarizes a number of randomized clinical trials that have been conducted with children with ASD between the ages of 2 and 5. The authors demonstrate that the results of these studies have tended to focus largely on cognitive gains and much less on the core symptoms of autism (e.g., social interaction and restricted interests/repetitive behaviors) and the impact of early interventions on current and future overall development. Furthermore, the lack of consistent replication trials and of studies that help us understand the mechanisms underlying current comprehensive models complicate the interpretation of these studies. The authors highlight the need for models that can be readily implemented in community settings, in addition to better outreach efforts. In trying to address the 2001 National Research Council goals for intervention, they note the importance of personalizing interventions, supporting and educating families, and developing more precise measurements of outcome.

In Chapter 5, Chawarska and her colleagues provide a timely update of the growing body of work on development of infant siblings of children with ASD. They focus primarily on the siblings' development during the first year of life, that is, before behavioral symptoms begin to emerge, and they provide a comprehensive summary of the work on prodromal markers of ASD in the behavioral and attentional domains. Importantly, the chapter focuses not only on the emergence of the core behavioral and attentional features of ASD but also on the development of emotional vulnerabilities among younger siblings. They identify important gaps in the literature regarding the links between early emotional vulnerabilities and later affective and behavioral problems, which are so common among children with ASD and their unaffected siblings, as well as the limited understanding of the relationship between social and emotional development in autism. The chapter highlights a number of limitations of the "high-risk siblings" approach, which the field will need to address as this research moves forward.

Sifre, Piven, and Elison address the complex issue of the neural basis of autism in Chapter 6, with particular attention to the sensorimotor, attentional, and reward networks. They consider the early development of high-risk infants and the way in which brain development in infants who are later diagnosed with ASD begins to diverge from the trajectories observed in unaffected siblings in the first 2 years of life. According to studies of the neural markers of early-emerging ASD, some markers are observable as early as 6 months, while others emerge over the first 2 years of life. Infants who are later diagnosed with ASD tend to increasingly diverge from unaffected siblings and low-risk peers, based on early markers of atypical brain development. From a behavioral standpoint, infants who are later diagnosed with ASD also diverge from low-risk peers in the first year of life in terms of early attentional mechanisms and aspects of visual social engagement. Early difficulties may impact other aspects of development, including semantic salience, attentional mechanisms, and reward processing. As a result, further work is needed on the differences in reward processing and salience-enhanced attention in both social and nonsocial contexts in ASD infants.

Miller and Ozonoff, in Chapter 7, then consider the critically important question of the longer-term outcomes of infants at risk for ASD. Given the evidence of elevated rates of the broader autism phenotype features, attention-deficit/hyperactivity disorder, and other atypical outcomes in siblings of children with ASD, the authors emphasize the need for longitudinal following of siblings who do not develop ASD but may exhibit atypical development in other domains. Their review also stresses the importance of focusing on additional areas for assessment of outcomes and incorporating measurements of functional domains appropriate to later developmental periods in investigating the processes underlying normative developmental mechanisms. At the same time, they also highlight the importance of using core measures across studies to ensure the comparability of findings.

In Chapter 8, Green tackles the important but complex question of preventive interventions during the prodromal stages of ASD. As he notes, many interventions can have a short-term effect, but evidence for sustained and developmentally meaningful effects is emerging, although it remains elusive. Future clinical trials focused on implementing interventions before definitive symptoms of autism begin to emerge will need to employ larger samples and be more explicitly focused on mechanisms of emerging developmental processes, paying careful attention to data collection and analysis methods. All such methods, to date, have been concerned with behavioral rather than biomedical interventions, and the feasibility of the latter remains a significant hurdle for future research. As Green discusses, engaging with all relevant stakeholders, including members of the autism community, advocates, and ethicists on the desired outcomes for early autism intervention, is a critically important issue.

In Chapter 9, Volkmar, Øien, and Wiesner summarize current knowledge and approaches to providing high-quality health care to infants and very young children at risk for ASD. They emphasize the importance and complexities inherent to providing comprehensive care, in addition to new models of care that have been developed specifically for children with special needs, such as the medical home, which strives to coordinate the care of specialists and other providers in a family-centered manner. Their chapter also underscores the importance of practitioner training in enabling parents to be informed participants in this process.

Shic and his colleagues, in Chapter 10, provide a broad review of the role of technology in the treatment, detection, and phenotyping of ASD. This chapter begins with a discussion of the needs and constraints imposed by the physical, cognitive, and developmental attributes of infants and toddlers with and without ASD, and then moves on to analysis of current research involving a vast array of technologies, including robots, mobile applications, gaming, wearables, and augmented and virtual reality. As they note, technology has advanced so rapidly that it is difficult to adequately evaluate its implications, at least using usual methods, and that in our enthusiasm, it is important to not only consider the advantages and promise of technology, but also its drawbacks and limitations. They end by discussing how an interdisciplinary perspective is, and will continue to be, a vital component of developing technologies to help the youngest individuals affected by autism.

In the final chapter of this volume, Abubakar and her colleagues review the steps needed to translate the results of all this work into usable approaches for developing countries, as well the challenges of adapting measures developed in western Europe and North America to resource-poor settings. Drawing on examples from East Africa, they focus on practical steps and solutions to ensure the validity of imported scales and highlight the need for culturally appropriate and contextually relevant screening and diagnostic tools to quantify the burden of ASD in Africa and ensure that children receive early diagnosis and intervention. Their chapter also underscores the importance of cultural sensitivity and sound practice in the development of instruments for applying results from studies to low- and middle-income countries.

The contributions in this book make it clear that the field of research and clinical care for infants and young children with autism, or infants who, as a result of genetic factors, are at risk for autism, has dramatically expanded. Outstanding issues have been identified, including the need for improving screening and diagnostic practices to take under consideration the vast phenotypic heterogeneity in syndrome expression present even at the earliest ages when ASD can be reliably identified. Another important issue is the need for better predictive and stratification biomarkers, more effective individualized early interventions, and better support for translating research advances into high-quality care for affected children and their families around the world.

In closing, we want to extend sincere thanks to our various contributors. We appreciate their willingness to contribute their outstanding work and their openness to editorial feedback. We also acknowledge the important assistance of Evelyn Pomichter and Monica Mleczek at the Yale Child Study Center; our colleagues Kelly Powell, PhD, Suzanne Macari, PhD, and Dustin Scheinost, PhD, who helped us review each chapter and provided feedback for the authors; and Ludivine Brunissen, BS, who provided exceptional assistance in editing the manuscript. We are also grateful to the V. & L. Marx Foundation and to the Jim Henson Foundation for their support of clinical research on young children with autism. At The Guilford Press, we thank Carolyn Graham for her editorial assistance, Kitty Moore for her overall stewardship of this project since its very beginning, and Seymour Weingarten for his help in our selection of a final title for this volume.

As always, we are grateful to our spouses, Marek and Lisa, as well as our children, Szymon, Julian, Lucy, and Emily, and our grandchildren, Chloe MacLeod and Henry Robert. We dedicate this volume to them.

REFERENCES

American Psychiatric Association. (1980). *Diagnostic and statistical manual of mental disorders* (3rd ed.). Washington, DC: Author.

American Psychiatric Association. (2013). *Diagnostic and statistical manual of mental disorders* (5th ed.). Arlington, VA: Author.

Bartak, L., & Rutter, M. (1973). Special educational treatment of autistic children: A comparative study. 1. Design of study and characteristics of units. *Journal of Child Psychology and Psychiatry and Allied Disciplines, 14*(3), 161–179.

Barton, M. L., Robins, D. L., Jashar, D., Brennan, L., & Fein, D. (2013). Sensitivity and specificity of proposed DSM-5 criteria for autism spectrum disorder in toddlers. *Journal of Autism and Developmental Disorders, 43*(5), 1184–1195.

Folstein, S., & Rutter, M. (1977). Genetic influences and infantile autism. *Nature, 265*(5596), 726–728.

Kanner, L. (1943). Autistic disturbances of affective contact. *Nervous Child, 2,* 217–250.

Kolvin, I. (1971). Studies in the childhood psychoses: I. Diagnostic criteria and classification. *British Journal of Psychiatry, 118*(545), 381–384.

Magiati, I., & Howlin, P. (2019). Adult life for people with autism spectrum disorders. In F. R. Volkmar (Ed.), *Autism and pervasve developmental disorders* (3rd ed., pp. 220–248). Cambridge, UK: Cambridge University Press.

National Research Council. (2001). *Educating young children with autism.* Washington, DC: National Academy Press.

Ritvo, E. R. (1977). Biochemical studies of children with the syndromes of autism, childhood schizophrenia and related developmental disabilities: A review. *Journal of Child Psychology and Psychiatry and Allied Disciplines, 18*(4), 373–379.

Rutter, M. (1972). Childhood schizophrenia reconsidered. *Journal of Autism and Childhood Schizophrenia, 2*(4), 315–337.

Siu, A. L., & the U.S. Preventive Services Task Force. (2016). Screening for autism spectrum disorder in young children: U.S. Preventive Services Task Force Recommendation Statement. *JAMA, 315*(7), 691–696.

Volkmar, F. R. (Ed.). (2019). *Autism and pervasive developmental disorders.* Cambridge, UK: Cambridge University Press.

Volkmar, F. R., & Nelson, D. S. (1990). Seizure disorders in autism. *Journal of the American Academy of Child and Adolescent Psychiatry, 29*(1), 127–129.

CHAPTER 1
• • • • • • •

The Evolution of Autism
as a Diagnostic Concept

Fred R. Volkmar and Roald A. Øien

More than 75 years have passed since Leo Kanner's classic (1943) description of the syndrome he called infantile autism. Over this period of time, many significant changes have occurred in our understanding of the condition and narrowed, or broadened, view of it. As we will discuss in this chapter, at present we paradoxically have two competing views—a narrow view more akin, in some ways, to Kanner's original paper and a broader view that reflects more generally an awareness that autism does shade off into normalcy (via the "broad autism phenotype"; Ingersoll & Wainer, 2014). The broader view has become, in many ways, more consistent with our evolving understanding of the genetics of autism.

These issues are of great relevance to the diagnosis of autism in infants and very young children. In Kanner's time, and for decades after that, it was not usual to see very young children who either seemed to have autism or to be at high risk for it. Indeed, on my (F.R.V.) first entry into the field in 1980, seeing a 4-year-old was equated with seeing a very young child with autism. Other chapters in this volume document the dramatic upsurge of interest in the first and earliest manifestations of the condition. Through studies of high-risk populations and use of new methods, considerable progress has been made in our attempt to see autism in its earliest form—before subsequent intervention and life circumstances and ongoing development have altered its course. In this chapter, we review the development of the concept from Kanner's original description to our current broad view of the autism spectrum, with particular emphasis on the diagnosis of ASD in infants and young children.

Issues in Diagnosis and Classification

Classification systems have different intended uses and purposes, including enhanced communication for clinical work, for facilitation research,

9

or for policy planning (Volkmar, Sukhodolsky, Schwab-Stone, & First, 2017). The consistent use of the same criteria for purposes of research has vastly increased the value of results obtained since, as a result, the critically important issues of generalization can be addressed forthrightly. In some countries, like the United States, use of specific diagnostic labels may also produce essential entitlements to services or treatments. This is especially so in the United States where the various states have a plethora of services and programs available (Doehring & Becker-Conttrill, 2013). Diagnostic systems that try to be both all-encompassing and useful for research as well as clinical purposes face unique challenges; such a task has been undertaken in the various DSMs since 1980. As noted elsewhere (e.g., see Jackson & Volkmar, 2019), alternatives are available, particularly the World Health Organization's approach of having different books for clinical and research use. Of course, for clinical work, establishing a working diagnosis is only one part of a broader diagnostic process that aims to decrease impairment and increase life choices and satisfaction. Other considerations also arise for comprehensive diagnostic approaches. Issues of reliability and validity are essential. That is, are there some independent validators that increase our concept in the basic diagnostic construct, and can the proposed criteria be meaningfully used by clinicians from different backgrounds and with different levels of experience?

Many tensions exist, for example, between clinical and research uses, between "lumping and splitting," and so forth. It is possible, for example, to increase diagnostic precision dramatically, but if the concept is too narrow, it cannot be generally applied. Conversely, it is possible that for research purposes a very narrow concept may facilitate identification of underlying pathophysiological processes. Another issue of importance for autism is the degree to which impairment (including, for children, interference in learning or development) must be viewed as an essential feature of the condition. Indeed, in some ways, Hans Asperger (1904–1980) himself explicitly raised this issue, for he viewed the condition he described more as a personality than as a developmental disorder, and he noted similar problems in the fathers of these children. As a practical matter, today this consideration arises in the issue of whether a person with social vulnerabilities, but who otherwise functions well, might be seen as having a disorder or a lifestyle/personality type. Some such persons might prefer to avoid feeling stigmatized by a categorical label, while others might wish to share their awareness of differences with others, including those with similar problems (Rutter, 2011).

A range of approaches to classification can be employed, including categorical and dimensional. In medicine, the dominant approach has been the categorical (presence/absence) model. Dimensional and categorical systems are not at all incompatible, however; it only becomes necessary to decide at what arbitrary point along a dimension a disorder is diagnosed. These distinctions apply both to common medical problems such as hypertension or hypocholesterolemia and to developmental disorders such as intellectual disability. Of course, the selection of such cutoffs can be complex.

Dimensional approaches provide more information than simple categorical ones. The use of screening, rating scales, and diagnostic instruments for autism are all good examples of these approaches. A specific categorical cutoff is somewhat arbitrary. For autism, screening instruments, rating scales, and diagnostic instruments have been developed (see Ibañez, Stone, & Coonrod, 2014; Lord, Corsello, & Grzadzinski, 2014). While several instruments are now essentially of mere historical interest, it is important to realize the challenges that developers face when they undertake to develop new such approaches. Issues involving development of these instruments are profoundly complex. For example: Who will endorse the information? Is direct observation used? How much training is needed? Does the instrument take various forms (e.g., depending on the child's ability level)? What is the intended age range and developmental level? Psychometric issues such as reliability, validity, and administration fidelity must be addressed. Practical issues of ease of use, performance, and administration are all important. Also, the question of whether the instrument can yield some categorical measure (e.g., of presence/absence or severity of autism) may also need to be addressed. Increasingly, diagnostic instruments have been used as "change" measures. This reflects both the paucity of such instruments for measuring treatment effects and the complexity of developing an instrument that is, on the one hand, supposed to be stable but, on the other hand, is measuring treatment efficacy.

A different approach has been adopted, for example, by the Childhood Autism Rating Scale, Second Edition (CARS-2; Schopler, Van Bourgondien, Wellman, & Love, 2010) which rates behaviors in 15 categories with a 4-point scale—from normal to severely autistic. The summary score can be translated into an estimate of the severity of autism—absent, mild, moderate, or severe. This test, frequently used in schools, strikes a balance between research and clinical tensions. Other approaches have used results from normative assessment instruments like the Vineland (Volkmar et al., 1987). Still others occur more on screening or more complex procedures for researched autism (see Volkmar, Booth, McPartland, & Wiesner, 2014a).

Developmental considerations in diagnostic classification schemes began in the late 1960s as it became more complex; for example, it was thought that multiaxial methods might be needed (Rutter et al., 1969). With some modifications, this approach continues to be used, although in the recent DSM-5 (American Psychiatric Association, 2013) the broader childhood-onset group has been largely eliminated and replaced with a shorter neurodevelopmental disorders section (including autism). This reflects the long-standing goal of minimizing the age-related "sections" of the manual. It remains to be seen how well this approach worked for other conditions.

The role of theory in guiding classifications has long been a thorny issue for classification schemes. Probably the primary lesson of the success of DSM-III (American Psychiatric Association, 1980) has been the importance of adopting a theoretical, but reliable, approach. Earlier versions of DSM were heavily theoretical, which posed problems at many levels. It is clear that for research purposes the research diagnostic criteria approach (American Psychiatric Association, 1980) has significantly advanced the study of many disorders, including autism.

For disorders like autism that are of very early onset, the fundamental nature of the particular condition and its impact on so many areas of development can markedly impact development in many ways. Understanding developmental factors, both typical and atypical, thus remains important. This importance is exemplified in the early impression that echolalia in autism was a maladaptive symptom and only later were its many potential adaptive functions recognized (Prizant & Rydell, 1984). Early-onset problems also increase the risk for comorbid conditions. In the study of individuals with intellectual deficiency, it became apparent that "diagnostic overshadowing" often led clinicians and investigators to fail to appreciate the presence of markedly increased rates of other disorders (Reiss, Levitan, & Szyszko, 1982). Conversely, longitudinal data also show the potential positive effects of environmental influence (e.g., lower rates of intellectual deficiency over time if the real-life acquisition of adaptive skills is considered; Rutter, 1991).

The role of etiology in the development of classification systems is an interesting one. Even when an etiology is known, for example, for a single-gene disorder, there usually is phenotypic heterogeneity. In some ways, tensions surrounding the issue of etiology are reflected in how Rett's disorder is approached in the DSMs. In DSM-IV (American Psychiatric Association, 1994), this syndrome was included in the overarching pervasive developmental disorder category but not because it was thought to be a form of autism (although this had been Rett's [1986] first impression). Instead, it was felt that this was the closest category and that, given its distinct course and clinical pattern, some etiology would likely be found. This was the case with the discovery of the MECP-2 gene (Moretti & Zoghbi, 2006). In DSM-5, the disorder was eliminated, although cases could still, in theory, meet the criteria for the ASD category (in reality, this is not likely). The consideration of how to best approach classification of disorders with behavioral and developmental features but also strong genetic etiologies remains a matter of some controversy.

Like any human construction, classification systems can be misused (e.g., Hobbs, 1975; Gould, 1996). One of the worst mistakes in this regard is to equate people with diagnostic labels (e.g., "the autistic" or "the schizophrenic" or "the diagnostic") rather than with person-centered language, which is always indicated. It is important to realize that categorical terms only capture a small fraction of the information relevant to the condition as it is expressed in that person, and much less the complexity of the individual in all of his or her facets. Scientifically, of course, it also presents a danger in that having a label can be assumed to be an explanation. Moreover, of course, having a categorical label should not be an obstacle to helping any person achieve his or her maximum potential in the home, school, and community settings.

Diagnostic Issues Specific to Classification of ASD

The history of autism research illustrates the importance of a robust and generally agreed-upon definition for research purposes. Before 1980, when DSM-III (American Psychiatric Association, 1980) was published, it was challenging to interpret research on what then was considered "childhood schizophrenia." After its official recognition in DSM-III, research on autism substantially increased; for example, in 2000 about 350 papers were published, while in 2010 this number had increased to 2,000 and during 2017, roughly 4,000 papers appeared! These numbers reflect the importance of diagnostic awareness and useful and generally agreed-upon definitions.

It is also important to reflect on the importance of such recognition for clinical purposes. Better awareness and classification can lead to better data to guide health policy and, of course, facilitate research on treatment. As we will discuss shortly, changes in diagnostic systems present opportunities as well as challenges. The opportunities arise given the possibility that data-based "tweaks" improved reliability. Conversely, if changes are significant, they may disrupt organizing research and may also have unintended consequences for service relative to eligibility.

From Kanner's Report to DSM-5

Kanner's Report

It is likely that reports of so-called "feral" children may represent the first reports of children with autism (Wolff, 2004; Candland, 1993). Although intellectual disability had been recognized since antiquity (Harris, 2006), interest in it and in child development, in general, began to increase with the Enlightenment and the debate of the role of nature versus nurture in child development (Hunt, 1961). By the mid-1800s, interest in psychiatric problems in children began to increase, and continuities with adult forms of mental illness were suggested (e.g., Maudsley, 1867), although little provision was made for recognizing the relevance of developmental factors in syndrome expression. The late 1800s were, in particular, a time of great activity in psychiatric taxonomy with the recognition of dementia praecox (now termed schizophrenia) and manic–depressive illness (bipolar disorder). These concepts were rapidly extended to children (e.g., "dementia praecossisima"; de Sanctis, 1906). The early tendency to equate severe psychiatric disturbance in childhood with adult schizophrenia later posed a difficulty in recognizing the validity of autism as a different diagnostic category.

Leo Kanner emigrated to the United States from Nazi Germany first to work in a state mental hospital, but he was then recruited to Johns Hopkins Hospital to bridge the gap between psychiatry and pediatrics. He had completed the first textbook in the field in the 1930s before publishing his seminal paper "Autistic Disturbances of Affective Contact" (Kanner, 1943).

In this original paper recognizing autism, Kanner presented 11 cases of children he believed to lack orientation to people and social interaction that characterizes typical development. He was careful to acknowledge the early development of social engagement as noted by Arnold Gesell at Yale in his studies of typical infants. He provided thoughtful, careful, and insightful descriptions of these first cases. He then synthesized his observations into an overall summary emphasizing two features he felt were essential for diagnosis: (1) autism—or the early lack of social interaction and engagement and (2) insistence on sameness, or, put another way, difficulties dealing with change in the nonsocial world. With the wisdom of hindsight (and the tremendous body of work on normal social development), we now recognize that these may be the flip sides of the same coin—that is, if you are ready to play the social game, you are also ready for constant change. Kanner's use of the term *resistance to change* or *insistence on sameness* was intended to note the significant problems these children had with a change in nonsocial work. Although not recognizing communication problems as a central diagnostic factor, Kanner did mention many of the unusual features of language/communicative development that we now consider hallmarks of autism. For the individuals who engaged in communicative speech, unusual prosody and difficulties with nonliteral language and pronoun use were noteworthy.

Kanner's report was prescient in many respects. It focused on the apparent paradox of overengagement with change in the nonsocial world and lack of interest in the social world (Klin, Jones, Schultz, & Volkmar, 2005; McPartland & Pelphrey, 2012). In his first paper, Kanner suggested that autism was congenital, and he particularly noted the attractive appearance of the children in his study group (i.e., unlike the appearance of those diagnosed with other syndromes associated with mental retardation or what we now term *intellectual disability.*

Unfortunately, a few aspects of this groundbreaking work ultimately caused confusion. First, Kanner's use of the word *autism* was meant to convey the socially isolated and isolationist quality of the child's existence, but also it harkened back to its early meaning as self-centered *thinking* in schizophrenia. Similarly, his observation of the fact that some of his subjects did well on some parts of IQ tests suggested that children with infantile autism, as he termed it, were not also intellectually disabled. Early reports of individuals with autism and savant skills also fueled this impression. It was assumed that good performance on some parts of the IQ tests (puzzles and other nonverbal activities) was typical of overall abilities and that poor performance on verbal tasks reflected lack of engagement or desire to cooperate. Similarly, his observation of a lack of unusual physical features (as in trisomy 21) and the ability of the children to do well on some parts of IQ tests suggested that children with infantile autism were not also mentally retarded. It took many decades to realize that this assumption was not correct and that many individuals also developed a co-occurring intellectual disability (see Goldstein, Naglieri, & Ozonoff, 2009; Klin, Saulnier, Tsatsanis, & Volkmar, 2005; Volkmar & Nelson, 1990). This led to the impression that parents *had* to be very successful to have a child with autism, and this impression, in turn, led to speculation in the 1950s that parents might actually *cause* autism. This thinking led to an entire generation of parents who were traumatized by being blamed for their child's condition and by following the recommendation of ineffective intensive therapy, which in the end did nothing at all for their child's problem. This issue was one of several that became clarified in the 1970s as longitudinal data became available and it became clear that children with autism were very much at risk for development of seizure disorder (epilepsy).

As mentioned earlier, Kanner noted the attractive appearance of his cases and emphasized that they were without obvious physical signs of conditions like Down syndrome. Only as the children were followed did it become clear that they were at increased risk for developing seizure disorder and that autism was associated with a small number of highly genetic conditions (see Rutter & Thapar, 2014). Finally, in his initial case series, parents tended to be highly successful and accomplished people, but there was little awareness of the potential for selection bias (i.e., that only well-informed and successful parents would be able to find the one child psychiatrist in the country). Indeed, Kanner's early report likely reflected the fact that it was educated parents who were most likely to be able to reach the likes of Leo Kanner in the decades long before the internet! As a result, the impression in the 1950s and 1960s was that autism was a disorder of higher status (educationally and occupationally) families, and this notion, in turn, led to an impression that potentially experienced or deviant parenting might play a role in pathogenesis (e.g., Bettelheim, 1974). Subsequently, autism was seen to be unrelated to parental education or socioeconomic status (SES; Wing, 1980).

From Kanner to DSM-III

Following Kanner's original description (1943), interest in autism gradually began to increase. Much of the work done relative to patients is, unfortunately, hard to interpret given the confusion with childhood schizophrenia. An entire line of work focused on parents as the "cause" of autism. This work (e.g., Bettelheim, 1974) suggested that separation from parents and psychodynamic therapy represented the only hope for remediation. This unfortunate thinking rested, in part, on Kanner's description of the parent's high levels of success and the very strong interest at the time in the effect of experience within a psychoanalytic theoretical framework. Several lines of work questioned the view of autism as a psychogenic disorder, and in addition, it was lumped in with the broad childhood schizophrenia/psychosis category.

In the United States, Rimland (1964), a psychologist and parent, provided a neurological model of autism; proposed some guidelines for diagnosis, along with the first screening/diagnostic instrument focused on new approaches to objective diagnosis; and provided a hypothetical neurobiological mechanism for autism (Rimland, 1964). Several lines of evidence also questioned the lumping of autism into the broader childhood psychosis category. In a series of studies, Kolvin and colleagues examined the clinical phenomenology of a large group of "psychotic children" (Kolvin, 1971). This work revealed a bimodal age of onset of "childhood psychosis," with a large group of cases identified as having difficulty in the first year of life, and then another group emerged with an onset in early and midadolescence. The first group of cases clinically resembled the children with autism described by Kanner, while the later-onset group had symptoms suggestive of schizophrenia (hallucinations, delusions, etc.). Family history data also suggested higher rates of schizophrenia in the later-onset than in the early-onset cases. Kolvin's study was convincing evidence that autism was a distinctive condition. Rutter (1972) summarized this work and suggested a reconsideration of autism as a distinctive condition.

Several other lines of evidence that emerged in the 1970s also provided valuable insights into autism. As children were followed over time, it appeared that the course of autism was also unusual (Kanner, 1971). As children were followed, a much higher than expected rate of epilepsy (seizure disorder) was seen (Volkmar & Nelson, 1990). While the early impression was that autism was not a strongly genetic condition, the first twin study (Folstein & Rutter, 1978) revealed substantial genetic contributions, with a very high rate of concordance in monozygotic twins (as compared to same-sex maternal twins) who also had a higher than expected rate of recurrence, but not nearly as high as in the identical twin pairs.

Finally, the first studies of treatment efficacy (e.g., Rutter & Bartak, 1973) observed that structured teaching was much more frequently associated with improvement than unstructured psychotherapy. It was around this time that the first behavioral intervention studies were conducted, leading to a vast body of work on applied behavioral analysis (e.g., Lovass & Smith, 1988; Ferster, 1972). In the United States and the United Kingdom, parents began to organize intervention programs based on these principles.

By the late 1970s, a consensus emerged that autism (then referred to as infantile autism, autism, or Kanner's autism) was a distinctive condition. Several attempts were made to provide better diagnostic guidelines. Rutter (1978) proposed a straightforward definition based on Kanner's work. Rutter's definition included social difficulties (not just due to associated developmental delay/intellectual disability [ID]), communication problems (again not just due to ID), and unusual behaviors of the type that Kanner had noted, for example, resistance to change, stereotyped mannerisms, and so forth. Rutter's definition also included a requirement for early onset (by age 30 months). In contrast, Ritvo and colleagues (National Society for Autistic Children [NSAC], 1978), working in conjunction with the newly organized National Autism Society, proposed a slightly different definition that included features such as unusual rates/patterns of development and hypo/hypersensitivity. Both definitions have had a substantial impact on subsequent official approaches to defining autism. At the same time, there was consideration of the best multiaxial diagnostic approaches to use. Importantly, the Washington University in St. Louis group pioneered the use of research diagnostic criteria in the definition of psychiatric disorder (Spitzer, Endicott, & Robbins, 1978). This approach avoided the conundrums of past, more theoretically based definitions by adhering strictly to the descriptive phenomenology of the condition.

DSM-III

The growing body of work led to the decision to include a new category for "infantile autism" as an officially recognized diagnosis in the groundbreaking DSM-III (American Psychiatric Association, 1980). A new term, *pervasive developmental disorder* (PDD), was coined as the class to which infantile autism and similar conditions were assumed to belong. Unfortunately, this term led to some confusion, and with the wisdom of hindsight, better terminology could have been employed. However, the critical accomplishment was the official recognition of autism as a distinctive condition.

At that time, autism was indeed regarded as one of the best examples of a "disorder" in psychiatry since it did not seem to shade off into normalcy

(Rutter & Garmezy, 1983). This view, of course, has now substantially changed (Ingersoll & Wainer, 2014). The definition provided for infantile autism was monothetic (i.e., all features have to be present), including social and communication features consistent with Rutter's (1978) definition as well as early onset. The social criterion of pervasive lack of response to others was not applicable to older individuals since children did develop some social skills over time, so a new category of "residual" infantile autism was included. Three other conditions were included in the new PDD class: (1) childhood-onset PDD (for children who developed autism after a period of normal development but then otherwise met the criteria for infantile autism); (2) residual childhood-onset PDD (a parallel to the residual infantile autism category); and (3) as was true throughout DSM-III, a new atypical pervasive developmental disorder for situations that did not meet all the features of a specific PDD, but the individual had problems suggestive of autism or a related condition. (This last-named category would morph into pervasive developmental disorder not otherwise specified [PDD-NOS] in DSM-III-R and DSM-IV.) Importantly, in many respects the foundation of the now recognized spectrum of difficulties associated with autism in some fundamental sense arose from this attempt, in DSM-III, to acknowledge that individuals had social and related difficulties that did not quite correspond to the official definitions provided.

DSM-III was a tremendous advance over its predecessors. For autism and related conditions, the official recognition of autism stimulated an already growing body of research. Given its rigorous approach, DSM-III was quickly adopted around the world, and, for autism, this further advanced international work on the condition. For autism and related conditions, several problems quickly became apparent the first time autism had been so recognized, and it is not surprising that some problems were quickly identified (Volkmar, Cohen, & Paul, 1986).

As noted earlier, the definition of "infantile" autism indeed focused on the most classic, presumably earliest, forms of the condition marked by little responsiveness to others. Clearly, any developmental approach was lacking, and the term *residual* infantile autism seemed highly inappropriate given the potentially very severe manifestations of the disorder in older individuals who no longer were "pervasively" unresponsive. As Wing and others have noted, social skills do develop, although often in unusual ways as children with autism age (Wing & Gould, 1979). The language (not communication) criteria were similarly somewhat narrow. The homothetic approach to the diagnosis of infantile autism was inflexible, and, somewhat paradoxically, the polythetic (various features could lead to a diagnosis) definition for childhood-onset PDD was much more flexible. The rationale for including this latter condition was also somewhat questionable: it appeared to be aimed specifically at the rare children who developed normally for a considerable period of time (usually 3 or 4 years) and then seemed to develop a particularly severe clinical presentation of autism. These children were first described by Heller (1908), and a few had been seen in Kolvin's case studies (Kolvin, 1971). Finally, use of the term *atypical* PDD has a somewhat unique history and complications relative to autism. Rank and colleagues had used an earlier term—atypical development—to describe children with unusual developmental patterns, some of which suggested features of autism (Rank, 1949; Rank & MacNaughton, 1949). Finally, given the long history of confusing autism with schizophrenia, it is perhaps not surprising that this was made an exclusionary criterion for autism. Of course, given the frequency of schizophrenia, there would be no reason to assume that adolescents or adults with autism were somehow protected from developing schizophrenia. Moreover, studies suggest that indeed this does occur at about the rate expected in the general population (Volkmar & Tsatsanis, 2002). Although DSM-III was a significant and clear advance problem in this and other categories, it prompted a relatively rapid revision in DSM-III-R (American Psychiatric Association, 1987).

DSM-III-R

Given the significant difficulties identified with the DSM-III definition, major revisions were undertaken with DSM-III-R (American Psychiatric Association, 1987). In some sense, these are summarized in the change of name of the main category—from *infantile autism* to *autistic disorder*. The emphasis was on providing a more flexible and developmentally oriented definition (see Siegel, Vukicevic, Elliott, & Kraemer, 1989; Waterhouse, Wing, Spitzer, & Siegel, 1993).

A polythetic definition was adopted, with *criteria/items* grouped into three domains: social development, communication and play, and restricted interests and repetitive behaviors (sometimes giving an example within the criteria). To achieve a diagnosis of autistic disorder, at least eight criteria had to be endorsed, with at least two social and one each from the other two categories. A field trial was used to help refine the DSM-III-R definition. Unfortunately, it suffered from several problems (cases were rated based on records, and the comparison group was highly inappropriate).

The pros and cons of the new definition quickly became evident. The positives included much better attention being given to issues of developmental change and developmental level (Volkmar, Cicchetti, Cohen, & Bregman, 1992b). At the same time, it also was noted that the new system appeared to have increased false-positive rates (Volkmar et al., 1992b; Factor, Freeman, & Kardash, 1989; Hertzig, Snow, New, & Shapiro, 1990).

The nature of the criteria was problematic in inclusion of examples within criteria. Clearly, the new approach focused more on present assessment than on history. Concern increased as it appeared that the new DSM-III-R was diverging substantially from the draft ICD-10 approach (Volkmar, Cicchetti, Bregman, & Cohen, 1992a).

The World Health Organization's *International Classification of Diseases, 10th edition* (ICD-10; World Health Organization, 1994) differed from DSM in several ways. At first a "two-books" approach was adopted, with clinical guidelines published separately from diagnostic criteria for research. Other issues were noted as well, for example, in the approach to dealing with comorbidity. Adopting the two-volume approach did mean that the research definition could be substantially more detailed. Clearly, significant differences between these two official systems had the potential for complicating research (Volkmar et al., 1992a). These issues were given serious consideration in the major revision of the diagnostic approach undertaken for DSM-IV (American Psychiatric Association, 1994).

DSM-IV and ICD-10

The revision process for DSM-IV was extensive. It included work groups for various diagnostic categories; these reviewed existing research and identified areas of consensus and controversy. Changes from DSM-III-R were made only when they could be justified and also in consideration of the pending changes with ICD-10 (Volkmar & Tsatsanis, 2002). For the autism/PDD categories, this included a series of commissioned literature reviews (see *Journal of Autism and Developmental Disorders*, December 1992 issue) that addressed a range of issues. One major problem was whether and how best to include other specified disorders (i.e., other than the atypical/not otherwise specified) category. The draft ICD-10 included Asperger syndrome (Sharma, Woolfson, & Hunter, 2012; Szatmari, 1991), Rett syndrome (Rutter, 1994; Gillberg, 1994; Tsai, 1992), and the apparently rare condition variously termed *disintegrative psychosis, Heller's syndrome,* or *childhood disintegrative disorder* (Volkmar, 1992). It was clear that, if possible, comparability of DSM-IV and ICD-10 was desired (Rutter & Schopler, 1992).

For the diagnosis of autistic disorder, a series of papers suggested that DSM-III-R was indeed more developmentally oriented but also overly broad (Volkmar et al., 1992b). Thus, a major issue was the balance of sensitivity and specificity of diagnostic approach while simultaneously maintaining a flexible and developmentally oriented definition of the condition. As a significant part of this process, an international field trial was conducted (Volkmar et al., 1994). This field trial included over 20 sites and over 100 raters, with nearly 1,000 cases rated. To avoid the problem of the DSM-III-R, field trial cases were included from clinics/clinicians only when the clinician felt that autism was a reasonable part of the differential diagnosis.

Information on raters, for example, level of experience, was also obtained. The criteria rates included previous DSM criteria as well as draft ICD-10 and new potential criteria. For most of the cases the raters in the field trial had multiple sources of information available to them (history, past examinations, current assessment). Clinicians were also asked to give their best estimate of the clinical diagnosis regardless of the criteria used.

The results of this field trial can be briefly summarized. Most importantly, the data suggested that DSM-III-R emerged as a diagnostic outlier (compared to DSM-III in the "lifetime" diagnostic sense or ICD-10 or clinician judgment). DSM-III-R had a high rate of false-positive cases, particularly in cases with greater intellectual impairment. The detailed draft ICD-10 research definition worked well but was more detailed and extensive than desired for DSM-IV. In concordance with the ICD-10 revision process and after extensive analysis, a new set of criteria were proposed that were conceptually identical in ICD-10 and DSM-IV.

Although reliability among clinicians has been questioned relative to clinical diagnosis (Lord et al., 2012), for the field trial data agreement among experienced raters on clinical diagnosis was excellent. For less experienced raters, reliability was increased by the use of the new diagnostic approach. Factor analysis produced several potential solutions, including the traditional three categories of criteria approach (social, communication, and restricted interests). A two-factor solution (social communication and restricted interests) and a five-factor solution (in which restricted interests criteria sorted into three groups) also were identified based on the various constraints imposed.

The field trial did not focus solely on the autistic disorder. As part of the field trial, data were collected on a potential "new" disorder tentatively included in ICD-10. These conditions, now seen as part of the broader autism phenotype, included Asperger syndrome, Rett syndrome, and childhood disintegrative disorder. Of these conditions, Asperger syndrome was probably the most widely recognized. The condition had been initially described by Hans Asperger (1944) a year after Kanner's paper was published. Asperger emphasized not only the autism and social vulnerability of the disorder but also its heritability. He noted that he had reviewed the condition more as a personality issue than as a developmental disorder—all issues that had been raised in recent years relative to the broader autism phenotype (Ingersoll & Wainer, 2014) and the growing body of work on the diverse genetic contributions to autism and related conditions (Rutter et al., 2014).

The DSM-IV field trial provided some data supporting the inclusion of Asperger's disorder in DSM-IV. Nearly 50 cases with this clinical diagnosis had been included, and these cases differed in important ways from both similarly cognitively able cases of autism and PDD-NOS (Volkmar et al., 1994). Interest in the condition increased dramatically from fewer than 100 scientific papers from 1944 to 1993 to about 1,700 after DSM-IV appeared. The decision to include Asperger syndrome was somewhat controversial, and the criteria finally proposed were, unfortunately, a compromise that, in retrospect, could have been better addressed with a more detailed and explicit definition, given that autistic disorder took precedence (see Rutter, 2011; Volkmar, Klin, and McPartland, 2014b). Based on the results of the field trial, support was also given to including Rett syndrome within the overarching PDD class—not so much because it was thought to be a form of autism (Rett's [1966] initial presumption) but because it was felt to be essential to include it somewhere. Cases with unusually late onset of autism were also explicitly sought for the field trial and provided some support for including a "new" category of childhood disintegrative disorder as well (Volkmar & Rutter, 1995).

As was true in DSM-III and DSM-III-R, a "subthreshold" condition was included in DSM-IV for cases with problems suggestive of autism, but it failed application of formal diagnostic criteria. In DSM-IV, this was termed *pervasive developmental disorder not otherwise specified* (PDD-NOS) and in ICD-10, *atypical autism*. As noted, this category previously had its own compelling history antedating DSM-III, and as the study of the broader phenotype has increased, this group of cases has assumed increasing importance (Ingersoll & Wainer, 2014). The DSM-IV and ICD-10 convergence lasted for almost two decades, when both systems began to be revised again.

DSM-5

The process was different for DSM-5 as compared to its immediate predecessors. The project was based at the headquarters of the American Psychiatric Association rather than at a university (as had been the case since DSM-III). The American Psychiatric Association also played a greater role in the organization and structure of the process. Some notable early decision was made, for example, to revamp the multiaxial categories, eliminate (as much as possible) subthreshold categories, and use large datasets collected in structured diagnostic instruments (i.e., rather than contemporaneous clinician ratings). Another important goal was, as much as possible, to include childhood-onset disorders within regular diagnostic groupings, rather than have a special child's section. For some conditions (including autism, intellectual deficiency, and related developmental problems), this was not possible, and so these conditions were grouped into a neurodevelopmental category to emphasize their special status. Goals included improving DSM-5 as much as possible over its predecessor. Of course, for autism there were some unique challenges: the DSM-IV/ICD-10 criteria had been used successfully around the world, and research and clinical interest had exploded since DSM-IV appeared. These criteria had themselves been translated into diagnostic assessment instruments, and the results of these assessments were now being used to inform the DSM-5 criteria.

In creating the DSM-5 criteria, the Neurodevelopmental Disorders Work Group sought to preserve the strengths of the DSM-IV approach while improving upon its limitations. The criteria provided in DSM-IV were highly effective in supporting the development of standardized assessment methods and in facilitating research, with scientific publications on autism increasing dramatically. Several criticisms of the DSM-IV approach could readily be made. The DSM-IV field trial was large and international in scope and included many individuals, but it was not based on an epidemiological sample. While young children had been included in that field trial, there had been an increased interest in making a diagnosis as early as possible (Chawarska, Klin, & Volkmar, 2008), and work using DSM-IV criteria suggests reduced diagnostic stability before age 3 (Lord, 1996).

More serious concerns were raised about the validity of the various additional subtypes of autism included in DSM-IV (e.g., Mayes, Calhoun, & Crites, 2001; Ozonoff & Griffith, 2000). Probably the greatest disagreement concerned the inclusion and definition of Asperger syndrome. The criteria included in DSM-IV were unsatisfactory in some respects, and given the very significant difference in the diagnostic approach, it is not surprising that this compromise definition proved controversial (see Volkmar et al., 2014b; Bennett et al., 2008). In a partial response to this dissatisfaction, the entire text of the Asperger syndrome category in DSM-IV was replaced in DSM-IV-TR (American Psychiatric Association, 2000). Lord et al. (2012) reported in a large multisite study that assessment location was more predictive of a diagnosis of Asperger syndrome than were characteristics of the individual child, suggesting the persistence of various specific approaches to diagnosis. For childhood disintegrative disorder, concerns were raised about the apparent rarity of the condition and its differences from autism (Hansen et al., 2008; Jones & Campbell, 2010; Kurita, Koyama, Setoya, Shimizu, & Osada, 2004; Luyster et al., 2005; Rogers, 2004).

For the broader PDD-NOS group, the growing body of genetic work suggests a reconceptualization of PDD-NOS as a milder end of the autism spectrum, that is, the broader autism phenotype (Piven, 2001; Wainer, Block, Donnellan, & Ingersoll, 2013).

In DSM-5 (American Psychiatric Association, 2013), a new term, *autism spectrum disorder* (ASD), was proposed for what had been the pervasive developmental disorder category. Within this category, the prior diagnosis was merged into a single ASD, and a new communication disorder was proposed as well: social communication disorder. Rett syndrome was eliminated unless a child with the syndrome also met the criteria for the new ASD category. Based on a factor analysis of a large set of data from standardized instruments, the traditional three sets of criteria (social, communication, and restricted interests/repetitive behavior) were reduced to two (social and communication features having been combined). The new social communication category became nomothetic; that is, it required that an individual demonstrate symptoms across all three clusters to meet the criteria for ASD. In contrast, the restricted and repetitive behaviors domain remained polythetic, requiring evidence of symptoms in two of four symptom groupings. A new criterion related to sensory difficulties was included in the latter category. The new diagnosis of social communication disorder was defined by pragmatic difficulties and problems in the use of verbal and nonverbal communication in social contexts. This condition, a communication disorder, was seen as distinct from ASD, although it had many similarities to the older PDD-NOS concept. The DSM-5 revision process was complicated and data-oriented (Guthrie, Swineford, Wetherby, & Lord, 2013; Huerta, Bishop, Duncan, Hus, & Lord, 2013; King, Veenstra-VanderWeele, & Lord, 2013; Lord & Gotham, 2014).

DSM-5 also introduced a series of specific conditions for ASD, reflecting a general effort to include themes and descriptors that apply transdiagnostically. For example, a first specifying condition marks the presence of any associated etiological condition; a second specifying condition, common across DSM-5 diagnostic categories, describes the required level of support and impact on a person's functioning in the two symptom domains; a third specifying condition notes the level of any associated intellectual disability; and, similarly, a fourth indicates whether language impairment is present. The final specifying condition indicates whether catatonia is present. As noted previously, the use of these specifying conditions is meant, in some ways, to replace the previous multiaxial system.

Questions about DSM-5 were raised even before DSM-5 appeared, and two studies had seriously questioned whether the new diagnostic label significantly narrowed the diagnosis concept and substantially reduced eligibility for service in children who were previously provided therapeutic interventions. The first of these studies, Mattila et al. (2011) used an earlier version of the draft DSM-5 criteria and found significant difficulties with the system not "capturing" the problems of higher functioning individuals on the spectrum (including both autism and Asperger syndrome). Since this study had used an early version of the criteria, the results were questioned. However, McPartland, Reichow, and Volkmar (2012) reanalyzed data from the DSM-IV field (essentially creating algorithms to "cross walk" between the old and new system). Their study used the most recent criterion set, but several problems were again raised about DSM-5. A notably large number of higher functioning (IQ > 70) individuals failed to meet the new criteria. The authors raised the issue of whether DSM-5's increased stringency was consistent with awareness of the problems faced by more cognitively able but socially disabled individuals. In their study, a large proportion of individuals with autism (as diagnosed in DSM-IV) who were high functioning lost their label, while a substantial majority of those with Asperger syndrome and PDD-NOS also lost their label and thus their eligibility for services. Given these concerns, a final criterion was added to DSM-5, allowing individuals with "well-established" diagnoses of autism, Asperger syndrome, and PDD-NOS to keep their diagnosis. While addressing the immediate problem, this solution created other issues since it effectively established the continuity of the old system while simultaneously creating a new and more stringent one.

Some 5 years after DSM-5, a reasonably large body of work appeared, generally supporting the results earlier obtained, for example, by Mattila et al. (2011) and McPartland et al. (2012) but with some notable additions. In one study of cognitively able adults compared on DSM-IV, ICD-10, and DSM-5 criteria (Wilson et al., 2013), over half of the cases with an ICD-10 PDD diagnosis also met DSM-5 criteria for ASD, with nearly 20% of those not meeting criteria for DSM-5 ASD meeting criteria for social communication. Worley and Matson (2012) demonstrated that individuals meeting proposed DSM-5 criteria tended to have more severe impairments than individuals meeting DSM-IV-TR criteria, a pattern replicated by Matson and colleagues (Matson, Beighley, & Turygin, 2012a; Matson, Hattier, & Williams, 2012b) who also reported that 47.8%—nearly half of toddlers meeting DSM-IV-TR ASD criteria—did not meet DSM-5 criteria. Another study noted some potential difficulties with DSM-5 criteria among females (Fraser et al., 2012, and see Matson et al., 2012a). A study of an existing dataset of adults indicated higher sensitivity to parent reports than observational assessment, highlighting the influence of the assessment method on ascertainment of cases (Mazefsky, McPartland, Gastgeb, & Minshew, 2013).

The utility of DSM-5 in toddlers has attracted considerable attention, given the increased emphasis on the presence of repetitive, restricted behaviors; these behaviors are generally believed to manifest robustly only somewhat later in development (Chawarska, Marcari, Volkmar, Kim, & Shic, 2014). Worley and Matson (2012) confirmed this concern, and it has been reported by other investigators as well (e.g., Barton, Dumont-Mathieu, & Fein, 2012). Other studies have raised concern that cases with a previous diagnosis of PDD-NOS often failed to exhibit the breadth of symptoms required by DSM-5 (Gibbs, Aldridge, Chandler, Witzlsperger, & Smith, 2012; Taheri & Perry, 2012).

In their recent meta-analysis of 25 papers, Smith, Reichow, and Volkmar (2015) found that most studies showed that between 50 and 75% of individuals would maintain their diagnosis. The significant difficulties related to higher functioning cases, and those—paradoxically, given the name change in DSM-5—are part of the broader autism spectrum. Many potential limitations were found in the studies reviewed, notably, use of historical data and reliance on specific assessment methods (i.e., clinician observation versus parent report). Methodological variations may have a significant impact on the results obtained (Mazefsky et al., 2013). In addition, most of the studies to date have been conducted within research settings so the question of how findings generalize to more traditional clinical settings remains unclear (Tsai, 2012). Somewhat paradoxically, highly relevant data relative to the validity of Asperger syndrome appeared after the decision to eliminate it from DSM-IV. For example, Chiang, Cheung, Brown, and Li's (2014) meta-analysis examining reported IQ profiles in 52 studies comparing cases with autism spectrum disorder and Asperger syndrome showed robust differences in patterns obtained across all studies. This suggested that they indeed represent distinctive subtypes on the autism spectrum. As a result, many of these cases will no longer qualify for a label and potentially for relevant services.

Several vital decisions likely had a deleterious impact on DSM-5. At a surface level, if one compares the over 2,200 ways a person could achieve a diagnosis of autistic disorder in DSM-IV to the 12 ways in DSM-5, one would reasonably assume that the latter is a stricter, less flexible diagnostic construct. Some aspects of the process were severely constrained by the American Psychiatric Association, presumably in the interest of streamlining the process but also to cut costs (Greenberg, 2013). For example, the use of data from excellently structured research interests may not capture the reality of real-world settings, and in contrast to DSM-IV, the field trials for DSM-5 focused primarily on aspects of reliability. Including sensory issues raises other problems in the slightly different approach of the DSM-IV field trial. This item had *not* worked well in differentiating autism from intellectual disability (Volkmar et al., 1994). The inclusion of a new communication disorder was not well justified in research, and it does not precisely correspond to the needs of individuals with Asperger syndrome or PDD-NOS in DSM-IV terms. Other aspects of the system are somewhat arbitrary. For example, use of catatonia as a specific modifier for ASD seems odd given the rarity of that association. The usefulness of the specifiers also remains to be clarified (Gardner, Campbell, Keisling, & Murphy, 2018).

The move from the traditional three-symptom clusters to two has some practical disadvantages. It rests on the results of a factor analytic study of a large set of data (Huerta et al., 2012). However, other studies (e.g., Sipes & Matson, 2014) note that several solutions are possible, and in DSM-IV, field trial factor analysis yielded reasonable two-, three-, or five-factor solutions (Volkmar et al., 1994). Any of these approaches might have been justified but the three-factor, polythetic solution yielded more flexible applications consistent with the notion of an autism spectrum.

Thus, paradoxically, despite the welcome name change of the overall category to autism spectrum disorder, the concept itself is now the narrower "Kanner's autism" that we had moved away from in the past. Perhaps the swing of the pendulum is welcome, but if it prevents early detection of cases or provision of services to individuals, it is quite problematic. Of course, the "grandfathering" in of cases from DSM-IV also creates issues for longitudinal and epidemiological research.

Dimensional Approaches to Diagnosis

Although dimensional instruments and dimensional assessments are not the primary focus of this chapter, they are highly relevant and, particularly with DSM-5, have had a significant role in the development of categorical criteria. Since Rimland's first development of a diagnostic checklist (Rimland, 1971), many such instruments have been developed—some for screening and others for diagnosis (see Lord & Gotham, 2014, and Ibañez et al., 2014, for comprehensive reviews). Some of these instruments focus on infants and younger children, other older individuals, or the more cognitively able; other instruments are based on parent or teacher reports and still others on direct observation; and most focus on autism but a few on Asperger syndrome (Campbell, 2005).

In some cases, instruments have been developed specifically to assess the range of issues relevant to the broader autism phenotype (e.g., Constantino & Todd, 2000). It is important to note that, particularly for the most psychometrically robust instruments, a high degree of training is needed (a topic relevant to their use in DSM-5). Other dimensional approaches, such as use of tests of intelligence, executive functioning, and adaptive skills, are, of course, also highly relevant to the assessment of persons with ASD. It is important to note that, unlike these normative approaches, those designed for use in ASD face unique challenges.

Challenges for dimensional assessment in autism/ASD include the broad range of syndrome expression, age, comorbidity, and IQ-related issues in syndrome expression; the relevance of historical information versus current examination; and the degree to which sometimes highly infrequent (but essential) behaviors are sampled. There are all the usual problems of reliability and so forth (see Lord and Gotham, 2014). Aspects of item administration or scoring can present challenges; we have seen examples in which motor tics were mistakenly coded as stereotyped mannerisms. The degree to which clinical judgment is essential also varies across instruments, as do flexibility in administration and the intended range of age or developmental level.

In theory, the potential for quantifying symptoms has essential research implications, providing measures of severity that can be assessed during treatment or providing potential new approaches to subtypes or consistency in genetic studies. These approaches have essential uses and limitations. An understandable tension exists between research and clinical use. Screening instruments present other complexities and sources of controversy (see Barton et al., 2012; Øien, et al., 2018a, 2018b) as compared to diagnostic instruments. The latter may focus either on parent report or direct observation (or both). Available diagnostic instruments also probably work best in school-age children with ASD who have some language and mild to moderate cognitive disability. Their use becomes more complex at other parts of the age and IQ range. The problems raised by comorbidity are major and substantial (see Miot et al., 2019; Hawks & Constantino, 2020) and are approached differently in official categorization schemes. For autism and related disorders, there is also a growing awareness that having such conditions increases the risk for other problems. In more cognitively able individuals with autism and Asperger syndrome, for example, higher than expected rates of mood and anxiety problems are noted (White, Bray, & Ollendick, 2012; Spiker, Lin, Van Dyke, & Wood, 2012; Stewart, Barnard, Pearson, Hasan, & O'Brien, 2006). These issues may have important implications for assessment and treatment, but sadly, basic data are lacking in many areas (e.g., there is more or less a total absence of work on rates of suicidal ideation/behavior in adolescents and adults with ASD). These issues become very relevant to DSM-5, given the decision to rely on data from tests rather than the results of field trials as in DSM-IV. Although the desire to make use of a considerable body of research on these instruments is commendable (Regier et al., 2012), there may be many challenges in translating them into "real-world" clinical practice.

Current Areas of Debate and Controversy

Several different areas are the source of some controversy or concern. As previously noted, DSM-5 apparently takes a much more stringent approach to a diagnosis of autism (at least for new cases as old cases are "grandfathered" in). This may present some challenges for newly diagnosed young children who in the past under DSM-IV would have had a diagnosis of autism, as well as for higher cognitively functioning individuals who often come to diagnosis somewhat later (and of course for higher functioning toddlers).

A second area of concern centers on the complex issues of comorbidity (Rutter, 1997). This issue has been dealt with in different ways by different systems. ICD-10, for example, had a preference for avoiding additional diagnosis and explicitly included several comorbid categories. DSM has historically been more welcoming of multiple diagnoses. These issues become more complex as children become older and are at risk for other problems—notably anxiety and depression—increases. Of course, even in young children comorbid diagnosis can be an issue, for example, within seizure disorder or intellectual disability. DSM-5 provides some, although limited, coding for certain possibilities, such as specific genetic diseases. It remains unclear as to what approach, over time, will prove the most help-ful.

Finally, relatively little research has been conducted to assess the potential biases in instruments used for purposes such as screening and assessment; such biases can be toward cultures, ethnicities, genders, and SES. The potential biases of such instruments are of great importance, as they often affect clinicians' judgments; thus, selecting the most appropriate one will be critical (Cicchetti, 1994).

Even though few studies are standardized across demographic vari-ables, such as age, gender, education, culture, ethnicity, and a range of other variables that could potentially affect the performance of such tools, it is important that we acknowledge such limitations to concurrent instru-ments, the so-called "gold-standard" instruments. Standardizing instru-ments according to such variables allows for norms relevant to a given nation, gender, or a specific culture. However, multiple factors affect the possibility of standardizing a given test for all potential biases.

Concurrent gold-standard instruments perform well in identifying ASD in most studies, especially when using ADOS (Autism Diagnostic Observation Schedule) and ADI-R (Autism Diagnostic Interview—Revised) (see Lord et al., 2014) to complement each other (Øien & Nordahl-Hansen, 2018). However, there is sparse knowledge of how screening and diagnostic instruments detect ASD in, for example, eastern cultures, different eth-nicities, or between sexes (Øien & Nordahl-Hansen, 2018). Many instru-ments specific to the identification and assessment of ASD are developed and standardized in the United States and Europe and are often translated into different languages for use in other populations. In many such cases, no validation study is conducted for each translation. On these grounds, it is increasingly important to be aware of and to develop new research on how culture, ethnicity, SES, and gender affect the performance of such instruments. A potential factor, such as sex, could affect how well screen-ing instruments perform across various cultures because humans, espe-cially parents, could rate behaviors differently based on their cultural views on normality.

A study by Vanegas and colleagues (Vanegas, Magaña, Morales, & McNamara, 2016) revealed that the sensitivity and specificity of the ADI-R were moderate in a U.S. Latino sample, but lower than previously reported. These authors argued that the tool needs to be standardized for differ-ent languages and cultures. Cross-cultural differences in ASD have been reported in earlier studies (Elsabbagh et al., 2012) and are thought to affect how ASD is perceived, diagnosed, and treated in different cultures (Freeth et al., 2014). An example comes from the ethnic Norwegian minority, the Sami population, among whom disorders such as ASD and other mental health issues have been less prevalent than in the majority community

(Nergård, 2006). It is also important to think about the concurrent validity of an instrument in the context of culture; for example, societal and cultural changes happen over time and might cause a gap between what was considered normative at the time of development and what is so considered currently. Furthermore, a range of other factors such as behaviors and temperament in males and females could affect how well instruments perform in detecting and diagnosing ASD (Dworzynski, Ronald, Bolton, & Happé, 2012; Øien et al., 2018a, 2018b). Some of the more complex issues in identifying and diagnosing autism at an early age are related to the heterogeneous presentation of the disorder. Heterogeneity in etiology, behaviors, core symptoms, cognitive skills, adaptive skills, language and communication, the patterns and time onset of diagnosis, and core symptom patterns elicits immense complexities in the clinical detection of the disorder and ultimately affects treatment and treatment planning (Ozonoff et al., 2010; Zwaigenbaum et al., 2015). Previous DSMs had a strict age-of-onset criterion, but it was removed from DSM-5 (American Psychiatric Association, 2013) because symptoms might not become evident until social demands exceed the child's capabilities (Ozonoff et al., 2015). Furthermore, symptom expression might also vary depending on verbal and nonverbal functioning (Chawarska et al., 2014). These challenges do not apply only to clinical detection, but potentially affects when parental concern emerges, consequently leading to diagnosis later rather than early.

Both categorical and diagnostic instruments face additional challenges relative to diagnosis of autism in infants and young children. These complexities include the marked potential for developmental change, the sometimes later development of autism (e.g., following regression), and challenges posed by the complex clinical presentation of other disorders such as language/communication problems and intellectual disability. In a study by Ozonoff et al. (2015), nearly half of the children with ASD outcomes were not so identified at age 2 and didn't receive a diagnosis until age 3. In her original longitudinal study, Lord (1996) noted that stereotyped mannerisms frequently developed in significant ways after the age of 2. Before 36 months of age, there is much more potential for diagnostic instability. After that time, however, this instability becomes much less common, and children who clearly have autism tend to retain this diagnosis (Ozonoff et al., 2015). However, truly major changes can be made in very young children, with some 3- and 4-year-olds dramatically responding to treatment.

These problems will, of course, be less problematic should good biomarkers for autism be identified. These might be genetic (Rutter et al., 2014), biochemical (Anderson, 2014), neurophysiological (McPartland, Dawson, Webb, Panagiotides, & Carver, 2004), neuroanatomical (Chawarska, Chang, & Campbell, 2015), or even behavioral (Chawarska, Ye, Shic, & Chen, 2016). But to date, no biomarker has been identified. Accordingly, in both clinical and research settings, it will be wise to be careful relative to the surety of early diagnostic assignment and to include an explicit follow-up aspect to both clinical diagnosis and research. For the latter, it is also critical that control and comparison groups include infants and young children with developmental delays *not* associated with vulnerability. Attention to the standardization of methods and stimuli is also critical, for major differences can be noted depending on the methods used (e.g., see Ozonoff et al., 2010; Rowberry et al., 2015; and Chawarska, Macari, & Shic, 2013). Work attempting to identify specific subtypes in early-age groups may be of great interest in this regard (Kim, Macari, Koller, & Chawarska, 2016).

Summary

In the more than 75 years that have passed since Kanner's classic description of infantile autism, noteworthy changes have taken place in our conceptualization of this disorder. The first decades of work on the condition were plagued with confusion about its relationship to other conditions (notably, schizophrenia), along with some noteworthy misconceptions about etiology, social class factors, cognitive abilities, and treatment approaches. During the 1970s, evidence emerged showing autism to be a unique condition that was distinctive in many ways. It had a strong brain and genetic basis, and it responded best to structured treatment designed to help the child compensate for the obstacles the syndrome poses for learning and development. The official recognition of the condition as "infantile autism" in 1980 by DSM-III was particularly important, and since that time the literature on autism has vastly increased.

As the same time, several tensions continue to the present. The first definition of autism in DSM-III focused on "infantile" autism—that is, in its most classic form, as it presumably exhibited itself in infancy. The issue of development was dealt with by including a "residual" category for those who had once met the criteria for the infantile form of the disorder. This approach was unsatisfactory, and so the next revision adopted an explicit orientation. The DSM-IV and ICD-10 convergence remained the gold standard for several decades. As noted above, with DSM-5 the pendulum has (somewhat paradoxically given the name change to autism spectrum disorder) swung backward to focus more on the prototypical cases of "Kanner's autism." As we note above, higher cognitive function cases are now more likely be excluded from the diagnosis, although, again paradoxically, those who had a diagnosis before DSM-5 are allowed to keep it!

The move in DSM-5 to autism spectrum disorder reflects an interesting and growing body of research on the autism spectrum. This had its origins in the recognition of atypical or "not otherwise specified" forms of the disorder. With time, a growing body of work suggests that autism does indeed shade off into normalcy. This work is consistent, in many ways, with what have become the rather complex genetic origins of the condition.

As we note in this chapter, for infants and young children, a growing awareness of the disorder and provision of new evidence-based treatments have presented important opposites for optimizing learning and eventual outcomes. As the same time, our lack of biological markers for the conditions and the rather variable performance of screening tests present important obstacles. As noted elsewhere in this volume, a range of new methodologies are being presented to focus on autism as it is first expressed. These studies will move to even earlier development, for example, looking for differences in utero. Clearly, while much work remains to be done, many advances have been made.

REFERENCES

American Psychiatric Association. (1980). *Diagnostic and statistical manual of mental disorders* (3rd ed.). Washington, DC: Author.

American Psychiatric Association. (1987). *Diagnostic and statistical manual of mental disorders* (3rd ed., rev.). Washington, DC: Author.

American Psychiatric Association. (1994). *Diagnostic and statistical manual of mental disorders* (4th ed.). Washington, DC: Author.

American Psychiatric Association. (2000). *Diagnostic and statistical manual of mental disorders* (4th ed., text rev.). Washington, DC: Author.

American Psychiatric Association. (2013). *Diagnostic and statistical manual of mental disorders* (5th ed.). Arlington, VA: Author.

Anderson, G. M. (2014). Biochemical biomarkers for autism spectrum disorder. In F. R. Volkmar, R. Paul, S. J. Rogers, & K. A. Pelphrey (Eds.), *Handbook of autism and pervasive developmental disorders* (4th ed., pp. 457–481). Hoboken, NJ: Wiley.

Asperger, H. (1944). Die "autistichen Psychopathen" im Kindersalter. *Archive für Psychiatrie und Nervenkrankheiten, 117,* 76–136.

Barton, M. L., Dumont-Mathieu, T., & Fein, D. (2012). Screening young children for autism spectrum disorders in primary practice. *Journal of Autism and Developmental Disorders, 42*(6), 1165–1174.

Bennett, T., Szatmari, P., Bryson, S., Volden, J., Zwaigenbaum, L., Vaccarella, L., . . . Boyle M. (2008). Differentiating autism and Asperger syndrome on the basis of language delay or impairment. *Journal of Autism and Developmental Disorders, 38*(4), 616–625.

Bettelheim, B. (1974). *A home for the heart.* New York: Knopf.

Campbell, J. M. (2005). Diagnostic assessment of Asperger's disorder: A review of five third-party rating scales. *Journal of Autism and Developmental Disorders, 35*(1), 25–35.

Candland, D. K. (1993). *Feral children and clever animals: Reflections on human nature.* New York: Oxford University Press.

Chawarska, K., Chang, J., & Campbell, D. (2015). Clinical correlates of early generalized overgrowth in autism spectrum disorder: In reply. *Journal of the American Academy of Child and Adolescent Psychiatry, 54*(11), 958–959.

Chawarska, K., Klin, A., & Volkmar, F. (Eds.). (2008). *Autism spectrum disorders in infants and toddlers: Diagnosis, assessment, and treatment.* New York: Guilford Press.

Chawarska, K., Macari, S., & Shic, F. (2013). Decreased spontaneous attention to social scenes in 6-month-old infants later diagnosed with autism spectrum disorders. *Biological Psychiatry, 74*(3), 195–203.

Chawarska, K., Macari, S., Volkmar, F. R., Kim, S., & Shic, F. (2014). ASD in infants and toddlers. In F. R. Volkmar, R. Paul, S. J. Rogers, & K. A. Pelphrey (Eds.), *Handbook of autism and pervasive developmental disorders* (4th ed., Vol. 1., pp. 121–147). Hoboken, NJ: Wiley.

Chawarska, K., Ye, S., Shic, F., & Chen, L. (2016). Multilevel differences in spontaneous social attention in toddlers with autism spectrum disorder. *Child Development, 87*(2), 543–557.

Chiang, H.-M., Cheung, Y. K., Brown, A., & Li, H. (2014). A meta-analysis of differences in IQ profiles between individuals with Asperger's disorder and high-functioning autism. *Journal of Autism and Developmental Disorders, 44*(7), 1577–1596.

Cicchetti, D. V. (1994). Guidelines, criteria, and rules of thumb for evaluating normed and standardized assessment instruments in psychology. *Psychological Assessment, 6*(4), 284–290.

Constantino, J. N., & Todd, R. D. (2000). Genetic structure of reciprocal social behavior. *American Journal of Psychiatry, 157*(12), 2043–2045.

de Sanctis, S. (1906). On some variations of dementia praecox. *Revista Sperimentali di Frenciatria, 32,* 141–165.

Doehring, P., & Becker-Conttrill, B. (2013). *Autism services across America.* Baltimore, MD: Brookes.

Dworzynski, K., Ronald, A., Bolton, P., & Happé, F. (2012). How different are girls and boys above and below the diagnostic threshold for autism spectrum disorders? *Journal of the American Academy of Child and Adolescent Psychiatry, 51*(8), 788–797.

Elsabbagh, M., Divan, G., Koh, Y.-J., Kim, Y. S., Kauchali, S., Marcín, C., . . . Fombonne, E. (2012). Global prevalence of autism and other pervasive developmental disorders. *Autism Research, 5*(3), 160–179.

Factor, D. C., Freeman, N. L., & Kardash, A. (1989). A comparison of DSM-III and DSM-III-R criteria for autism. *Journal of Autism and Developmental Disorders, 19*(4), 637–640.

Ferster, C. B. (1972). Clinical reinforcement. *Seminars in Psychiatry, 4*(2), 101–111.

Folstein, S., & Rutter, M. (1978). Genetic influences and infantile autism. *Annual progress in child psychiatry and child development* (pp. 437–441). New York: Brunner/Mazel.

Fraser, R., Cotton, S., Gentle, E., Angus, B., Allott, K., & Thompson, A. (2012). Non-expert clinicians' detection of autistic traits among attenders of a youth mental health service. *Early Intervention in Psychiatry, 6*(1), 83–86.

Freeth, M., Milne, E., Sheppard, E., & Ramachandran, R. (2014). Autism across cultures: Perspectives from non-western cultures and implications for research. In F. R. Volkmar, R. Paul, S. J. Rogers, & K. A. Pelphrey (Eds.), *Handbook of autism and pervasive developmental disorders, Vol. 2* (4th ed., pp. 997–1013). Hoboken, NJ: Wiley.

Gardner, L. M., Campbell, J. M., Keisling, B., & Murphy, L. (2018). Correlates of DSM-5 autism spectrum disorder levels of support ratings in a clinical sample. *Journal of Autism and Developmental Disorders, 48*(10), 3513–3523.

Gibbs, V., Aldridge, F., Chandler, F., Witzlsperger, E., & Smith, K. (2012). An exploratory study comparing diagnostic outcomes for autism spectrum disorders under DSM-IV-TR with the proposed DSM-5 revision. *Journal of Autism and Developmental Disorders, 42*(8), 1750–1756.

Gillberg, C. (1994). Debate and argument: Having Rett syndrome in the ICD-10 PDD category does not make sense [Comment]. *Journal of Child Psychology and Psychiatry and Allied Disciplines, 35*(2), 377–378.

Goldstein, S., Naglieri, J. A., & Ozonoff, S. (Eds.). (2009). *Assessment of autism spectrum disorders.* New York: Guilford Press.

Gould, S. J. (1996). *The mismeasure of man.* New York: Norton.

Greenberg, G. (2013). *The book of woe: The DSM and the unmaking of psychiatry.* New York, Penguin.

Guthrie, W., Swineford, L. B., Wetherby, A. M., & Lord, C. (2013). Comparison of DSM-IV and DSM-5 factor structure models for toddlers with autism spectrum disorder. *Journal of the American Academy of Child and Adolescent Psychiatry, 52*(8), 797–805.

Hansen, R. L., Ozonoff, S., Krakowiak, P., Angkustsiri, K., Jones, C., Deprey, L. J., . . . Hertz-Picciotto, I. (2008). Regression in autism: Prevalence and associated factors in the CHARGE Study. *Ambulatory Pediatrics, 8*(1), 25–31.

Harris, J. C. (2006). *Intellectual disability: Understanding its development, causes, classification, evaluation, and treatment.* New York: Oxford University Press.

Hawks, Z. W., & Constantino, J. N. (2020). Neuropsychiatric "comorbidity" as causal influence in autism. *Journal of the American Academy of Child and Adolescent Psychiatry, 59*(2), 229–235.

Heller, T. (1908). Dementia infantilis. *Zeitschrift fur die erforschung und behandlung des jugenlichen schwachsinns, 2,* 141–165.

Hertzig, M. E., Snow, M. E., New, E., & Shapiro, T. (1990). DSM-III and DSM-III-R diagnosis of autism and pervasive developmental disorder in nursery school children. *Journal of the American Academy of Child and Adolescent Psychiatry, 29*(1), 123–126.

Hobbs, N. (1975). *Issues in the classification of children.* San Francisco: Jossey-Bass.

Huerta, M., Bishop, S. L., Duncan, A., Hus, V., & Lord, C. (2013). Response to Ritvo and Ritvo letter: Commentary on the application of DSM-5 criteria for autism spectrum disorder. *American Journal of Psychiatry, 170*(4), 445–446.

Hunt, J. M. (1961). *Intelligence and experience.* New York: Ronald Press.

Ibañez, L. V., Stone, W. L., & Coonrod, E. E. (2014). Screening for autism in young children. In F. R. Vollkmar, S. J. Rogers, R. Paul, & K. A. Pelphrey (Eds.), *Handbook of autism and pervasive developmental disorders* (4th ed., Vol. 2, pp. 585–608). Hoboken, NJ: Wiley.

Ingersoll, B., & Wainer, A. (2014). The broader autism phenotype. In F. R. Vollkmar, S. J. Rogers, R. Paul, & K. A. Pelphrey (Eds.), *Handbook of autism and pervasive developmental disorders* (4th ed., Vol. 1, pp. 28–56). Hoboken, NJ: Wiley.

Jackson, S. L., & Volkmar, F. R. (2019). Diagnosis and definition of autism and other pervasive developmental disorders. In F. Volkmar (Ed.), *Autism and pervasive developmental disorders* (3rd ed., pp. 1–24). Cambridge, UK: Cambridge University Press.

Jones, L. A., & Campbell, J. M. (2010). Clinical characteristics associated with language regression for children with autism spectrum disorders. *Journal of Autism and Developmental Disorders, 40*(1), 54–62.

Kanner, L. (1943). Autistic disturbances of affective contact. *Nervous Child, 2,* 217–250.

Kanner, L. (1971). Follow-up study of eleven autistic children originally reported in 1943. *Journal of Autism and Childhood Schizophrenia, 1*(2), 119–145.

Kim, S. H., Macari, S., Koller, J., & Chawarska, K. (2016). Examining the phenotypic heterogeneity of early autism spectrum disorder: Subtypes and short-term outcomes. *Journal of Child Psychology and Psychiatry, 57*(1), 93–102.

King, B. H., Veenstra-VanderWeele, J., & Lord, C. (2013). DSM-5 and autism: Kicking the tires and making the grade. *Journal of the American Academy of Child and Adolescent Psychiatry, 52*(5), 454–457.

Klin, A., Jones, W., Schultz, R., & Volkmar, F. R. (2005). The enactive mind—from actions to cognition: Lessons from autism. In F. R. Volkmar, A. Klin, R. Paul, & D. J. Cohen (Eds.), *Handbook of autism and pervasive developmental disorders: Diagnosis, development, neurobiology, and behavior* (3rd ed., Vol. 1, pp. 682–703). Hoboken, NJ: Wiley.

Klin, A., Saulnier, C., Tsatsanis, K., & Volkmar, F. R. (2005). Clinical evaluation in autism spectrum disorders: Psychological assessment within a transdisciplinary framework. In F. R. Volkmar, A. Klin, R. Paul, & D. J. Cohen (Eds.), *Handbook of autism and pervasive developmental disorders* (3rd ed., Vol. 2, pp. 772–798). Hoboken, NJ: Wiley.

Kolvin, I. (1971). Studies in childhood psychoses: I. Diagnostic criteria and classification. *British Journal of Psychiatry, 118,* 381–384.

Kurita, H., Koyama, T., Setoya, Y., Shimizu, K., & Osada H. (2004). Validity of childhood disintegrative disorder apart from autistic disorder with speech loss. *European Child and Adolescent Psychiatry, 13*(4), 221–226.

Lord, C. (1996). Follow-up of two-year-olds referred for possible autism. *Journal of Child Psychology and Psychiatry, 36*(8), 1065–1076.

Lord, C., Corsello, C., & Grzadzinski, R. (2014). Diagnostic instruments in autistic spectrum disorders. In F. R. Volkmar, S. J. Rogers, R. Paul, & K. A. Pelphrey (Eds.), *Handbook of autism and developmental disorders* (pp. 610–650). Hoboken, NJ: Wiley.

Lord, C., & Gotham, K. (2014). DSM-5 and ASD: Reflections and commentary. In T. E. Davis, III, S. W. White, & T. H. Ollendick (Eds.), *Handbook of autism and anxiety* (pp. 247–261). Cham, Switzerland: Springer International.

Lord, C., Petkova, E., Hus, V., Gan, W., Lu, F., Martin, D. M., . . . Risi, R. (2012). A multisite study of the clinical diagnosis of different autism spectrum disorders. *Archives of General Psychiatry, 69*(3), 306–313.

Lovass, O. I., & Smith, T. (1988). Intensive behavioral treatment for young autistic children. In B. B. Lahey & A. E. Kazdin (Eds.), *Advances in clinical child psychology* (Vol. 11, pp. 285–324). New York: Plenum Press.

Luyster, R., Richler, J., Risi, S., Hsu, W.-L., Dawson, G., Bernier, R, . . . Lord, C. (2005). Early regression in social communication in autism spectrum disorders: A CPEA study. *Developmental Neuropsychology, 27*(3), 311–336.

Matson, J. L., Beighley, J., & Turygin, N. (2012a). Autism diagnosis and screening: Factors to consider in differential diagnosis. *Research in Autism Spectrum Disorders, 6*(1), 19–24.

Matson, J. L., Hattier, M. A., & Williams, L. W. (2012b). How does relaxing the algorithm for autism affect DSM-V prevalence rates? *Journal of Autism and Developmental Disorders, 42*(8), 1549–1556.

Mattila, M. L., Kielinen, M., Linna, S. L., Jussila, K., Ebeling, H., Bloigu, R., . . .
Moilanen, I. (2011). Autism spectrum disorders according to DSM-IV-TR and
comparison with DSM-5 draft criteria: An epidemiological study. *Journal of the
American Academy of Child and Adolescent Psychiatry, 50*(6), 583–592.

Maudsley, H. (1867). *The physiology and pathology of mind.* New York: Appleton & Co.

Mayes, S. D., Calhoun, S. L., & Crites, D. L. (2001). Does DSM-IV Asperger's disorder
exist? *Journal of Abnormal Child Psychology, 29*(3), 263–271.

Mazefsky, C., McPartland, J., Gastgeb, H., & Minshew, N. (2013). Brief report: Comparability of DSM-IV and DSM-5 ASD research samples. *Journal of Autism and
Developmental Disorders, 43*(5), 1236–1242.

McPartland, J., Dawson, G., Webb, S. J., Panagiotides, H., & Carver, L. J. (2004).
Event-related brain potentials reveal anomalies in temporal processing of faces
in autism spectrum disorder. *Journal of Child Psychology and Psychiatry, 45*(7),
1235–1245.

McPartland, J. C., & Pelphrey, K. A. (2012). The implications of social neuroscience
for social disability. *Journal of Autism and Developmental Disorders, 42*(6),
1256–1262.

McPartland, J. C., Reichow, B., & Volkmar, F. R. (2012). Sensitivity and specificity of
proposed DSM-5 diagnostic criteria for autism spectrum disorder. *Journal of the
American Academy of Child and Adolescent Psychiatry, 51*(4), 368–383.

Miot, S., Akbaraly, T., Michelon, C., Couderc, S., Crepiat, S., Loubersac, J., . . . Bagh-
dadli, A. (2019). Comorbidity burden in adults with autism spectrum disorders
and intellectual disabilities—a report from the EFAAR (Frailty Assessment in
Aging Adults with Autism Spectrum and Intellectual Disabilities) study. *Frontiers
in Psychiatry Frontiers Research Foundation, 10,* 617.

Moretti, P., & Zoghbi, H. Y. (2006). MeCP2 dysfunction in Rett syndrome and related
disorders. *Current Opinion in Genetics and Development, 16*(3), 276–281.

National Society for Autistic Children. (1978). Definition of the syndrome of autism.
Journal of Autism and Childhood Schizophrenia, 8(2), 162–169.

Nergård, J. I. (2006). *Den levende erfaring: En studie i samisk kunnskapstradisjon.*
Oslo: Cappelen Akademisk.

Øien, R. A., & Nordahl-Hansen, A. (2018). Bias in assessment instruments for autism.
In *Encyclopedia of autism spectrum disorders* (Vol. 51, pp. 1–2). New York:
Springer.

Øien, R. A., Schjolberg, S., Volkmar, F. R., Shic, F., Cicchetti, D. V., Nordahl-Hansen,
A., . . . Chawarska, K. (2018a). Clinical features of children with autism who
passed 18-month screening. *Pediatrics, 141*(6), 6.

Øien, R. A., Vambheim, S. M., Hart, L., Nordahl-Hansen, A., Erickson, C., Wink,
L., . . . Grodberg, D. (2018b). Sex-differences in children referred for assessment:
An exploratory analysis of the Autism Mental Status Exam (AMSE). *Journal of
Autism and Developmental Disorders, 48*(7), 2286–2292.

Ozonoff, S., & Griffith, E. M. (2000). Neuropsychological function and the external
validity of Asperger syndrome. In A. Klin, F. R. Volkmar, & S. S. Sparrow (Eds.),
Asperger syndrome (pp. 72–96). New York: Guilford Press.

Ozonoff, S., Iosif, A.-M., Baguio, F., Cook, I. C., Hill, M. M., Hutman, T., . . . Young,
G. S. (2010). A prospective study of the emergence of early behavioral signs of

autism. *Journal of the American Academy of Child and Adolescent Psychiatry, 49*(3), 256–266.

Ozonoff, S., Young, G. S., Landa, R. J., Brian, J., Bryson, S., Charman, T., . . . Iosif, A.-M. (2015). Diagnostic stability in young children at risk for autism spectrum disorder: A Baby Siblings Research Consortium study. *Journal of Child Psychology and Psychiatry, 56*(9), 988–998.

Piven, J. (2001). The broad autism phenotype: A complementary strategy for molecular genetic studies of autism. *American Journal of Medical Genetics, 105*(1), 34–35.

Prizant, B. M., & Rydell, P. J. (1984). Analysis of functions of delayed echolalia in autistic children. *Journal of Speech and Hearing Research, 27*(2), 183–192.

Rank, B. (1949). Adaptation of the psychoanalytic technique for the treatment of young children with atypical development. *American Journal of Orthopsychiatry 19,* 130–139.

Rank, B., & MacNaughton, D. (1949). A clinical contribution to early ego development. In A. Freud & H. Hartmann (Eds.), *The psychoanalytic study of the child* (Vol. 3, pp. 53–65). Oxford, UK: International Universities Press.

Regier, D. A., Narrow, W. E., Clarke, D. E., Kraemer, H. C., Kuramoto, S. J., Kuhl, E. A., & Kupfer, D. J. (2012). DSM-5 field trials in the United States and Canada: Part II. Test-retest reliability of selected categorical diagnoses. *American Journal of Psychiatry, 170*(1), 59–70.

Reiss, S., Levitan, G., & Szyszko, J. (1982). Emotional disturbance and mental retardation: Diagnostic overshadowing. *America Journal of Mental Deficiency, 86,* 567–574.

Rett, A. (1966). Uber ein eigenartiges hirntophisces Syndroem bei hyperammonie im Kindersalter. *Wein Medizinische Wochenschrift, 118,* 723–726.

Rett, A. (1986). Rett syndrome: History and general overview. *American Journal of Medical Genetics, 1986*(Suppl 1), 21–25.

Rimland, B. (1964). *Infantile autism: The syndrome and its implications for a neural theory of behavior.* New York: Appleton-Century-Crofts.

Rimland, B. (1971). The differentiation of childhood psychoses: An analysis of checklists for 2,218 psychotic children. *Journal of Autism and Childhood Schizophrenia, 1*(2), 161–174.

Rogers, S. J. (2004). Developmental regression in autism spectrum disorders. *Mental Retardation and Developmental Disabilities Research Reviews, 10*(2), 139–143.

Rowberry, J., Macari, S., Chen, G., Campbell, D., Leventhal, J. M., Weitzman, C., & Chawarska, K. (2015). Screening for autism spectrum disorders in 12-month-old high-risk siblings by parental report. *Journal of Autism and Developmental Disorders, 45*(1), 221–229.

Rutter, M. (1972). Childhood schizophrenia reconsidered. *Journal of Autism and Childhood Schizophrenia, 2*(4), 315–337.

Rutter, M. (1978). Diagnosis and definitions of childhood autism. *Journal of Autism and Developmental Disorders, 8*(2), 139–161.

Rutter, M. (1991). Isle of Wight revisited: Twenty-five years of child psychiatric epidemiology. In S. Chess & M. E. Hertzig (Eds.), *Annual progress in child psychiatry and child development, 1990* (pp. 131–179). Philadelphia: Brunner/Mazel.

Rutter, M. (1994). Debate and argument: There are connections between brain and mind and it is important that Rett syndrome be classified somewhere [comment]. *Journal of Child Psychology and Psychiatry and Allied Disciplines, 35*(2), 379–381.

Rutter, M. (1997). Comorbidity: Concepts, claims and choices. *Criminal Behaviour and Mental Health, 7*(4), 265–285.

Rutter, M. (2011). Research review: Child psychiatric diagnosis and classification: Concepts, findings, challenges and potential. *Journal of Child Psychology and Psychiatry and Allied Disciplines, 52*(6), 647–660.

Rutter, M., & Bartak, L. (1973). Special educational treatment of autistic children: A comparative study: II. Follow-up findings and implications for services. *Journal of Child Psychology and Psychiatry and Allied Disciplines, 14*(4), 241–270.

Rutter, M., & Garmezy, N. M. (1983). Developmental psychopathology. In E. M. Hetherington (Ed.), *Mussen's handbook of child psychology: Socialization, personality and child development* (Vol. 4, pp. 755–911). New York: Wiley.

Rutter, M., Lebovici, S., Eisenberg, L., Sneznevskij, A. V., Sadoun, R., Brooke, E., & Lin, T. Y. (1969). A tri-axial classification of mental disorders in childhood: An international study. *Journal of Child Psychology and Psychiatry and Allied Disciplines, 10*(1), 41–61.

Rutter, M., & Schopler, E. (1992). Classification of pervasive developmental disorders: Some concepts and practical considerations [comments]. *Journal of Autism and Developmental Disorders, 22*(4), 459–482.

Rutter, M., & Thapar, A. (2014). Genetics of autism spectrum disorders. In F. R. Volkmar, R. Paul, S. J. Rogers, & K. A. Pelphrey (Eds.), *Handbook of autism and pervasive developmental disorders* (4th ed., pp. 411–423). Hoboken, NJ: Wiley.

Schopler, E., Van Bourgondien, M. E., Wellman, G. J., & Love, S. R. (2010). *Childhood Autism Rating Scale, Second edition (CARS2).* Torrance, CA: Western Psychological Services.

Sharma, S., Woolfson, L. M., & Hunter, S. C. (2012). Confusion and inconsistency in diagnosis of Asperger syndrome: A review of studies from 1981 to 2010. *Autism, 16*(5), 465–486.

Siegel, B., Vukicevic, J., Elliott, G. R., & Kraemer, H. C. (1989). The use of signal detection theory to assess DSM-III-R criteria for autistic disorder. *Journal of the American Academy of Child and Adolescent Psychiatry, 28*(4), 542–548.

Sipes, M., & Matson, J. L. (2014). Factor structure for autism spectrum disorders with toddlers using DSM-IV and DSM-5 criteria. *Journal of Autism and Developmental Disorders, 44*(3), 636–647.

Smith, I. C., Reichow, B., & Volkmar, F. R. (2015). The effects of DSM-5 criteria on number of individuals diagnosed with autism spectrum disorder: A systematic review. *Journal of Autism and Developmental Disorders, 45*(8), 2541–2552.

Spiker, M. A., Lin, C., Van Dyke, M., & Wood, J. J. (2012). Restricted interests and anxiety in children with autism. *Autism, 16*(3), 306–320.

Spitzer, R. L., Endicott, J. E., & Robbins, E. (1978). Resarch diagnostic criteria. *Archives of General Psychiatry, 35,* 773–782.

Stewart, M. E., Barnard, L., Pearson, J., Hasan, R., & O'Brien, G. (2006). Presentation of depression in autism and Asperger syndrome: A review. *Autism, 10*(1), 103–116.

Szatmari, P. (1991). Asperger's syndrome: Diagnosis, treatment, and outcome. *Psychiatric Clinics of North America, 14*(1), 81–93.

Taheri, A., & Perry, A. (2012). Exploring the proposed DSM-5 criteria in a clinical sample. *Journal of Autism and Developmental Disorders, 42*(9), 1810–1817.

Tsai, L. (1992). Is Rett syndrome a subtype of pervasive developmental disorder? *Journal of Autism and Developmental Disorders, 22,* 551–561.

Tsai, L. Y. (2012). Sensitivity and specificity: DSM-IV versus DSM-5 criteria for autism spectrum disorder. *American Journal of Psychiatry, 169*(10), 1009–1011.

Vanegas, S. B., Magaña, S., Morales, M., & McNamara, E. (2016). Clinical validity of the ADI-R in a U.S.-based Latino population. *Journal of Autism and Developmental Disorders, 46*(5), 1623–1635.

Volkmar, F. R. (1992). Childhood disintegrative disorder: Issues for DSM-IV. *Journal of Autism and Developmental Disorders, 22*(4), 625–642.

Volkmar, F. R., Booth, L. L., McPartland, J. C., & Wiesner, L. A. (2014a). Clinical evaluation in multidisciplinary settings. In F. R. Volkmar, S. J. Rogers, R. Paul, & K. A. Pelphrey (Eds.), *Handbook of autism and pervasive developmental disorders: Assessment, interventions, and policy* (4th ed., Vol. 2, pp. 661–672). Hoboken, NJ: Wiley.

Volkmar, F. R., Cicchetti, D. V., Bregman, J., & Cohen, D. J. (1992a). Three diagnostic systems for autism: DSM-III, DSM-III-R, and ICD-10. Special Issue: Classification and diagnosis. *Journal of Autism and Developmental Disorders, 22*(4), 483–492.

Volkmar, F. R., Cicchetti, D. V., Cohen, D. J., & Bregman, J. (1992b). Brief report: Developmental aspects of DSM-III-R criteria for autism. *Journal of Autism and Developmental Disorders, 22*(4), 657–662.

Volkmar, F. R., Cohen, D. J., & Paul, R. (1986). An evaluation of DSM-III criteria for infantile autism. *Journal of the American Academy of Child Psychiatry, 25*(2), 190–197.

Volkmar, F. R., Klin, A., & McPartland, J. C. (2014b). Asperger syndrome: An overview. In J. C. McPartland, A. Klin, & F. R. Volkmar (Eds.), *Asperger syndrome: Assessing and treating high-functioning autism spectrum disorders* (2nd ed., pp. 1–42). New York: Guilford Press.

Volkmar, F. R., Klin, A., Siegel, B., Szatmari, P., Lord, C., Campbell, M., . . . Towbin, K. (1994). Field trial for autistic disorder in DSM-IV. *American Journal of Psychiatry, 151*(9), 1361–1367.

Volkmar, F. R., & Nelson, D. S. (1990). Seizure disorders in autism. *Journal of the American Academy of Child and Adolescent Psychiatry, 29*(1), 127–129.

Volkmar, F. R., & Rutter, M. (1995). Childhood disintegrative disorder: Results of the DSM-IV autism field trial. *Journal of the American Academy of Child and Adolescent Psychiatry, 34*(8), 1092–1095.

Volkmar, F. R., Sparrow, S. S., Goudreau, D., Cicchetti, D. V., Paul, R., & Cohen, D. J. (1987). Social deficits in autism: An operational approach using the Vineland Adaptive Behavior Scales. *Journal of the American Academy of Child and Adolescent Psychiatry, 26*(2), 156–161.

Volkmar, F. R., Sukhodolsky, D., Schwab-Stone, M., & First, M. B. (2017). Diagnostic classification. In A. Martin, M. Bloch, & F. R. Volkmar (Eds.), *Lewis's child and adolescent psychiatry: A comprehensive textbook* (pp. 354–363). Philadelphia: Wolters-Kluwer.

Volkmar, F. R., & Tsatsanis, K. (2002). Psychosis and psychotic conditions in childhood and adolescence. In D. T. Marsh & M. A. Fristad (Eds.), *Handbook of serious emotional disturbance in children and adolescents* (pp. 266–283). New York: Wiley.

Wainer, A. L., Block, N., Donnellan, M. B., & Ingersoll, B. (2013). The broader autism phenotype and friendships in non-clinical dyads. *Journal of Autism and Developmental Disorders, 43*(10), 2418–2425.

Waterhouse, L., Wing, L., Spitzer, R. L., & Siegel, B. (1993). Diagnosis by DSM-III-R versus ICD-10 criteria. *Journal of Autism and Developmental Disorders, 23*(3), 572–573.

White, S. W., Bray, B. C., & Ollendick, T. H. (2012). Examining shared and unique aspects of social anxiety disorder and autism spectrum disorder using factor analysis. *Journal of Autism and Developmental Disorders, 42*(5), 874–884.

Wilson, C., Gillan, N., Spain, D., Robertson, D., Roberts, G., Murphy, C. M., . . . Murphy, D. G. (2013). Comparison of ICD-10R, DSM-IV-TR and DSM-5 in an adult autism spectrum disorder diagnostic clinic. *Journal of Autism and Developmental Disorders, 43*(11), 2515–2525.

Wing, L. (1980). Childhood autism and social class: A question of selection? *British Journal of Psychiatry 137*, 410–417.

Wing, L., & Gould, J. (1979). Severe impairments of social interaction and associated abnormalities in children: Epidemiology and classification. *Journal of Autism and Developmental Disorders, 9*(1), 11–29.

Wolff, S. (2004). The history of autism. *European Child and Adolescent Psychiatry, 13*(4), 201–208.

World Health Organization. (1994). *International classification of diseases* (10th ed.). Geneva, Switzerland: Author.

Worley, J. A., & Matson, J. L. (2012). Comparing symptoms of autism spectrum disorders using the current DSM-IV-TR diagnostic criteria and the proposed DSM-V diagnostic criteria. *Research in Autism Spectrum Disorders, 6*(2), 965–970.

Zwaigenbaum, L., Bauman, M. L., Stone, W. L., Yirmiya, N., Estes, A., Hansen, R. L., . . . Wetherby, A. (2015). Early identification of autism spectrum disorder: Recommendations for practice and research. *Pediatrics, 136*(4, Suppl. 1), S10–S40.

CHAPTER 2

• • • • • • • •

Screening for Autism Spectrum Disorder and Developmental Delays in Infants and Toddlers

Emily Campi, Catherine Lord, and Rebecca Grzadzinski

History of Screening Recommendations

In 1892, the largest medical screening facility in the history of the United States, Ellis Island, began universal health and IQ screenings for immigrants as they entered the country (Birn, 1997). A few decades later, the U.S. Army began screening enlisted recruits for psychological challenges, marking the first widespread screening implementation for mental health concerns. However, it was not until half a century later that the U.S. Commission of Chronic Illness defined screening as the "application of tests" to "rapidly identify unrecognized disease" (Morabia & Zhang, 2004, p. 463). Screening has since become common practice across a range of medical conditions and is intended to differentiate those who need further evaluation from those who are well (Gould, 1996).

The development of screening procedures, however, has been infused with Western bias. For example, the majority of commonly studied screening tools are written in English, and items are based on Western cultural norms, making these tools difficult to apply to diverse populations (Camp, 2007). Many of the early attempts to develop screening tools, therefore, were unlikely to address the needs of children from diverse cultures or whose families spoke languages other than English. For example, Hyman, Chafey, and Smith (1977) argued that assessment bias in psychological practices (e.g., failure to norm assessments on minority groups, socioeconomic differences in access to assessment) led to increases in socioeconomic and health disparities. These biases, inherent in the development of screening tools, have also been widely studied in cancer and perinatal depression screening procedures; this suggests a widespread need in the health care community to increase responsivity to cultural needs in patient populations (Altpeter, Mitchell, & Pennell, 2005; Ka'opua, 2008; Price & Handrick,

2009). Although the concept of screening arguably began as part of the eugenics movement and has, therefore, been historically fraught with ethical problems (Gould, 1996), there is currently a movement toward adopting culturally and linguistically responsive screening procedures that demonstrate accuracy in diverse populations in order to promote access to services for all in need. Screening research is working toward culturally responsive tools through adaptations and inclusion of cultural concerns to expand the research focus beyond tool performance (Soto et al., 2015; Harris, Barton, & Albert, 2014). See Chapter 11 for more information regarding challenges of screening in diverse settings.

Today, screening begins prenatally and continues throughout the lifespan. Within the first year of life, children are routinely screened for a variety of medical concerns. Before their first birthday, children receive hearing and vision screening, growth (height, weight, and head circumference) tracking, and testing for anemia and the presence of high levels of lead in the blood. These efforts are intended to identify possible illness even before overt symptoms are present to initiate treatment and improve long-term outcomes. More recently, screening within the first few years of life for developmental disabilities, including autism spectrum disorder (ASD), has been considered with the same goals in mind.

Although ASD was first identified by Leo Kanner in 1943, the history of recommendations for screening is relatively brief. The most recent estimates by the Centers for Disease Control and Prevention (CDC) suggest that the prevalence of ASD is 1 in 59 children (Baio et al., 2018), highlighting the need for awareness of early signs of the disorder and implementation of universal standard screening. See Chapter 1 for more information regarding the history of ASD. The American Academy of Pediatrics (AAP), the American Academy of Neurology (AAN), the American Academy of Child and Adolescent Psychiatry (AACAP), the Child Neurology Society (CNS), and the U.S. federal government have made recommendations regarding early screening for ASD (AAP, Committee on Children with Disabilities, 2001; AAP, Council on Children with Disabilities, 2006; Volkmar et al., 1999, 2014). The first major legislative action to be taken regarding early identification of developmental disabilities was a 1997 amendment to the federal Individuals with Disabilities Education Act (IDEA, 1990). This amendment mandated that pediatricians refer children to appropriate professionals for further evaluation in a timely manner when developmental concerns, including concerns for ASD, arise (AAP, Committee on Children with Disabilities, 2001). The IDEA amendment marked the first legislative action related to evaluations for developmental disabilities.

A few years later, the AAN and the CNS collaborated to produce a recommendation that standardized developmental screening be conducted during well-child visits for any child for whom developmental concerns were raised (Filipek et al., 2000). However, the presence of early developmental delay in children with ASD is inconsistent, sometimes subtle, and may be overlooked in young children (Baird, Douglas, & Murphy, 2011; Brian et al., 2014; Kim et al., 2018). Identifying delays in young children is especially challenging since the timing of developmental milestones varies, even in typical development. In addition, children with ASD may display heterogeneous developmental profiles in which some developmental milestones are met but others, such as directed vocalizations, pointing, and response to name, are delayed or inconsistent to varying degrees (Baranek et al., 2013; Colgan et al., 2006; Ozonoff et al., 2010). See Chapter 6 for more details regarding development of children at risk for ASD. Given this heterogeneity, in 2001, the AAP recommended universal standard screening for possible developmental delays (ASD and otherwise), regardless of whether concerns had been raised (AAP, Committee on Children with Disabilities, 2001).

The AAP released another statement in 2006 that distinguished surveillance from screening and defined specific recommendations for detection of delays throughout infancy and toddlerhood. The AAP defined surveillance as a general awareness of potential developmental concerns, while defining screening as the use of standardized measures to detect developmental disorders (AAP, Council on Children with Disabilities, 2006). This 2006 statement recommended that pediatricians survey each child by asking parents about concerns, keeping a log of developmental history for each patient, making informed observations of the child during each well-child visit, and documenting these observations in medical charts. This well-documented surveillance was recommended to occur in conjunction with the administration of standardized developmental screening at 9-, 18-, 24-, and 30-month well-child visits (AAP, Council on Children with Disabilities, 2006).

In 2011, the National Institute for Health and Care Excellence (NICE) in Britain also issued an official ASD screening recommendation. In this statement, NICE recommended screening whenever concerns were raised and provided a table of potential red flags for ASD to be used as a reference for health care professionals (Baird et al., 2011). NICE did not recommend screening unless concerns were raised. However, this recommendation warned professionals that ASD may still be present even if children showed certain skills that are usually lacking in children with ASD, such as pretend play, eye contact, or smiling (Baird et al., 2011). Since the publication of this NICE recommendation, European screening procedures have remained nonuniversal, with procedural variations from country to country (Garcia-Primo et al., 2014). Concerns over evaluation of screening tools for clinical and research purposes in diverse populations across European regions, as well as the need for testing in large-scale community samples, including those with widely varying socioeconomic statuses and cultural backgrounds, may inhibit adoption of widespread screening practices (Garcia-Primo et al., 2014). Further, early screening in the community brings logistical challenges, including managing clinic flow, coordinating implementation during busy seasons, providing adequate staffing and staff training, giving useful feedback on false-negative results, and ensuring effective referrals (King et al., 2010; Ojen et al., 2018). Despite these challenges, development of screening tools to accurately detect risk for ASD in diverse infants and toddlers remains a priority (Bolte, Marschik, Falck-Ytter, Charman, & Roeyers, 2013; Janvier, Coffield, Harris, Mandell, & Cidav, 2018; Marlow, Servili, & Tomlinson, 2019). Screening tools for developmental delay and/ or ASD that are currently available or in development are outlined below, as well as the psychometric properties of each tool.

Screening Tools

The heterogeneity of ASD symptoms in early childhood requires screening tools that not only address a wide variety of symptoms, but also identify symptoms that vary in severity. This can be challenging given the AAP recommendation that screening be completed and scored quickly at brief, routine well-child visits (AAP, Council on Children with Disabilities, 2006). In developing effective, practical screening tools for ASD, researchers must balance reliability of the measure with speed and ease of implementation.

When selecting appropriate screening tools, it is also important to consider populations in which the tool was validated, as well as cultural and linguistic characteristics of the measure in order to reduce barriers related to culture, literacy, and socioeconomic status. Research supports specific items on some developmental measures, parent report on ASD-specific questionnaires, and trained clinical observation as the most effective screening modalities (Hardy, Haisley, Manning, & Fein, 2015; Wiggins, Bakeman, Adamson, & Robins, 2007; Wetherby, Brosnan-Maddox, Peace, & Newton, 2008; Bishop et al., 2017; Robins et al., 2014; Stone, Coonrod, & Ousley, 2000). For ASD-specific screening, the most effective tools or items are often those that measure indicators of core ASD symptoms, including social communication, restricted and repetitive behavior, and sensory regulation (Bishop et al., 2017; Hardy et al., 2015; Reznick, Baranek, Reavis, Watson, & Crais, 2007; Robins, Fein, Barton, & Green, 2001; Wetherby et al., 2008; Wiggins et al., 2007). For example, the communication items on the Ages and Stages Questionnaire—3rd Edition (ASQ-3) and the Withdrawn and Pervasive Developmental Problems scales on the Child Behavior Checklist (CBCL) were found to be most predictive of ASD as compared to other items on these broadband developmental screening tools (Hardy et al., 2015; Muratori et al., 2011).

Screening measures are commonly divided into two types of tools: Level 1 and Level 2. Level 1 screening tools are short, easy to administer, broad-based, and intended to determine if any developmental concerns are present, ASD or otherwise. Level 2 screening tools are longer, require more training to administer, have a narrower focus, and are intended for use when developmental concerns about a child have already been raised. Level 1 screening tools might be most appropriate in primary care practice settings where time and staff are limited resources (King et al., 2010). Level 2 screening tools may be best implemented as a secondary, more specialized step in screening once a child has been flagged to be at risk for developmental concerns. A positive result on either type of screener should lead to referral for further diagnostic evaluation. Because Level 1 tools require less time and training to administer than Level 2 screeners, they are more practical for use at every well-child visit, making universal standard screening easier. Level 2 screeners, reserved for children who present with parent or clinician concerns, help clinicians tailor referrals for diagnostic evaluations.

The utility of a screening tool is determined by assessing various psychometric properties that indicate the tool's ability to detect symptoms and distinguish concerns specific to ASD from other developmental concerns. These properties include sensitivity, specificity, positive predictive value (PPV), and negative predictive value (NPV). The balance between sensitivity and specificity is particularly important, both of which some scholars suggest should remain above 80% for a tool to be considered psychometrically sound (Wetherby et al., 2008). Sensitivity is the ability of a test to detect a true case of ASD, whereas specificity is the ability of a test to detect a true lack of ASD. PPV refers to the proportion of true ASD cases out of all those who screen positive, whereas NPV refers to the proportion of children who do not have ASD out of all those who screen negative. In this way, PPV and NPV are related to the prevalence of ASD in the sample. Across Level 1 and Level 2 screeners, sensitivity and PPV are perhaps most important when determining the utility of a screening tool. High sensitivity indicates a high rate of true positives, while strong PPV considers these true positives in light of population prevalence. However, psychometric properties may vary based on the developmental and chronological age of the child being tested, so accommodation of developmental differences across the recommended age range for any given tool must be considered when establishing cutoff scores that determine risk (Sturner, Howard, Bergmann, Stewart, & Afarian, 2017). Given the purpose of screening, it is generally considered more appropriate for a screening tool to yield false positives that can be clarified after further evaluation than to have false negatives that ultimately miss referrals for further evaluation. However, the potential for unnecessary emotional burden on families increases with greater rates of false-positive screening results (Gurian, Kinnamon, Henry, & Waisbren, 2006; Hewlett & Waisbren, 2006; Siu & the U.S. Preventive Services Task Force, 2016).

Screening tools are available in a variety of formats, including caregiver questionnaires, parent interviews, and trained observation by a clinician. See Table 2.1 for a summary of screening tools. Descriptions of

TABLE 2.1. Summary of Screening Tools

	Psychometric properties				Level	Age range (months)	Format	Administration			Cost
	Sensitivity	Specificity	PPV	NPV				Level of expertise	Time to administer	Language availability	
Ages and Stages Questionnaire (ASQ)	70–95%	70–100%[a]			1	1–66	Parent questionnaire	Participation in training via DVD or on-site	10–15 min	English, Spanish, French	One-time $225 purchase; photocopies can be made of the questionnaires
Autism Behavior Checklist (ABC)	54–92%	93–96%			2	24–168	Parent questionnaire	Minimal	10–20 min	English, Albanian, Arabic, Chinese, Portuguese, Spanish, and 19 others	$29 for 25 protocols
Autism Detection in Early Childhood (ADEC)	79–100%	52–100%	74–95%	82–100%	2	12–36	Trained observation	Training in the manual	10–25 min	English, Spanish	One-time $777 purchase; $47 for 10 score sheets
Autism Observation Scale for Infants (AOSI)	38%	86%	Research under way	Research under way	2	6–18	Clinician observation	Experience with infants and ASD	20 min	English	For research purposes only
Autism Symptom Interview (ASI)	63–91%	35–62%			1	24–59	Parent interview	Minimal	15–20 min	English	Still in development

46

Baby and Infant Screen for Children with aUtism Traits: Part 1 (BISCUIT: Part 1)	66–94%	72–98%			2	17–37	Parent interview	Minimal	20–30 min	English, Chinese, Arabic, Serbian, Italian, Spanish, Dutch, Greek	Not clinically available
Checklist for Early Signs of Developmental Disorders	68%	96%	10%	99%	1	3–39	Caregiver questionnaire	Minimal	5–10 min		Not clinically available
Child Behavior Checklist (CBCL)	58–96%	27–92%	50–64%	62–90%	1	18–60	Parent questionnaire	Minimal	10–15 min	English, Spanish, French, and 42 others	$30 for 50 questionnaires
Childhood Autism Rating Scale (CARS)	94–100%	85%	85%	73–100%	2	18–72	Clinician observation	Specific CARS training	5–10 min	English, Bulgarian, Italian	$46.25 for 25 questionnaires
Developmental Behaviour Checklist—Early Screen (DBC-ES)	68–88%	48–69%	74–77%	43–83%	2	18–48	Parent questionnaire	Minimal	5–10 min	English, Arabic, Chinese, French, German, and 17 others	Not clinically available
Early Screening of Autistic Traits Questionnaire (ESAT)	90–94%	25–100%	25–40%	98%	1	8–20	Parent questionnaire and follow-up observation	Minimal for the questionnaire, significant training for the observation	10–15 min for the questionnaire, 1.5 hr for the observation	English, Serbian	Free online download

(continued)

TABLE 2.1. (continued)

	Psychometric properties				Level	Age range (months)	Format	Administration			
	Sensitivity	Specificity	PPV	NPV				Level of expertise	Time to administer	Language availability	Cost
Early Video-Guided Autism Screener (E-VAS)	83–92%	38–77%			2	18–48	Parent questionnaire with video clips of typical development and ASD symptoms	Minimal	<30 min	English	Still in development
First Year Inventory (FYI)	92%	78%	74–85%	93%	1	12	Parent questionnaire	Minimal	15–20 min	English, Spanish, Hebrew, Dutch-Flemish, Italian, Chinese	Only available for research purposes
Infant-Toddler Checklist (ITC)	89–94%	89–94%	>70%	>70%	1	6–24	Parent questionnaire	Minimal	5–10 min	English and Spanish	Free online download
Modified Checklist for Autism in Toddlers (M-CHAT)	34–97%	83–99%	36–80%	99%	1	16–30	Parent questionnaire with a follow-up interview for screen-positive cases	Minimal	<5 min for the questionnaire, 5–10 min for the interview	English, Chinese, French, Italian, Spanish, and 54 others	Free online download
Observation Scale for Autism (OSA)	92%	100%			2	24–30	Clinician observation	Specific OSA training	10 min	English	Still in development
Parent Observation of Early Markers Scale (POEMS)	25–100%	65–87%	10–29%		2	1–24	Parent questionnaire	Minimal	10 min	English	Not clinically available

Parent's Observations of Social Interaction	54–89%	74–83%			1	18–48	Parent questionnaire	Minimal	<5 min	English	Free online download
PDD Behavior Inventory (PDD-BI)	74–92%	50–81%			2	18–221	Parent or teacher questionnaire	Minimal	30–45 min	English	$103 for 25 questionnaires and scoring sheets
Pervasive Developmental Disorders Screening Test—Second Edition (PDDST-II)	58–92%	49–91%			1	18–48	Parent questionnaire	Minimal	10–20 min	English and Spanish	$50 for 25 questionnaires
Screen for Social Interaction—Younger (SSI-Y)	87%	71%			1	24–42	Parent questionnaire	Minimal	10–15 min	English	Free online download
Screening Tool for Autism in Two-Year-Olds (STAT)	83–100%	83–86%	68–86%	90–97%	2	13–36	Structured interaction	Specific STAT training	20 min	English	$25 for 25 protocols and a one-time $500 purchase of the testing kit
Social Communication Questionnaire (SCQ)	47–89%	75–89%	65–93%	55%	1	>18	Parent questionnaire	Minimal	<10 min	English, German, Italian, and 12 others	$44 for 20 questionnaires

[a]Autism-specific statistic was not reported, so specificity for any developmental disorder is listed.

measures in the following sections are organized based on each tool's aim of development. That is, screening tools that have been developed specifically to identify ASD are separated from general developmental tools that have also been applied to measure risk for ASD.

Caregiver Questionnaires: ASD Specific

Autism Behavior Checklist

The Autism Behavior Checklist (ABC) is a 57-item parent questionnaire in which parents answer whether specific behaviors in each of six areas (sensory behaviors, relating, stereotypies and object use, language, self-help, and social behaviors) are present or absent in their child (Rellini, Tortolani, Trillo, Carbone, & Montecchi, 2004). Each item reported as "present" receives a score between 1 and 4 depending on its level of consistency with ASD symptoms (Rellini et al., 2004). The ABC takes approximately 10–20 minutes to complete and is intended for use in children ages 2–14 years (Krug, Arick, & Almond, 1978).

In one sample of children ages 6 to 15 years with ASD and other developmental disorders, the ABC was found to have 87% sensitivity and 96% specificity for ASD (Wadden, Bryson, & Rodger, 1991). Furthermore, in a study of Brazilian children with ASD, nonautism language disorders, and typical development, the ABC was found to have 92% sensitivity and 93% specificity (Marteleto & Pedromônico, 2005). However, in one study of a clinical sample of younger children (ages 18 months to 11 years), the ABC had a sensitivity of only 54% (Rellini et al., 2004), suggesting that the ABC may not be an appropriate screening tool for young children at risk for ASD.

Checklist for Early Signs of Developmental Disorders

The Checklist for Early Signs of Developmental Disorders (CESDD) is a 25-item checklist based on the most prevalent early markers for ASD, and it is intended to be completed in 5–10 minutes by daycare providers regarding children ages 3–39 months (Dereu, Roeyers, Raymaekers, Meirsschaut, & Warreyn, 2012). Items consider many ASD-specific behaviors, such as "lack of gestures," "abnormal eye contact," "lack of functional play," and "use of someone's hand as an instrument to obtain a desired object" (Dereu et al., 2012). The cutoff for concern is two or more checked items for children under 12 months and four or more checked items for children over 12 months (Dereu et al., 2010).

The CESDD was initially validated in Belgium in a prospective study of a community-based sample of children ages 3–39 months, with a mean age of 17 months (Dereu et al., 2010). This study found the CESDD to have sensitivity and specificity values of 68% and 96%, respectively (Dereu et al., 2010). The PPV and NPV were measured at 10% and 99%, respectively (Dereu et al., 2010). Although the specificity and NPV values are strong, the sensitivity and PPV values suggest that the CESDD may require more research and development before it is recommended for widespread use. This measure has yet to be evaluated in the United States and is not clinically available.

Developmental Behaviour Checklist—Early Screen

The Developmental Behaviour Checklist—Early Screen (DBC-ES) is a 17-item parent questionnaire derived from a longer questionnaire, the DBC, which focused primarily on emotional disturbance in children ages 4–18 years with intellectual disability (ID; Gray & Tonge, 2005). However, the DBC-ES differs from the original DBC in that it is used to distinguish young children (ages 18–48 months) with ASD from their peers with ID (Gray & Tonge, 2005). Questions are answered on a scale from 0 (not true) to 2 (very true), and total scores range from 0 to 34 (Gray & Tonge, 2005). This tool takes 5–10 minutes to complete and was evaluated as an ASD screener in two independent Australian clinical samples of children ages 18–48 months (Gray & Tonge, 2005; Gray, Tonge, Sweeney, & Einfeld, 2008). A suggested cutoff score of 11 out of 34 points was established (Gray & Tonge, 2005; Gray et al., 2008). Sensitivity and specificity were reported to be 88% and 69%, respectively, and PPV and NPV were reported to be 74% and 83%, respectively (Gray & Tonge, 2005; Gray et al., 2008). While the full-length DBC is available in many languages, the DBC-ES is not clinically available and requires more research before it is recommended for use as an ASD screener.

Early Screening of Autistic Traits Questionnaire

The Early Screening of Autistic Traits Questionnaire (ESAT) is a 14-item yes-or-no questionnaire that addresses a child's play, interests, social communication, and joint attention skills (Swinkels et al., 2006). This measure can be completed in 10–15 minutes by a parent, or it can be completed by a clinician after a 90-minute in-home observation of the child (Dietz, Swinkels, van Daalen, van Engeland, & Buitelaar, 2006). The ESAT was found to be most sensitive and specific when using a cutoff point of three or more "no" responses on a scale of 0–14 (Swinkels et al., 2006). This cutoff point was initially validated in a population-based sample of children ages 8–20 months in the Netherlands (Swinkels et al., 2006). This study yielded 90% sensitivity, 100% specificity as compared with typically developing children, and 81% specificity as compared to children with attention-deficit/hyperactivity disorder (ADHD; Swinkels et al., 2006). Additionally, a short four-item version of the ESAT was found to have a sensitivity of 94%, indicating that the short version can be used as a pre-screening tool to determine which families should complete a full-length screening (Swinkels et al., 2006). However, poor specificity on the four-item version suggested that it was not a reliable screening tool to determine if a full diagnostic evaluation was necessary, but only to determine whether a full-length ESAT screening was appropriate (Swinkels et al., 2006). Furthermore, a follow-up study of a clinical sample of children ages 13–23 months was conducted using the four-item prescreening version of the ESAT followed by the 14-item full-length ESAT completed by a trained observer after a 90-minute, in-home observation of children who received positive results on the prescreening (Dietz et al., 2006). This study found that the two-step ESAT had only 25% specificity for ASD but identified ASD and other developmental disorders 82% of the time (Diet et al., 2006). Therefore, while the full-length ESAT with clinician observation was not found to be specific to ASD, the 14-item parent questionnaire (without the lengthy clinician observation) is a promising tool for ASD screening.

First Year Inventory

The First Year Inventory (FYI) is a parent questionnaire with 63 items intended to detect early signs of ASD in 12-month-olds. This measure takes parents 15–20 minutes to complete. Items on the FYI were chosen based on extensive analysis of videos of young children who later developed ASD, retrospective parent reports of children's behaviors in infancy, and prospective research on children who had older siblings with ASD (Reznick et al., 2007). Commonalities such as language delays, withdrawal from social interaction, lack of joint attention and imitative behaviors, and failure to make eye contact at appropriate times were observed among infants who later developed ASD (Adrien et al., 1992; Gillberg et al., 1990; Hoshino et al., 1982; Lord, 1995; Osterling & Dawson, 1994; Zwaigenbaum et al., 2005). These and other symptoms were grouped into two domains on the FYI: Social Communication and Sensory-Regulatory Functions (Reznick et al., 2007). The FYI requires parents to answer several types of questions. Forty-six questions have the answer choices "never," "seldom," "sometimes," and "often"; 14 questions are multiple choice; and 1 question asks parents what specific consonant sounds their child produced (Reznick et al., 2007). Higher scores on the FYI indicated more atypical behavior, and certain responses were weighted as higher-risk responses in scoring, such that behaviors that were more symptomatic of ASD were assigned 2 points, behaviors that were potentially symptomatic of ASD were assigned 1 point, and typical behaviors were assigned 0 points (Reznick et al., 2007).

The FYI was initially tested in a sample of 12-month-old infants selected from birth records within a 20–30 mile radius of Chapel Hill, North Carolina (Reznick et al., 2007). This initial study provided a normative scoring sample and found that the FYI was easy for parents to understand and complete (Reznick et al., 2007). The tool can also provide individual profiles of children that illustrate specific areas of concern and level of risk for ASD (Reznick et al., 2007). This initial study developed a risk score scale of 0–50 on which 90% of the normative sample scored below 15 (Reznick et al., 2007). As a result, a score of 15 was established as a cutoff for ASD risk (Reznick et al., 2007). The FYI was further validated in a study of toddlers who were recruited from local preschools and had ASD, other developmental disabilities, or typical developmental trajectories (Watson et al., 2007). With the established cutoff score of 15, the FYI showed 92% sensitivity and 78% specificity for ASD (Watson et al., 2007). In the same sample, the PPV was reported at 74%, and the NPV was reported at 93% (Watson et al., 2007). Furthermore, in a longitudinal follow-up of children screened in toddlerhood, 31% of children with an ASD diagnosis by age 3 years were in the high-risk group on the FYI at 12 months, and 85% of children with ASD or another developmental problem that warranted services had been in the high-risk group at age 12 months (Turner-Brown, Baranek, Reznick, Watson, & Crais, 2012). The FYI is still under development and not yet available for clinical use.

Modified Checklist for Autism in Toddlers

The Modified Checklist for Autism in Toddlers (M-CHAT) is the most widely studied and cited screening tool for developmental concerns. It consists of 23 written yes-or-no questions regarding sensory, social communication, and play behaviors in toddlers, and it is intended to detect ASD symptoms in children 16–30 months old (Robins et al., 2001). This tool was developed based on the Checklist for Autism in Toddlers (CHAT; Baron-Cohen, Allen, & Gillberg, 1992) and a list of ASD symptoms found in very young children. Caregivers can complete the measure in less than 5 minutes. A child receives a point for each answer that is considered a symptom of ASD, and a cutoff point of 3 on a scale of 0–23 indicates reason for administration of the M-CHAT follow-up interview (M-CHAT/F; Robins et al., 2001), which was developed to increase the specificity of the measure and takes 5–10 minutes (Robins et al., 2001). Research on the M-CHAT supports its use as a general developmental screener, but various studies have conflicting results regarding its utility as an ASD-specific screener.

The M-CHAT was first validated in a prospective study of a community-based sample (n = 1,293) of children who were screened at their 24-month well-child pediatrician visits (Robins et al., 2001). This study found that the measure had a sensitivity of 97%, specificity of 95%, PPV of 36%, and NPV of 99% for ASD in this community-based sample (Robins et al., 2001). However, specificity rose to 99%, PPV rose to 68%, and NPV and sensitivity remained the same when the M-CHAT/F interview was included to determine screening results (Robins et al., 2001). These improvements in psychometrics suggested that the M-CHAT/F is a beneficial step to maximize the efficacy of the measure in children whose results on the M-CHAT indicate moderate risk. However, if a child scores 7 or more on the M-CHAT questionnaire, he or she can be considered to have high risk for developmental disorders, and referral for evaluation is recommended even without administration of the M-CHAT/F (Chlebowski, Robins, Barton, & Fein, 2013). The high rate of children who screened positive and went on to receive developmental delay (DD) or ASD diagnoses suggested that the M-CHAT/F was a reliable screening tool for developmental disorders, including ASD (Chlebowski et al., 2013).

In 2014, the M-CHAT-Revised with Follow-Up (M-CHAT-R/F), which uses simpler wording than the M-CHAT/F, was validated in a clinical sample of n = 16,071 children at 18- and 24-month well-child visits (Robins et al., 2014). This prospective study divided M-CHAT-R initial screening results into three categories: scores from 0 to 2 were low risk and did not require any follow-up; scores from 3 to 7 were medium risk and pediatricians should follow up with the M-CHAT-R/F; and scores above 7 were high risk, indicating that the child should be directly referred to specialized evaluation (Robins et al., 2014). Alternative cut-point analyses were conducted and showed that lowering the cutoff for medium risk to 2 yielded the best psychometric properties as compared to cutoff scores set at any other value from 1 to 9 (Robins et al., 2014). The cutoff score of 2 provided 94% sensitivity and 83% specificity for ASD, though PPV and NPV were not reported (Robins et al., 2014). Another prospective study, which included the follow-up interview for all children scoring above the risk cutoff on the M-CHAT, even those scoring at high risk (> 7), found the M-CHAT/F to have 97–98% sensitivity, specificity and PPV in a clinical sample of children (n = 5,071) ages 14–40 months (Sturner et al., 2016). However, one study of a population-based sample of 18-month-old children recruited from the Norwegian Mother and Child Cohort found the M-CHAT to have 93% specificity but only 34% sensitivity for ASD, indicating that, while the M-CHAT is a valuable general developmental screening tool, it may not be effective in detecting ASD at 18 months of age (Stenberg et al., 2014). The M-CHAT has also been examined in large, community-based samples. Ojen and colleagues (2018) examined developmental outcomes in n = 68,197 cases that screened negative and found only

228 of these to be false negatives. Additionally, Sturner et al. (2017) compared the utility of the M-CHAT in children younger than 20 months and children older than 20 months, with a total sample size of $n = 73,564$. The younger group of children failed more items on the M-CHAT, although there were fewer confirmed cases of ASD in this group, indicating a need to consider developmental changes throughout toddlerhood when scoring the M-CHAT (Sturner et al., 2017). Despite some mixed results, most research on this measure suggests that it is a valuable population-based screening tool that is easy to administer and interpret.

Parent Observation of Early Markers Scale

The Parent Observation of Early Markers Scale (POEMS) is a 61-item parent questionnaire intended for use in children ages 1–24 months (Feldman et al., 2012). The questionnaire asks parents to consider children's behavior in the areas of social communication, restricted and repetitive behaviors, behavioral problems, and emotional problems over the previous week and answer questions on a scale from 1 to 4 on which higher scores indicate more problematic behaviors (Feldman et al., 2012). Scores on the POEMS range from 61 to 244, and a cutoff score of 70 indicates risk for ASD (Feldman et al., 2012).

The POEMS was initially validated in a prospective study of high-risk infants (with older siblings diagnosed with ASD) ages 1 to 24 months at the start of the study (Feldman et al., 2012). The questionnaire was administered to parents an average of 8 times over 2 years and found to have sensitivity and specificity values of 25 to 100% and 65 to 87%, respectively, using ASD diagnoses at age 3 (Feldman et al., 2012). PPV ranged from 10 to 29% (Feldman et al., 2012). Sensitivity increased as children got older, while specificity decreased over time and PPV remained relatively stable (Feldman et al., 2012). The POEMS applicability to infants as young as 1 month is promising, but more research is necessary before the measure is available for clinical use.

Parent's Observations of Social Interaction

The Parent's Observations of Social Interaction (POSI) is a seven-item parent questionnaire that takes less than 5 minutes to complete. The POSI requires a minimum fifth-grade literacy level, so it increases accessibility for families with lower levels of education (Smith, Sheldrick, & Perrin, 2012). Items require responses on a Likert-type scale regarding frequency of a child's behaviors, such as showing interest in other children and responding to his or her name (Smith et al., 2012). Three or more responses in the neutral or atypical range indicate reason for concern (Smith et al., 2012). The POSI was initially developed based on a two-stage retrospective study of a clinical sample of children ages 18–48 months (Stage 1) and 16–30 months (Stage 2; Smith et al., 2012). This study yielded sensitivity values of 54–89% and specificity values of 74–83% with higher sensitivity in Stage 1 of the study and higher specificity in stage 2 (Smith et al., 2012). The POSI is available for free online, but it requires further research in a larger population-based sample before it can be recommended for widespread clinical use.

PDD Behavior Inventory

The PDD Behavior Inventory (PDD-BI) is a 188-item parent or teacher questionnaire that takes approximately 30 to 45 minutes to complete (Cohen & Sudhalter, 2005). The PDD-BI assesses maladaptive behaviors and social communication skills in 1 year, 6 month- to 18 years, 5 month-old children based on parents' or teachers' answers to each item on a four-point Likert-type scale ranging from never to often (Cohen et al., 2010; Cohen & Sudhalter, 2005). The teacher version of the PDD-BI has fewer items than the parent version as it only includes items that can be assessed within a school setting (Cohen, Schmidt-Lackner, Romanczyk, & Sudhalter, 2003). This tool was initially developed as a measure to describe change over time, but it has also been studied as a screening tool. The recommended cutoff for risk for ASD is a T-score of 45 or below on the Autism Composite, a subset of items that is most sensitive and specific to ASD (Reel, Lecavalier, Butter, & Mulick, 2012).

In one clinical sample, the PDD-BI was found to have 74% sensitivity and 62% specificity, which led researchers to recommend against using the PDD-BI as an ASD screening tool (Reel et al., 2012). However, the sensitivity rose to 92% and the specificity to 67% when only children with nonverbal IQs lower than 70 were included in analyses (Reel et al., 2012). Furthermore, one study found the parent version of the PDD-BI to have 80% sensitivity and 81% specificity, while the teacher version had 84% sensitivity and 50% specificity for ASD (Cohen et al., 2010). Conflicting results in studies on the PDD-BI as an autism-specific screener indicate that more research in larger samples is necessary.

Pervasive Developmental Disorders Screening Test— Second Edition

The Pervasive Developmental Disorders Screening Test—Second Edition (PDDST-II) is a screening tool that consists of three sequential parent questionnaires that range from 16 to 18 yes-or-no questions (Eaves & Ho, 2004). Children receive a point for each affirmative answer on all stages of the screener (Eaves & Ho, 2004). A score of 3 or higher on a scale of 0 to 18 on the first stage, which can be used as a stand-alone Level one screening tool, indicates risk for ASD and reason to administer the second stage

(Eaves & Ho, 2004). Likewise, a score of 4 or higher on a scale of 0–17 in Stage 2 indicates reason to administer Stage 3, and a score of 6 or higher on a scale of 0–16 necessitates a full diagnostic evaluation (Eaves & Ho, 2004). The PDDST-II is appropriate for children ages 18–48 months, and it takes 10–20 minutes to complete all three stages (Siegel, 2013).

The sensitivity and specificity of the PDDST-II in a clinic-based sample of children ages 18–48 months varied by stage of the screener. Stage 1 was found to have a sensitivity of 92% and a specificity of 91% (Siegel, 2013); Stage 2 had a sensitivity of 73% and a specificity of 49%; and Stage 3 had a sensitivity of 58% and specificity of 60% (Siegel, 2013). These data suggest that Stage 1 of the PDDST-II is the most effective screener for ASD in young children, though the utility of the other stages is limited.

Screen for Social Interaction—Younger

The Screen for Social Interaction—Younger (SSI-Y) is a 54-item parent questionnaire that takes 10–15 minutes to complete (Ghuman, Leone, Lecavalier, & Landa, 2011). This measure asks questions about social interaction and joint attention in preschool-age children (24–42 months). Answer choices range from 0 (almost never) to 3 (almost all the time; Ghuman et al., 2011). If a child scores fewer than 45 out of a total possible 162 points, he or she is considered to be at risk for ASD (Ghuman et al., 2011). The SSI-Y was initially validated in a clinical sample of children ages 24–61 months, and the measure yielded a sensitivity value of 87% and a specificity value of 71% (Ghuman et al., 2011). The SSI-Y has promising initial results and is available as a free online download, thereby increasing accessibility. However, more research in a larger, younger, more diverse sample is necessary before it can be recommended for widespread clinical use.

Social Communication Questionnaire

Developed to parallel the longer, more in-depth parent interview, the Autism Diagnostic Interview–Revised (ADI-R; Lord, Rutter, & Le Couteur, 1994), the Social Communication Questionnaire (SCQ) asks parents to answer 40 yes-or-no questions regarding their child's behavior, play, and social skills over the child's lifespan (Lifetime version) or in the past three months (Current version; Rutter, Bailey, & Lord, 2003). The SCQ requires less than 10 minutes to complete. Answers that may indicate signs of ASD receive a score of 1, and responses that do not indicate concern for ASD receive a score of 0. As such, higher scores indicate greater risk for ASD. A cutoff score of 15 on a scale from 0 to 40 was recommended as indication of concern for ASD that should be followed up with further assessment (Wiggins et al., 2007).

Although the SCQ is primarily intended for school-age children, one study found 89% sensitivity and specificity in a sample of children ages

17–45 months who were recruited from an early intervention program (Wiggins et al., 2007). This study also found that a cutoff score of 11 in this younger sample provided the best sensitivity and specificity as compared to the original recommended cutoff of 15, which provided only 47% sensitivity (Wiggins et al., 2007). However, prospective research on the use of the SCQ as an ASD screening tool in toddlers in the United Kingdom who were referred for speech and language services found 64% sensitivity and 75% specificity, which led researchers to recommend the SCQ as a supplemental tool to be used in conjunction with clinical judgment regarding autism symptoms (Charman et al., 2016), but not as a stand-alone screener for young children.

Caregiver Questionnaires: Applied to ASD

Ages and Stages Questionnaire

The original Ages and Stages Questionnaire (ASQ) was a general developmental screener intended to catch potential concerns or delays in children ages 5–66 months (Squires & Bricker, 2009). It is most useful as a first step in the screening process to determine whether a child shows developmental concerns, though it is not intended for use as an ASD-specific tool (Hardy et al., 2015). This questionnaire takes 10–15 minutes for parents to complete and assesses motor, communication, and social functioning through a series of questions with the answer choices "yes," "sometimes," and "not yet." The ASQ organizes results into varying degrees of concern: typically developing, monitoring zone, or requiring further assessment. Children who fall in the typically developing range are not recommended for any follow-up evaluation or increased monitoring, while children in the monitoring zone are recommended to participate in continued screening and surveillance (Squires & Bricker, 2009). On the ASQ, a lower score indicates more reason for concern (Squires & Bricker, 2009).

The ASQ-3 is the most recent version of the ASQ. It was modified for use in children ages 1 month to 5½ years (Squires & Bricker, 2009). Like the original ASQ, the ASQ-3 is intended for use as a general developmental screener; however, researchers have begun to explore the utility of the ASQ-3 as a screening tool for ASD specifically. The cutoff point for further assessment on the ASQ-3 yielded 70% sensitivity for ASD in a prospective study of a community-based sample of children ages 16–30 months who attended well-child visits at 20 different pediatrician's offices; however, when children who scored in the monitoring zone on the communication domain were included, this number rose to 95% (Hardy et al., 2015). This increase in sensitivity suggested that using the monitoring zone in the communication domain as a cutoff point for positive screening results in children under the age of 3 may be advantageous for identification of early cases of ASD. This study also showed that the ASQ-3 provided low specificity for ASD, such that the ASQ-3 identified 1,038 screen-positive cases, only 21 of whom went on to receive a diagnosis of ASD (Hardy et al., 2015). However, the social and motor domains on the ASQ effectively distinguished among true- and false-negative results on the M-CHAT in a large community sample of 18-month-olds, thereby operating as an effective counterpart to a psychometrically sound tool (Ojen et al., 2018). As such, the ASQ-3's utility as a stand-alone screener for ASD is limited, though it may be useful as a general developmental screener or in concert with other psychometrically sound measures.

Child Behavior Checklist

The Child Behavior Checklist (CBCL) is a 100-item parent questionnaire regarding general behavior problems and has a version for 1.5- to 5-year-old children and a version for 6- to 18-year-old children. Parents are asked to respond "not true (as far as you know)," "somewhat or sometimes true," or "very true or often true" to each question, and the questionnaire takes 10–15 minutes to complete. The version for younger children addresses internalizing and externalizing behaviors in the following domains: emotional reactivity, anxious/depressed behavior, somatic complaints, withdrawn behavior, attention problems, pervasive developmental problems, and aggressive behavior (Achenbach & Rescorla, 2001). The CBCL is available as a general developmental screening tool in 45 languages (Achenbach & Rescorla, 2001), increasing its utility in diverse populations.

Researchers in Italy, Korea, and the United States have analyzed the reliability of the CBCL as a screening tool to identify children with ASD (Muratori et al., 2011; Rescorla, Kim, & Oh, 2015; Havdahl, von Tetzchner, Huerta, Lord, & Bishop, 2016). In Italy, the Withdrawn and Pervasive Developmental Problems scales were found to identify preschoolers with ASD at high sensitivity (89% for the Withdrawn scale, 85% for the Pervasive Developmental Problems scale) and distinguish them from those who are typically developing or have other psychiatric disorders at high specificity (92% and 90%; Muratori et al., 2011). Similarly, the Withdrawn, Attention Problems, and Pervasive Developmental Problems scales differentiated Korean preschoolers with ASD from their typically developing peers (Rescorla et al., 2015). Although the CBCL may be useful in distinguishing ASD from typical development, a recent study of children ages 2–13 in the United States found sensitivity and specificity values of 63% and 65%, respectively (Havdahl et al., 2016). Many children who met cutoff scores for ASD on the Withdrawn and Pervasive Developmental Problems scales had general emotional/behavioral problems, not ASD (Havdahl et al., 2016). While the CBCL is widely supported as a general developmental screening tool, some evidence suggests that it may not be appropriate for ASD-specific screening.

Infant–Toddler Checklist

The Infant–Toddler Checklist (ITC) is a broadband screening tool intended to pick up communication delays in children ages 6–24 months. This tool consists of 24 questions regarding various modes of communication, including gestures, vocalizations, eye contact, and emotional expression (Wetherby & Prizant, 2002), and takes 5–10 minutes to complete. Caregivers answer each question with "not yet," "sometimes," or "often" and have the option to write general comments concerning developmental issues. One prospective study screened a diverse community-based sample of children between the ages of 12 and 24 months (*n* = 5,385; 59% Caucasian, 30% African American, 3% Hispanic, 2% Asian), then invited families back for a full ASD evaluation if children screened positive or families reported concerns via a follow-up questionnaire mailed after the child's fourth birthday (Wetherby et al., 2008). Results showed that the ITC had PPV and NPV that both exceeded 70% for children with communication delays, though sensitivity and specificity were not reported (Wetherby et al., 2008). The same study found that the ITC was less effective in distinguishing children with ASD from children with general communication disorders (Wetherby et al., 2008). A prospective study that compared the ITC results of children with ASD (*n* = 18), typically developing children (*n* = 18), and children with DD (*n* = 18) drawn from a larger community sample (*n* = 3,026; 83% Caucasian) found sensitivity and specificity for ASD to be 89% (Wetherby et al., 2004). This number rose to 94% when ITC scores were paired with video observation by a trained clinician and identification of 13 red flags for ASD. Together these findings indicated that the ITC might be a useful stand-alone primary screener or supplement to other measures as a secondary screening tool, but research to determine the utility of the ITC in detecting ASD specifically in a larger sample is necessary (Wetherby et al., 2004).

Parent Interview

Autism Symptom Interview

Unlike many other Level 1 screening tools, the Autism Symptom Interview (ASI) is a measure that relies on parent interview with a clinician (face to face or by telephone) rather than parent questionnaire. This measure is similar to the SCQ in its origin in the ADI-R, but it differs in that it requires a 15–20 minute parent interview that can be administered by a clinician without significant ASD experience (Bishop et al., 2017). The ASI has two versions: one for children ages 2 years to 4 years, 11 months (ASI–Preschool) and one for children ages 5–12 years (ASI–School Age), and both provide scores in the domains of Communication, Reciprocal Social Interaction, and Restricted and Repetitive Behaviors and Interests (Bishop et al., 2017). The ASI targets current behaviors that are consistent with ASD symptoms by asking parents to report their child's behavior in the last 3 months (Bishop et al., 2017). Higher scores on the ASI are indicative of behavior that is more consistent with ASD symptoms. The recommended cutoff point is 27 on a scale of 0–72 for verbal children and 14 on a scale of 0–39 for nonverbal children (Bishop et al., 2017; Newschaffer et al., 2017).

In one prospective study of a convenience sample of children ages 24–39 months, the ASI was found to have sensitivity of 91% and specificity of 35% when the recommended cutoff score was used to determine results (Newschaffer et al., 2017). Participant demographics and assessor level of ASD experience had no significant effects on the screening results, suggesting that the ASI may be useful for screening in a variety of populations by relatively naive clinicians (Newschaffer et al., 2017). The ASI may be a promising new tool, but it is not currently available for clinical use because research into its utility is ongoing.

Baby and Infant Screen for Children with aUtIsm Traits: Part 1

The Baby and Infant Screen for Children with aUtIsm Traits: Part 1 (BISCUIT: Part 1) is an interview in which parents of children ages 17–37 months are asked 62 questions with answers on a 3-point Likert-type scale (Matson, Wilkins, & Fodstad, 2010). Parents are asked to compare their child to a typically developing peer and answer whether their child is not different/has no impairment, is somewhat different/has mild impairment, or is very different/has severe impairment. The measure requires minimal interviewer training and takes approximately 20–30 minutes to administer (Matson et al., 2010).

The BISCUIT: Part 1 was initially validated as an ASD screening tool in a sample of children ages 17–37 months who were enrolled in a program for children who had or were at risk for DD (Matson et al., 2009). This study found sensitivity for ASD ranging from 66 to 94% and specificity ranging from 72 to 98% using varying cutoff points (Matson et al., 2009). Mean scores of children without any developmental diagnosis and with ASD were 10 and 59, respectively (Matson et al., 2009). These results led to a final cut-point of 39 on a scale of 0–124, which provided sensitivity of 84% and specificity of 83% in this sample (Matson et al., 2009). Based on these results, the BISCUIT: Part 1 may be a reliable screening tool for ASD, though more research in a diverse population is required to confirm its utility.

Clinician Observation

Autism Detection in Early Childhood

The Autism Detection in Early Childhood (ADEC) is intended to screen children ages 12–36 months based on a 16-item questionnaire to be filled out by a clinician after a 10- to 25-minute play-based observation of a child (Young, 2007). Each item is scored between 0 and 2, with a higher score indicating greater risk for ASD (Young, 2007). Total scores range from 0 to 32, and scores of 0–10 indicate low risk, 11–13 indicate moderate risk, 14–19 indicate high risk, and 20–32 indicate very high risk for ASD (Young, 2007). The ADEC has been validated in Australia, Mexico, and the United States (Hedley et al., 2015; Hedley, Young, Angelica, Gallegos, & Salazar, 2010; Nah, Young, Brewer, & Berlingeri, 2014).

The ADEC was validated in Australia in a prospective population-based study of children ages 12–36 months (Nah et al., 2014). This study found that a cutoff of 11 out of 32 points provided a sensitivity of 100% and a specificity of 74–90%; however, when cases with severe DD were excluded from analyses, specificity was 89–96% (Nah et al., 2014). PPV and NPV were calculated to be 84–95% and 100%, respectively (Nah et al., 2014). A study of a similar sample in Mexico found the Spanish ADEC to have sensitivity values of 79–94% and specificity values of 88–100% (Hedley et al., 2010). The ADEC was most recently validated in a prospective study of a clinical sample of children ages 14–37 months in the United States (Hedley et al., 2015). This study found sensitivity and specificity values ranging from 87 to 93% and 52 to 82%, respectively (Hedley et al., 2015). PPVs and NPVs were reported to be 74–87% and 82–94%, respectively (Hedley et al., 2015). A brief version of the ADEC is currently under development with promising initial data: sensitivity of 81%, specificity of 78%, PPV of 81%, and NPV of 78% (Nah, Young, & Brewer, 2018). Overall, though findings on specificity were mixed, results of these studies suggest that the ADEC is a valid screening tool for ASD in toddlers.

Autism Observation Scale for Infants

The Autism Observation Scale for Infants (AOSI) is intended to assess ASD symptoms in children between 6 and 18 months of age. The AOSI is a semi-structured free-play interaction that lasts approximately 20 minutes. It is expected that the clinician who administers the AOSI has experience with infants and with ASD (Bryson, Zwaigenbaum, McDermott, Rombaugh, & Brian, 2008). After the interaction, the clinician is required to complete an 18-item questionnaire regarding social communication behavior, transitional skills, and motor skills observed during the interaction (Bryson et al., 2008) and to code each item on a scale of 0–3, in which a higher score indicates more atypical behavior (Bryson et al., 2008).

The AOSI was initially validated in samples of infants ages 6 months, 12 months, and 18 months who were recruited through self-referrals to an ongoing prospective study (Bryson et al., 2008). This study primarily focused on interrater and test–retest reliability and found that interrater reliability was above 0.65 and that test–retest reliability ranged from 0.61 to 0.68 (Bryson et al., 2008). A later prospective study found the AOSI to have 38% sensitivity and 86% specificity in a clinical sample of high-risk and low-risk infants (Bryson & Zwaigenbaum, 2014). These values were not improved by use of alternate cutoff scores on the measure (Bryson & Zwaigenbaum, 2014). Because of its low sensitivity, the AOSI is only recommended for research purposes (Bryson & Zwaigenbaum, 2014).

Childhood Autism Rating Scale

The Childhood Autism Rating Scale (CARS) is intended to screen children ages 2–6 years based on a questionnaire filled out by a trained observer. Children over age 6 can also be rated using the CARS if they have an IQ of 79 or lower or a significant communication impairment. This screening tool has 15 items that address communication, relation to others, displays of emotion, physical movement, play skills, reactions to change, and sensory behaviors (Schopler, Reichler, & Renner, 1988). The observer answers each question on a scale from no apparent abnormality to severe concern based on a 5- to 10-minute unstructured observation of the child. A version of the CARS is also available for parents to fill out, in which items can be marked "not a problem," "mild to moderate problem," "severe problem," "not a problem now, but was in the past," or "don't know." Children receive higher scores for more severely problematic behavior that may be indicative of ASD (Schopler et al., 1988). Total scores below 30 on a scale of 1–60 indicate that a child is not at risk for ASD; scores between 30 and 36.5 indicate a moderate concern for ASD; and scores above 36.5 indicate high concern for ASD (Rellini et al., 2004). A more recent edition of the CARS, the CARS-2, includes the same criteria as the CARS but has a different format to increase ease of use (Moulton, Bradbury, Barton, & Fein, 2019).

In one study of children who had been referred for developmental concerns, the CARS had 100% sensitivity for ASD (Rellini et al., 2004). A study published the following year used the CARS as a screening tool for children ages 2–6 years who had been referred for general developmental evaluation as a result of concerns (Perry, Condillac, Freeman, Dunn-Geier, & Belair, 2005). This study resulted in 94% sensitivity and 85% specificity to distinguish ASD from other developmental problems (Perry et al., 2005), suggesting that the CARS may be a reliable tool for use in clinical settings. The utility of the CARS for children under 2 years of age is unknown.

Observation Scale for Autism

The Observation Scale for Autism (OSA) requires a 10-minute clinician observation period during which the clinician focuses on reciprocal communication, social interaction (especially between the caregiver and the child), reciprocal play, and spontaneous language (Haglund, Dahlgren, Källén, Gustafsson, & Råstam, 2015). After the observation period, the clinician fills out a 12-item questionnaire in which the child receives a point for behavior in each item that does not align with developmentally appropriate behavior for a 24- to 30-month-old child (Haglund et al., 2015). Therefore, a higher score corresponds to more concern for ASD. The OSA was initially tested in a culturally diverse sample of children with ASD, Down syndrome, and typical development (Haglund et al., 2015). This initial validation found that nine items showed the most significant differences between the group of children with ASD and the other groups, and, with a cutoff score of 3 (out of nine items), the OSA had 92% sensitivity and 100% specificity for ASD (Haglund et al., 2015). However, since the OSA is a new tool designed to detect ASD symptoms in children after their second birthday, or around 30 months of age, the utility of the measure in younger children has not yet been studied.

Screening Tool for Autism in Two-Year-Olds

The Screening Tool for Autism in Two-Year-Olds (STAT) is a 20-minute structured interaction between a trained clinician and a 13- to 24-month-old child (Stone & Ousley, 1997). The STAT is intended to elicit specific behaviors through a series of play interactions targeting imitation, joint attention, and communication skills (Stone et al., 2000). The STAT is scored based on 12 items that a child can "pass" or "fail" (Stone et al., 2000). Each "pass" receives a score of 1 and a "fail" receives a score of 0. A lower score is indicative of more concern for ASD. The items are divided into three different areas, and a score lower than 2 on a scale of 0–4 in any area indicates that a child failed that area (Stone et al., 2000). The cutoff for ASD concern on this measure is failing any two of the three areas (Stone et al., 2000).

In a validation sample of children ages 24–35 months recruited from a developmental evaluation center, the STAT yielded 83% sensitivity and 86% specificity (Stone et al., 2000). However, these statistics were found in a clinical sample, and mental ages of the children in the ASD group were significantly different than mental ages of the children in the typically developing group, a discrepancy that may have affected the screening results (Stone et al., 2000). Another study addressed this issue by using the STAT with children ages 24–35 months recruited from a developmental evaluation center and divided into matched pairs (a child with ASD and a child without ASD) based on chronological and mental age (Stone, Coonrod, Turner, & Pozdol, 2004). This study found excellent interrater reliability, excellent test–retest reliability, 100% sensitivity, and 85% specificity (Stone et al., 2004). Furthermore, a prospective study of a clinical sample examined the utility of the STAT to screen children under 2 years of age (Stone, McMahon, & Henderson, 2008). This study found that a cutoff point of 2.75 on a scale of 0–4 for failure in any area was appropriate for children ages 13–23 months (Stone et al., 2008). This cutoff yielded 93% sensitivity and 83% specificity in this younger sample (Stone et al., 2008). Together, the results of these studies indicate that the STAT is a reliable tool for screening children for ASD between the ages of 1 and 3 years, though it requires the time and expertise of a trained and skilled clinician.

Technology-Based Screening

As technology becomes increasingly present in the day-to-day lives of many families and telehealth gains traction as a viable method to increase access to health care services, many scientists are shifting their focus to video and application-based care. Telehealth is emerging as a potential avenue for reducing health care costs and socioeconomic barriers and increasing access in remote areas via home computers and mobile devices (Dorsey & Topol, 2016). Additionally, machine learning techniques are emerging strategies that are beginning to be employed to enhance effectiveness of early screening (Achenie et al., 2019; Thabtah & Peebles, 2020).

Efforts such as the Autism Navigator (*http://autismnavigator.com*), led by Dr. Amy Wetherby and supported by the National Institute of Mental Health (NIMH), are extending ASD awareness to families across the United States. This program includes electronic screening using the Early Screening for Autism and Communication Disorders (ESAC; not yet commercially available). ESAC sensitivity ranges from 81 to 84% and specificity ranges from 70 to 89%, with variation in results depending on the child's age at the time of screening (Schrader et al., 2020). The ESAC results can be sent directly to primary care physicians, and families can then be provided with referrals to professionals who can perform thorough diagnostic evaluations. Similarly, efforts out of La Trobe University in Australia have created ASDetect (*ASDetect.org*), a free application that uses video-based examples of early social and communication milestones and ASD symptoms to promote parental and professional awareness. Based on the results of two early detection studies (Barbaro & Dissanayake, 2010, 2012), ASDetect guides parents through a series of questions, videos, and activities completed with the child in order to alert the parent to any concerning symptoms that might require additional assessment. ASDetect is not a screening tool for autism but rather a method designed to increase parental awareness of potential symptoms (Barbaro & Dissanayake, 2012). Efforts such as these aim to increase knowledge about ASD, increase the widespread use of surveillance and screening, and decrease socioeconomic gaps in diagnosis and intervention. Limited research is currently available on such tools, but they are emerging as a new direction for efficient screeners that are responsive to the changing needs and priorities of families in the 21st century. See Chapter 10 for further information regarding applications of technology to support children and families impacted by ASD.

Early Video-Guided Autism Screener

The Early Video-Guided Autism Screener (E-VAS) is a newly developed online tool that includes videos of typical and atypical behavior in children ages 18–48 months to educate caregivers on symptomatic behavior before asking them to complete a 29-item questionnaire regarding their child's behavior (Newschaffer et al., 2017). The measure takes less than 30 minutes to complete (Newschaffer et al., 2017). The goal of this format is to increase awareness of early ASD symptoms in play, flexibility, sharing, facial expressions, gestures, and unusual body movements and help caregivers accurately identify those symptoms in their own children (Newschaffer et al., 2017). Parents answer each item on a scale of 0–4, with a higher score indicating greater symptom severity (Newschaffer et al., 2017). The cutoff for concern for ASD is 53 on a scale of 0–116 points (Newschaffer et al., 2017).

In a prospective study of a convenience sample of children ages 24–39 months who had been referred for neurodevelopmental evaluations, the E-VAS yielded 92% sensitivity and 38% specificity for ASD with the recommended cutoff score (Newschaffer et al., 2017). However, this tool provided 83% sensitivity and 49% specificity, with the cutoff score set at 62 in the same sample (Newschaffer et al., 2017). These findings suggest that, with further research and development to improve specificity, this new tool may attain widespread use as an ASD screener.

Summary of Available Screening Tools

A wide variety of screening tools are available for clinical and research use. A measure's cost, accessibility, ease of use, cultural responsivity, and required time and training necessary for administration and scoring must be considered along with psychometric properties when deciding which tools to use. Due to the need for culturally and linguistically responsive screening tools that demonstrate efficacy in diverse populations, further research should focus on cultural adaptations and establishing norms in a variety of populations and cultures. The responsible practitioner or researcher must also attend to ethical considerations, such as balancing sensitivity and specificity, in order to identify as many cases as possible while eliminating unnecessary family stress during the screening process. Therefore, the developmental screening process will benefit from continued efforts to optimize psychometric performance of existing measures or create innovative procedures with more sensitive and specific outcomes.

Of the existing Level 1 screeners that are available for clinical use, the best balance of all these factors can be found with the ITC and the M-CHAT. These measures are available for free online and perform well in high-risk populations, indicating their utility as widely accessible early screening measures. The M-CHAT has been translated into numerous languages and is perhaps the most widely used screening tool, making it more accessible to a range of populations (Chlebowski et al., 2013). In addition, both the M-CHAT initial questionnaire and the ITC can be completed in less than 10 minutes. Even if a child receives a positive screening result on the initial M-CHAT questionnaire, the follow-up interview only adds another 10 minutes. A benefit of the ITC is that it is appropriate for screening children as young as 6 months of age. Yet, each measure has its disadvantages. It is important to consider that some of the research on these tools reported psychometric properties with regard to identifying developmental or communication disorders in general, so accuracy with regard to ASD specifically may be somewhat lower. The M-CHAT is not applicable for children under 16 months of age—too late for some parents who have concerns even earlier and a disadvantage as we attempt to lower the age of initial identification. The ITC is only available in English and Spanish, decreasing its accessibility in diverse populations.

None of the Level 2 screeners are freely available, limiting feasibility as universal screening measures. However, Level 2 screeners are more useful in specialized settings, and most established screening tools for other health issues come at a cost. Considering the experiential and financial commitments necessary for administration, the CARS and the STAT have the best sensitivities. Several measures, including the E-VAS and the OSA, are still under development but may eventually be viable options for Level 2 screening that requires less time and fewer financial resources than the CARS and the STAT.

The Current State of Screening for ASD

The U.S. Preventive Services Task Force Recommendation

In 1984, a group of 16 medical experts were mandated to form the U.S. Preventive Services Task Force (USPSTF) to review evidence and make recommendations regarding prevention of diseases and disorders (*www.uspreventiveservicestaskforce.org*). This group is now composed of experts in prevention, primary care, family medicine, internal medicine, pediatrics, behavioral health, nursing, and obstetrics and gynecology. The USPSTF collaborates with the Agency for Healthcare Research and Quality to weigh the costs and benefits of various preventive care measures and to produce recommendations for care and continued medical research. It is important to note that the task force intends its recommendations to apply solely to individuals who show no signs or symptoms of the disorder under consideration (Coury, 2015). In 2016, the USPSTF provided screening recommendations regarding depression, cardiovascular disease, pulmonary disease, and various cancers.

In addition to the aforementioned recommendations, in February 2016, the USPSTF published a twofold recommendation regarding standardized screening for ASD in very young children. First, the task force supported the continued use of standardized screening tools to confirm the presence of developmental problems if parents or pediatricians were concerned about a child (Siu & the USPSTF, 2016). Second, "the USPSTF conclude[d] that the current evidence is insufficient to assess the balance of benefits and harms of screening for ASD in young children for whom no concerns of ASD have been raised by their parents or a clinician" (Siu & the USPSTF, 2016, p. 691). The task force acknowledged the availability of high-quality screening tools but questioned the evidence for benefits from widespread use of these tools (Siu & the USPSTF, 2016). Specifically, the USPSTF argues that early universal screening may not be useful since studies showing the benefits of intervention have focused mostly on older children, with limited long-term evidence for early intervention outcomes, and that children who have ASD are typically identified by family members or primary care physicians, not through screening processes (Siu & the USPSTF, 2016). The task force called for more research to find adequate evidence for the direct impact of early universal standard screening on outcomes, particularly in children for whom no concerns had been raised prior to screening (Siu & the USPSTF, 2016). Additionally, the USPSTF stated that children identified by screening tools alone could have milder ASD symptoms than those who were identified by parent or clinician concern (Siu & the USPSTF, 2016). Further, these mildly affected children could have positive outcomes even with a later age of diagnosis and start of intervention, negating the need for standardized screening before parent or clinician concern arises (Siu & the USPSTF, 2016).

Responses to the USPSTF Recommendation

Although the USPSTF recommendation was "not a recommendation for or against screening" (Siu & the USPSTF, 2016, p. 693), it gave the impression that universal standard screening was not encouraged (Pierce, Courchesne, & Bacon, 2016; Veenstra-VanderWeele & McGuire, 2016). Many experts in ASD, including the major advocacy and scientific groups Autism Speaks, the Autism Science Foundation, and the Baby Siblings Research Consortium, reacted to this recommendation with concern about the contradictions present in the USPSTF's screening recommendation, gaps in review of available evidence, and potential implications of the USPSTF statement for the ASD community (Fein et al., 2016; Pierce et al., 2016; Veenstra-VanderWeele & McGuire, 2016). The USPSTF also disputed the ability of universal standard screening procedures to increase opportunities for participation in early intervention, reduce average age at first diagnosis, and lower the rate of cases missed by parents and pediatricians who rely on concern alone (Pierce et al., 2016). However, evidence (e.g., from Miller et al., 2011; Oosterling et al., 2010; Robins et al., 2014) suggests that early universal screening may, in fact, produce these benefits, among others.

Benefits of Early Screening and Intervention

The primary purpose of screening is to provide diagnosis as early as possible under the assumption that earlier diagnosis leads to earlier intervention and better outcomes. (See Chapters 4 and 8 for extensive reports on early intervention for children with ASD or prodromal risk signs.) The implementation of universal standard screening has been shown to decrease the age of diagnosis by almost 2 years (Oosterling et al., 2010; Robins et al., 2014)—2 years during which early intervention services can be provided that would otherwise not be available. Evidence suggests that the younger a child is at the start of intensive early intervention, the more social, communication, and adaptive skills the child will acquire (Granpeesheh, Dixon, Tarbox, Kaplan, & Wilke, 2009; Rogers et al., 2012). Thus, a decrease in age at first diagnosis provided by widespread implementation of universal standard screening may be a critical first step toward effective intervention. The task force stated that, in a risk-benefit analysis of universal standard screening for ASD, there was not enough evidence to show that the benefits of screening outweigh the potential harms (Siu & the USPSTF, 2016). However, benefits of early universal screening include widespread identification and referral to evaluation and services for young children at risk for ASD (Oosterling et al., 2010; Robins et al., 2014). While research is ongoing to determine the long-term effects of early intervention, access to which is facilitated by early screening procedures, there is mounting evidence of its benefits (Anderson, Liang, & Lord, 2014; Bradshaw, Steiner, Gengoux, & Koegel, 2015; Dawson et al., 2010; Granpeesheh et al., 2009; Green et al., 2010, 2013; Rogers et al., 2012), suggesting that the potential benefit of increased access to intervention through early screening may outweigh the potential harms of screening. The USPSTF also ignored other possible benefits of screening. Universal standard screening provides an opportunity to identify non-ASD neurodevelopmental disorders, significant language delays, or other global developmental delays that may warrant early intervention. In research studies, nearly all children who screened positive had a neurodevelopmental disorder, albeit not all ASD, that necessitated a referral for early intervention services (Robins et al., 2014). Yet, whether general screening for developmental delay is sufficient to detect early cases of ASD or whether ASD-specific screening tools are necessary is still unclear.

The USPSTF argued that children who are identified later in life, and about whom parents and physicians did not raise concerns during early childhood, may have milder cases of ASD than those who are identified in early childhood by screening tools and are more likely to have positive outcomes regardless of age of diagnosis (Siu & the USPSTF, 2016). While there is research suggesting that individuals with higher cognitive functioning and milder ASD symptoms have better outcomes in general (Sigman & McGovern, 2005; Szatmari et al., 2015), there is little evidence for the USPSTF's claim that children who have milder symptoms do not benefit as much from early diagnosis and intervention as their peers with more severe symptoms (Turner & Stone, 2007). See Chapter 7 for more information regarding the long-term outcomes of infants at risk for ASD.

The Complex Nature of ASD Symptoms

Throughout their recommendation, the USPSTF failed to acknowledge the unique nature of ASD in that it cannot currently be diagnosed through biological measures, such as blood tests or brain scans (Veenstra-VanderWeele & McGuire, 2016). Instead, the task force reviewed research on ASD in the same way they might consider studies on cancer or other diseases that have known, identifiable biological markers (Veenstra-VanderWeele & McGuire, 2016). This perspective led the task force to recommend that standardized screening for ASD only be implemented when parents or clinicians have concerns about a child's potential ASD symptoms (Veenstra-VanderWeele & McGuire, 2016). While parental concern is highly valuable and should always warrant screening, evidence suggests that children should be screened with or without parental concern. In fact, some children who receive positive screening results have parents and physicians who raised no developmental concerns prior to screening (Miller et al., 2011). Miller et al. (2011) found that 30% of children who screened positive and received an ASD diagnosis had not presented with prior concerns. Further, only 20% of these children with true positive screening results had both providers and parents who were concerned prior to screening and diagnosis (Miller et al., 2011). This finding indicates that screening tools are vital in identifying children who may be at risk for ASD and are not being identified via other methods, such as qualitative parent or professional concerns.

Additionally, the task force assumes that parents understand normal developmental trajectories and early symptoms of ASD and that clinicians have an adequate opportunity to observe signs and symptoms in short, routine visits. Due to the complexity and heterogeneity of early ASD symptoms, these assumptions promote a nonsystematic, unreliable method of deciding when and whom to screen (Coury, 2015; Pierce et al., 2016; Veenstra-VanderWeele & McGuire, 2016). Many early ASD symptoms are subtle, such as failure to respond to one's name or other bids for social engagement, decreased or lack of nonverbal communication (e.g., pointing, facial expressions, eye gaze), decreased initiations for social engagement, and diminished joint attention skills (Reznick et al., 2007). Recognizing these red flags can be complicated due to the heterogeneity of these behaviors across children. Furthermore, these behaviors are rarely completely absent, but rather are reduced or inconsistent, making it more challenging to notice a deficit. For example, toddlers with ASD respond to their name about half of the time, and, while typically developing children respond more consistently, they still do not *always* respond (Gabrielsen et al., 2015). Research also suggested that during an average 10-minute period, 89% of the behavior of a child with ASD aligned with typical behavior (Gabrielsen et al., 2015). This finding indicated that the symptoms that may raise concern for early ASD are often the minority of a child's behaviors and may not be apparent during a brief medical visit. In fact, professionals with substantial experience with ASD were only able to identify 61% of children with ASD after a 10-minute observation (Gabrielsen et al., 2015). Therefore, it can be expected that pediatricians without specific expertise in ASD will be even less likely to notice behaviors of concern during short, routine appointments. See Chapters 3 and 6 for more information on development of children with ASD.

This issue is further complicated because symptoms of ASD are sometimes inconsistent in the first few years of life (Brian et al., 2014; Kim et al., 2018). Onset of symptoms is yet more complicated by developmental regressions that may occur in children with ASD, such that a child may not meet the criteria for concern on a screener at an early age but may meet these criteria when screening is administered again at a later age (Rogers, 2004; Brown & Prelock, 1995). The results of these studies suggest that, despite the USPSTF recommendation to screen only when concerns are present, screening tools should be implemented early to identify cases that may be missed by clinical impressions alone and should continue to be implemented throughout the first 3 years of life to ensure that children whose ASD symptoms develop later are still identified as early as possible.

Other Factors That Affect Screening

Although the AAP, the AAN, and the CNS have historically recommended universal standard screening for ASD, truly universal screening has not yet been implemented in the United States owing to inconsistencies in physician implementation, resources for screening procedures, and access to screening tools (King et al., 2010; Liptak et al., 2008; Radecki, Sand-Loud, O'Connor, Sharp, & Olson, 2011; Arunyanart et al., 2012; Zuckerman et al., 2014; Khowaja, Hazzard, & Robins, 2015). From 2002 to 2009, the percentage of pediatricians who used screening tools at well-child visits across North America increased from 23 to 48%, a statistic that rose just slightly to 50% by 2012 (Radecki et al., 2011; Arunyanart et al., 2012). Furthermore, pediatricians whose patient population was largely composed of nonwhite or Medicaid-insured families were less likely to use standardized screening tools for ASD (Arunyanart et al., 2012). Therefore, use of screening tools at all pediatrician visits, including emergency or sick visits, is imperative in identifying ASD cases in uninsured families, who are less likely than insured families to attend well-child visits (Miller et al., 2011). Unfortunately, the USPSTF determination might drive the field backward by further reducing the likelihood that practitioners will implement universal standard screening (Veenstra-VanderWeele & McGuire, 2016).

Beyond variability in practitioners' implementation of screening, there are many barriers to families' access to screening procedures, including racial and cultural factors, primary language, geographic location, literacy levels, parent education, and socioeconomic status (Antezana, Scarpa, Valdespino, Albright, & Richey, 2017; Zuckerman et al., 2014). Although prevalence of ASD may not differ significantly among racial groups, parents in Latino and black communities are less likely to report ASD symptoms displayed by their children (Liptak et al., 2008), and Latino and black children tend to receive later diagnoses (Jo, Schieve, Rice, Yeargin-Allsopp, & Tian, 2015; Mandell, Listerud, Levy, & Pinto-Martin, 2002). This discrepancy may be related to a lack of awareness of ASD symptoms; language barriers when trying to express concerns to appropriate professionals; limited access to culturally and linguistically appropriate screening measures; and/or the cultural stigma associated with raising concerns about psychiatric conditions (Zuckerman et al., 2014). For example, the questions included in some parent-report screeners written in English are difficult for parents whose preferred language is not English or for those with literacy challenges (Khowaja et al., 2015). Families with lower levels of parental education may lack knowledge of typical and atypical development, so they might be less able to accurately answer pediatricians' questions during developmental surveillance (Khowaja et al., 2015). Evidence also showed that families with lower maternal education, lower socioeconomic status, and minority backgrounds were less likely to attend follow-up evaluations after receiving positive screening results (Herlihy et al., 2014; Khowaja et al., 2015). These challenges in screening completion and follow-up, along with concerns regarding geographic and policy-related barriers, led to later ASD diagnosis and loss of opportunities for early intervention in these populations (Daniels & Mandell, 2014; Herlihy et al., 2014; Khowaja et al., 2015). Similar cultural considerations must be examined with regard to ASD screening in developing countries with limited access to screening, professional consultation, and services for developmental disorders (Samadi & McConkey, 2011). See Chapter 11.

The variety of factors that impact each step of the screening process highlights the need to, at the very least, increase implementation of standard screening to known high-risk populations, such as younger siblings of children with ASD or infants born before term. Further, screening tools that can be completed in a variety of languages, orally, on paper, or online must be made available to optimize access to screening services. Efforts are required to ensure that standard screening is accessible to diverse populations in order to decrease the disparity in age of first identification among minority, undereducated, and low-socioeconomic-status families. Recruiting early childcare providers to administer screening is one proposed method to attenuate the impact of these social determinants of health on screening and referral procedures (Janvier et al., 2016). If pediatricians follow the 2016 USPSTF recommendation, screening only when concerns have been raised and if no further measures to address these barriers are explored, children in minority or undereducated families are more likely to be missed. See Figure 2.1 for a summary of the screening process.

Summary of Responses

Although the USPSTF screening recommendation did not *explicitly* recommend against screening for ASD, the contradictions, gaps, and potential implications of the task force's statement left universal standard screening with little support. While more research may be necessary to determine the long-term outcomes of universal standard screening, the overwhelming response of the research and clinical ASD community to the USPSTF's recommendation was that health care professionals should continue to use ASD screening tools for all patients even as research continues, especially since the USPSTF determination was in direct contrast to the precedent set by the AAP, the AAN, and the CNS (Coury, 2015; Pierce et al., 2016; Veenstra-VanderWeele & McGuire, 2016).

Because the USPSTF is a well-respected committee that has contributed to significant improvements in many areas of preventive care, their recommendations regarding ASD screening may have widespread influence on ASD research and diagnosis. The task force called for more research regarding intervention outcomes in samples of children who were identified by screening tools only to determine the utility of screening (Siu & the USPSTF, 2016). However, evidence for long-term outcomes of early diagnosis and treatment is not easily gathered due to the effects of ASD on the entire family, the challenges in quantifying ASD symptoms, and the difficulties in truly randomizing intensive treatment conditions (Pierce et

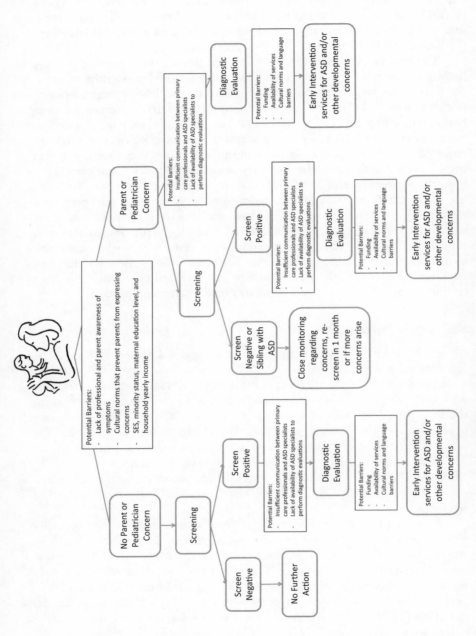

FIGURE 2.1. Decision tree: Screening to diagnosis.

al., 2016; Bolte & Diehl, 2013). Thus, researchers fear that autism research funding may be misallocated, focusing more on whether to screen and less on development of effective treatments for children who receive an ASD diagnosis (Pierce et al., 2016). A shift in research focus back to the utility of screening could "trigger a step backward" (Veenstra-VanderWeele & McGuire, 2016, p. 328) in the gains that have been made toward earlier diagnosis and effective intervention. This in turn could potentially perpetuate the already troubling disparity in age at first diagnosis due to race, familial education levels, socioeconomic status, and household yearly income (Coury, 2015; Veenstra-VanderWeele & McGuire, 2016).

Future Directions for Screening

As the USPSTF noted, perhaps the largest barrier to understanding the utility of early screening is the lack of research on longer-term effects of early intervention in samples identified by screening (Siu & the USPSTF, 2016). Additionally, the task force presented concerns about the impact of screening on the early intervention process, such as limited resources for evaluation and treatment and the complicated process that links screening and access to services (Siu & the USPSTF, 2016). These concerns are present in findings from one qualitative study of a purposive sample of families who received early intervention referrals and followed up, families who received early intervention referrals and did not follow up, and early intervention providers (Jimenez, Barg, Guevara, Gerdes, & Fiks, 2012). Jimenez and colleagues (2012) found that barriers to service access included communication issues, parent reliance on their own concerns to determine whether to seek services, a "wait and see" attitude, and logistical barriers. These barriers indicate the need to improve total service access, ranging from screening to diagnostic assessment to implementation of interventions.

Disciplines providing ASD supports will also need to invest in longitudinal research that tracks children from initial screening through adulthood. This research should focus on a family's ability to access care as well as on whether early intervention is implemented, the intensity and focus of this treatment, and the type of treatment provided. Of course, compared to other study designs (e.g., cross-sectional), longitudinal designs are inherently more costly and time consuming. Therefore, retrospective research regarding the screening process and type and intensity of early intervention that was received by school-age children and adults with ASD when they were children may be a more feasible way to address the USPSTF's concerns regarding methods for identification that ultimately yield optimal outcomes, though these types of studies might not meet typical epidemiological standards. For example, these studies would rely on parent or participant recall regarding participation in early intervention. Furthermore, recent developments in early intervention practices may yield significantly different long-term results than were achieved by interventions implemented a decade ago. Alternatively, much information can continue to be gleaned through cross-sectional studies. Although the implications may be limited, the lower cost makes these studies more feasible.

Research on screening could also benefit from greater focus on implementation and feasibility of screening procedures. For example, identification of novel methods through which to implement screening consistently in populations that vary in language preference, level of literacy, access to health care services, race, and socioeconomic status is important. New methods should be designed for implementation in a variety of community-based settings, such as schools or daycare centers, in order to increase accessibility for families without regular access to primary care (Janvier et al., 2016). If new screening tools are developed for use in primary care settings, training nurse practitioners and other staff on the early signs of developmental delay and ASD in order to increase the number of professionals who already have contact with the patients and knowledge of unusual patterns of development and considering the challenges in implementation in real-world settings may prove useful (Barbaro & Dissanayake, 2010; King et al., 2010). Additionally, telehealth and application-based screening, such as E-VAS and Autism Navigator, may be ways to use modern technology to adapt to the needs of a diverse population. See Chapter 10.

Increasing both physician and parent awareness regarding early developmental milestones and ASD symptoms will promote early identification and treatment. Organizations such as the CDC (*www.cdc.gov*), Autism Speaks (*www.autismspeaks.org*), and the Autism Science Foundation (*https://autismsciencefoundation.org*) are already working toward increasing awareness through their free and accessible websites with accurate information regarding developmental milestones and disorders, including ASD. While there is plenty of work to be done, research on the benefits of screening and the availability of adequate screening measures indicates that efficient, accurate screening is a worthwhile endeavor.

REFERENCES

Achenbach, T. M., & Rescorla, L. A. (2001). *Manual for the ASEBA School-Age Forms and Profiles*. Burlington: University of Vermont, Research Center for Children, Youth, and Families.

Achenie, L. E. K., Scarpa, A., Factor, R. S., Wang, T., Robins, D. L., & McCrickard, D. S. (2019). A machine learning strategy for autism screening in toddlers. *Journal of Developmental and Behavioral Pediatrics, 40*(5), 369–376.

Adrien, J. L., Perrot, A., Sauvage, D., Leddet, I., Larmonde, C., Hameury, L., & Barthelemy, C. (1992). Early symptoms in autism from family home movies: Evaluation and comparison between 1st and 2nd year of life using I.B.S.E. scale. *Acta Paedopsychiatrica, 55*(2), 71–75.

Altpeter, M., Mitchell, J., & Pennell, J. (2005). Advancing social workers' responsiveness to health disparities: The case of breast cancer screening. *Health and Social Work, 30*(3), 221–232.

American Academy of Pediatrics, Committee on Children with Disabilities. (2001). Developmental surveillance and screening of infants and young children. *Pediatrics, 108*(1), 192–196.

American Academy of Pediatrics, Council on Children with Disabilities. (2006). Identifying infants and young children with developmental disorders in the medical home: An algorithm for developmental surveillance and screening. *Pediatrics, 118*(1), 405–420.

Anderson, D. K., Liang, J. W., & Lord, C. (2014). Predicting young adult outcome among more and less cognitively able individuals with autism spectrum disorders. *Journal of Child Psychology and Psychiatry, 55*(5), 485–494.

Antezana, L., Scarpa, A., Valdespino, A., Albright, J., & Richey, J. A. (2017). Rural trends in diagnosis and services for autism spectrum disorder. *Frontiers in Psychology, 8*(590), 1–5.

Arunyanart, W., Fenick, A., Ukritchon, S., Imjaijitt, W., Northrup, V., & Weitzman, C. (2012). Developmental and autism screening: A survey across six states. *Infants and Young Children, 25*(3), 175–187.

Baio, J., Wiggins, L., Christensen, D. L., Maenner, M. J., Daniels, J., Warren, Z., . . . Dowling, N. F. (2018). Prevalence of autism spectrum disorder among children aged 8 years—Autism and developmental disabilities monitoring network, 11 sites, United States, 2014. *Surveillance Summaries, 67*(6), 1–23.

Baird, G., Douglas, H. R., & Murphy, S. M. (2011). Recognising and diagnosing autism in children and young people: Summary of NICE guidance. *Practice, 343*, 900–902.

Baranek, G. T., Watson, L. R., Boyd, B. A., Poe, M. D., David, F. J., & McGuire, L. (2013). Hyporesponsiveness to social and nonsocial sensory stimuli in children with autism, children with developmental delays, and typically developing children. *Development and Psychopathology, 25*(2), 307–320.

Barbaro, J., & Dissanayake, C. (2010). Prospective identification of autism spectrum disorders in infancy and toddlerhood using developmental surveillance: The social attention and communication study. *Journal of Developmental and Behavioral Pediatrics, 31*, 376–385.

Barbaro, J., & Dissanayake, C. (2012). Early markers of autism spectrum disorders in infants and toddlers prospectively identified in the Social Attention and Communication Study. *Autism, 17*(1), 64–86.

Baron-Cohen, S., Allen, J., & Gillberg, C. (1992). Can autism be detected at 18 months?: The needle, the haystack, and the CHAT. *British Journal of Psychiatry, 161*(6), 839–843.

Birn, A. E. (1997). Six seconds per eyelid: The medical inspection of immigrants at Ellis Island, 1892–1914. *Dynamis: Acta Hispanica ad Medicinae Sceintiarumque, Historiam Illustrandam, 17*, 281–316.

Bishop, S. L., Huerta, M., Gotham, K., Havdahl, K. A., Pickles, A., Duncan, A., . . . Lord, C. (2017). The Autism Symptom Interview, School-Age: A brief telephone interview to identify autism spectrum disorders in 5- to 12-year-old children. *Autism Research, 10*(1), 78–88.

Bolte, E. E., & Diehl, J. J. (2013). Measurement tools and target symptoms/skills used to assess treatment response for individuals with autism spectrum disorder. *Journal of Autism and Developmental Disorders, 43*(11), 2491–2501.

Bolte, S., Marschik, P. B., Falck-Ytter, T., Charman, T., & Roeyers, H. (2013). Infants at risk for autism: A European perspective on current status, challenges, and opportunities. *European Child and Adolescent Psychiatry, 22*(6), 341–348.

Bradshaw, J., Steiner, A. M., Gengoux, G., & Koegel, L. K. (2015). Feasibility and effectiveness of very early intervention for infants at-risk for autism spectrum disorder: A systematic review. *Journal of Autism and Developmental Disorders, 45*, 778–794.

Brian, A. J., Roncadin, C., Duku, E., Bryson, S. E., Smith, I. M., Roberts, W., . . . Zwaigenbaum, L. (2014). Emerging cognitive profiles in high-risk infants with and without autism spectrum disorder. *Research in Autism Spectrum Disorders, 8*(11), 1557–1566.

Brown, J., & Prelock, P. A. (1995). Brief report: The impact of regression on language development in autism. *Journal of Autism and Developmental Disorders, 25*(3), 305–309.

Bryson, S. E., & Zwaigenbaum, L. (2014). Autism Observation Scale for infants. *Comprehensive Guide to Autism*, 299–310.

Bryson, S. E., Zwaigenbaum, L., McDermott, C., Rombough, V., & Brian, J. (2008). The Autism Observation Scale for Infants: Scale development and reliability data. *Journal of Autism and Developmental Disorders, 38*(4), 731–738.

Camp, B. W. (2007). Evaluating bias in validity studies of developmental/behavioral screening tests. *Journal of Developmental and Behavioral Pediatrics, 28*(3), 234–240.

Charman, T., Baird, G., Simonoff, E., Chandler, S., Davison-Jenkins, A., Sharma, A., . . . Pickles, A. (2016). Testing two screening instruments for autism spectrum disorder in UK community child health services. *Developmental Medicine and Child Neurology, 58*(4), 369–375.

Chlebowski, C., Robins, D. L., Barton, M. L., & Fein, D. (2013). Large-scale use of the Modified Checklist for Autism in Low-Risk Toddlers. *Pediatrics, 131*(4), 1121–1127.

Cohen, I. L., Gomez, T. R., Gonzalez, M. G., Lennon, E. M., Karmel, B. Z., & Gardner, J. M. (2010). Parent PDD Behavior Inventory profiles of young children classified according to Autism Diagnostic Observation Schedule–Generic and Autism Diagnostic Interview–Revised criteria. *Journal of Autism and Developmental Disorders, 40*(2), 246–254.

Cohen, I. L., Schmidt-Lackner, S., Romanczyk, R., & Sudhalter, V. (2003). The PDD Behavior Inventory: A rating scale for assessing response to intervention in children with pervasive developmental disorder. *Journal of Autism and Developmental Disorders, 33*(1), 31–45.

Cohen, I. L., & Sudhalter, V. (2005). *The PDD Behavior Inventory*. Lutz, FL: Psychological Assessment Resources.

Colgan, S. E., Lanter, E., McComish, C., Watson, L. R., Crais, E. R., & Baranek, G. T. (2006). Analysis of social interaction gestures in infants with autism. *Child Neuropsychology, 12*(4–5), 307–319.

Coury, D. L. (2015). Babies, bathwater, and screening for autism spectrum disorder: Comments on the USPSTF recommendations for autism spectrum disorder screening. *Journal of Developmental and Behavioral Pediatrics, 36*(9), 661–663.

Daniels, A. M., & Mandell, D. S. (2014). Explaining differences in age at autism spectrum disorder diagnosis: A critical review. *Autism, 18*(5), 583–597.

Dawson, G., Rogers, S., Munson, J., Smith, M., Winter, J., Greenson, J., . . . Varley, J. (2010). Randomized, controlled trial of an intervention for toddlers with autism: The early start Denver model. *Pediatrics, 125*(1), 17–23.

Dereu, M., Roeyers, H., Raymaekers, R., Meirsschaut, M., & Warreyn, P. (2012). How useful are screening instruments for toddlers to predict outcome at age 4?: General development, language skills, and symptom severity in children with a false positive screen for autism spectrum disorder. *European Child and Adolescent Psychiatry, 21*(10), 541–551.

Dereu, M., Warreyn, P., Raymaekers, R., Meirsschaut, M., Pattyn, G., Schietecatte, I., & Roeyers, H. (2010). Screening for autism spectrum disorders in Flemish daycare centres with the checklist for early signs of developmental disorders. *Journal of Autism and Developmental Disorders, 40*, 1247–1258.

Dietz, C., Swinkels, S., van Daalen, E., van Engeland, H., & Buitelaar, J. K. (2006). Screening for autistic spectrum disorder in children aged 14–15 months: II. Population screening with the Early Screening of Autistic Traits Questionnaire (ESAT): Design and general findings. *Journal of Autism and Developmental Disorders, 36*, 713–722.

Dorsey, E. R., & Topol, E. J. (2016). State of telehealth. *New England Journal of Medicine, 375*, 154–161.

Eaves, L. C., & Ho, H. H. (2004). The very early identification of autism: Outcome to age 4½–5. *Journal of Autism and Developmental Disorders, 34*(4), 367–378.

Fein, D., Carter, A., Bryson, S. E., Carver, L. J., Charman, T., Chawarska, K., . . . Iverson, J. M. (2016). Commentary on USPSTF final statement on universal screening for autism. *Journal of Developmental and Behavioral Pediatrics, 37*(7), 573–578.

Feldman, M. A., Ward, R. A., Savona, D., Regehr, K., Parker, K., Hudson, M., . . . Holden, J. J. A. (2012). Development and initial validation of a parent report measure of the behavioral development of infants at risk for autism spectrum disorders. *Journal of Autism and Developmental Disorders, 42*, 13–22.

Filipek, P. A., Accardo, P. J., Ashwal, S., Baranek, G. T., Cook, E. H., Jr., Dawson, G., . . . Volkmar, F. R. (2000). Practice parameter: Screening and diagnosis of autism. *Neurology, 55*(4), 468–479.

Gabrielsen, T. P., Farley, M., Speer, L., Villalobos, M., Baker, C. N., & Miller, J. (2015). Identifying autism in a brief observation. *Pediatrics, 135*, 330–338.

Garcia-Primo, P., Hellendoorn, A., Charman, T., Roeyers, H., Dereu, M., Roge, B., . . . Canal-Bedia, R. (2014). Screening for autism spectrum disorders: State of the art in Europe. *European Child and Adolescent Psychiatry, 23*(11), 1005–1021.

Ghuman, J. K., Leone, S. L., Lecavalier, L., & Landa, R. J. (2011). The Screen for Social Interaction (SSI): A screening measure for autism spectrum disorders in preschoolers. *Research in Developmental Disabilities, 32*, 2519–2529.

Gillberg, C., Ehlers, S., Shaumann, H., Jakobsson, G., Dahlgren, S., Lindblom, R., . . . Blidner, E. (1990). Autism under age 3 years: A clinical study of 28 cases referred for autistic symptoms in infancy. *Journal of Child Psychology and Psychiatry and Allied Disciplines, 21*, 921–934.

Gould, S. J. (1996). *The mismeasure of man.* New York: Norton.

Granpeesheh, D., Dixon, D. R., Tarbox, J., Kaplan, A. M., & Wilke, A. E. (2009). The effects of age and treatment intensity on behavioral intervention outcomes for children with autism spectrum disorders. *Research in Autism Spectrum Disorders, 3,* 1014–1022.

Gray, K. M., & Tonge, B. J. (2005). Screening for autism in infants and preschool children with developmental delay. *Australian and New Zealand Journal of Psychiatry, 39,* 378–386.

Gray, K. M., Tonge, B. J., Sweeney, D. J., & Einfeld, S. L. (2008). Screening for autism in young children with developmental delay: An evaluation of the Developmental Behaviour Checklist: Early Screen. *Journal of Autism and Developmental Disorders, 38,* 1003–1010.

Green, J., Charman, T., McConachie, H., Aldred, C., Slonims, V., Howlin, P., . . . & Barrett, B. (2010). Parent-mediated communication-focused treatment in children with autism (PACT): A randomised controlled trial. *The Lancet, 375*(9732), 2152–2160.

Green, J., Wan, M. W., Guiraud, J., Holsgrove, S., McNally, J., Slonims, V., . . . BASIS Team. (2013). Intervention for infants at risk of developing autism: A case series. *Journal of Autism and Developmental Disorders, 43*(11), 2502–2514.

Gurian, E. A., Kinnamon, D. D., Henry, J. J., & Waisbren, S. E. (2006). Expanded newborn screening for biochemical disorders: The effect of a false-positive result. *Pediatrics, 117*(6), 1915–1921.

Haglund, N., Dahlgren, S. O., Källén, K., Gustafsson, P., & Råstam, M. (2015). The Observation Scale for Autism (OSA): A new screening method to detect autism spectrum disorder before age three years. *Journal of Intellectual Disability, 3,* 230–237.

Hardy, S., Haisley, L., Manning, C., & Fein, D. (2015). Can screening with the Ages and Stages Questionnaire detect autism? *Journal of Developmental and Behavioral Pediatrics, 36,* 536–543.

Harris, B., Barton, E. E., & Albert, C. (2014). Evaluating autism diagnostic and screening tools for cultural and linguistic responsiveness. *Journal of Autism and Developmental Disorders, 44,* 1275–1287.

Havdahl, K. A., von Tetzchner, S., Huerta, M., Lord, C., & Bishop, S. L. (2016). Utility of the Child Behavior Checklist as a screener for autism spectrum disorder. *Autism Research, 9,* 33–42.

Hedley, D., Nevill, R. E., Monroy-Moreno, Y., Fields, N., Wilkins, J., Butter, E., & Mulick, J. A. (2015). Efficacy of the ADEC in identifying autism spectrum disorder in clinically referred toddlers in the US. *Journal of Autism and Developmental Disorders, 45,* 2337–2348.

Hedley, D., Young, R., Angelica, M., Gallegos, J., & Salazar, C. M. (2010). Cross-cultural evaluation of the Autism Detection in Early Childhood (ADEC) in Mexico. *Autism, 14*(2), 93–112.

Herlihy, L. E., Brooks, B., Dumont-Mathieu, T., Barton, M. L., Fein, D., Chen, C. M., & Robins, D. L. (2014). Standardized screening facilitates timely diagnosis of autism spectrum disorders in a diverse sample of low-risk toddlers. *Journal of Developmental Behavioral Pediatrics, 35*(2), 85–92.

Hewlett, J., & Waisbren, S. E. (2006). A review of the psychosocial effects of false-positive results on parents and current communication practices in newborn screening. *Journal of Inherited Metabolic Disease, 29*(5), 677–682.

Hoshino, Y., Kumashiro, H., Yashima, Y., Tachinbana, R., Watanabe, M., & Furukawa, H. (1982). Early symptoms of autistic children and its diagnostic significance. *Folia Psychiatrica et Neurologica Japonica, 36,* 367–374.

Hyman, I. A., Chafey, E., & Smith, K. (1977). *Developing criterion referenced assessment for Head Start: Theoretical and practical considerations.* Paper presented at the meeting of the American Psychological Association.

Janvier, Y. M., Coffield, C. N., Harris, J. F., Mandell, D. S., & Cidav, Z. (2018). The developmental check-in: Development and initial testing of an autism screening tool targeting young children from underserved communities. *Autism, 23*(3), 689–698.

Janvier, Y. M., Harris, J. F., Coffield, C. N., Louis, B., Xie, M., Cidav, Z., & Mandell, D. S. (2016). Screening for autism spectrum disorder in underserved communities: Early childcare providers as reporters. *Autism, 20*(3), 364–373.

Jimenez, M. E., Barg, F. K., Guevara, J. P., Gerdes, M., & Fiks, A. G. (2012). Barriers to evaluation for early intervention services: Parent and early intervention employee perspectives. *Academic Pediatrics, 12*(6), 551–557.

Jo, H., Schieve, L. A., Rice, C. E., Yeargin-Allsopp, M., & Tian, L. H. (2015). Age at autism spectrum disorder (ASD) diagnosis by race, ethnicity, and primary household language among children with special health care needs, United States, 2009–2010. *Maternal and Child Health Journal, 19*(8), 1687–1697.

Ka'opua, L. S. (2008). Developing a culturally responsive breast cancer screening promotion with native Hawaiian women in churches. *Health and Social Work, 33*(3), 169–177.

Khowaja, M. K., Hazzard, A. P., & Robins, D. L. (2015). Sociodemographic barriers to early detection of autism: Screening and evaluation using the M-CHAT, M-CHAT-R, and follow-up. *Journal of Autism and Developmental Disorders, 46*(6), 1797–1808.

Kim, S. H., Bal, V. H., Benrey, N., Choi, Y. B., Guthrie, W., Colombi, C., & Lord, C. (2018). Variability in autism symptom trajectories using repeated observations from 14 to 36 months of age. *Journal of the American Academy of Child and Adolescent Psychiatry, 57*(11), 837–848.

King, T. M., Tandon, D., Macias, M. M., Healy, J. A., Duncan, P. M., Swigonski, N. L., . . . Lipkin, P. H. (2010). Implementing developmental screening and referrals: Lessons learned from a national project. *Pediatrics, 125*(2), 350–360.

Krug, D. A., Arick, J. R., & Almond, P. J. (1978). Autism screening instrument for educational planning: Background and development. In J. Gillam (Ed.), *Autism: Diagnosis, instruction, management and research.* Austin: University of Texas Press.

Liptak, G. S., Benzoni, L. B., Mruzek, D. W., Nolan, K. W., Thingvoll, M. A., Wade, C. M., & Fryer, G. E. (2008). Disparities in diagnosis and access to health services for children with autism: Data from the National Survey of Children's Health. *Journal of Developmental and Behavioral Pediatrics, 29,* 152–160.

Lord, C. (1995). Follow-up of two-year-olds referred for possible autism. *Journal of Child Psychology and Psychiatry and Allied Disciplines, 36,* 1365–1382.

Lord, C., Rutter, M., & Le Couteur, A. (1994). Autism Diagnostic Interview—Revised: A revised version of a diagnostic interview for caregivers of individuals with possible pervasive developmental disorders. *Journal of Autism and Developmental Disorders, 24*(5), 659–685.

Mandell, D. S., Listerud, J., Levy, S. E., & Pinto-Martin, J. (2002). Race differences in age at diagnosis among Medicaid-eligible children with autism. *Journal of the American Academy of Child and Adolescent Psychiatry, 41*(12), 1447–1453.

Marlow, M., Servili, C., & Tomlinson, M. (2019). A review of screening tools for the identification of autism spectrum disorders and developmental delay in infants and young children: Recommendations for use in low- and middle-income countries. *Autism Research, 12*(2), 176–199.

Marteleto, M. R. F., & Pedromônico, M. R. M. (2005). Validity of Autism Behavior Checklist (ABC): Preliminary study. *Revista Prasileira de Psiquiatria, 27*(4), 295–301.

Matson, J. L., Wilkins, J., & Fodstad, J. C. (2010). The validity of the Baby and Infant Screen for Children with aUtIsm Traits: Part 1 (BISCUIT: Part 1). *Journal of Autism and Developmental Disorders, 41,* 1139–1146.

Matson, J. L., Wilkins, J., Sharp, B., Knight, C., Sevin, J. A., & Boisjoli, J. A. (2009). Sensitivity and specificity of the Baby and Infant Screen for Children with aUtIsm Traits (BISCUIT): Validity and cutoff scores for autism and PDD-NOS in toddlers. *Research in Autism Spectrum Disorders, 3,* 924–930.

Miller, J. S., Gabrielsen, T., Villalobos, M., Alleman, R., Wahmhoff, N., Carbone, P. S., & Segura, B. (2011). The Each Child Study: Systematic screening for autism spectrum disorders in a pediatric setting. *Pediatrics, 127,* 866–871.

Morabia, A., & Zhang, F. F. (2004). History of medical screening: From concepts to action. *Postgraduate Medical Journal, 80,* 463–469.

Moulton, E., Bradbury, K., Barton, M., & Fein, D. (2019). Factor analysis of the Childhood Autism Rating Scale in a sample of two year olds with an autism spectrum disorder. *Journal of Autism and Developmental Disorders, 49*(7), 2733–2746.

Muratori, F., Narzisi, A., Tancredi, R., Cosenza, A., Calugi, S., Saviozzi, I., . . . Calderoni, S. (2011). The CBCL 1.5–5 and the identification of preschoolers with autism in Italy. *Epidemiology and Psychiatric Sciences, 20*(4), 329–338.

Nah, Y., Young, R. L., & Brewer, N. (2018). Development of a brief version of the Autism Detection in Early Childhood. *Autism, 23*(2), 494–502.

Nah, Y., Young, R. L., Brewer, N., & Berlingeri, G. (2014). Autism Detection in Early Childhood (ADEC): Reliability and validity data for a Level 2 screening tool for autistic disorder. *Psychological Assessment, 26*(1), 215–226.

Newschaffer, C. J., Schriver, E., Berrigan, L., Landa, R., Stone, W. L., Bishop, S., . . . Warren, Z. E. (2017). Development and validation of a streamlined autism case confirmation approach for use in epidemiologic risk factor research in prospective cohorts. *Autism Research, 10*(3), 485–501.

Ojen, R. A., Schjolberg, S., Volkmar, F. R., Shic, F., Cicchetti, D. V., Nordahl-Hansen, A., . . . Chawarska, K. (2018). Clinical features of children with autism who passed 18-month screening. *Pediatrics, 141*(6), 1–10.

Oosterling, I. J., Wensing, M., Swinkels, S. H., van der Gaag, R. J., Visser, J. C., Woudenberg, T., . . . Buitelaar, J. K. (2010). Advancing early detection of autism spectrum disorder by applying an integrated two-stage screening approach. *Journal of Child Psychology and Psychiatry, 51*(3), 250–258.

Osterling, J., & Dawson, G. (1994). Early recognition of children with autism: A study of first birthday home videotapes. *Journal of Autism and Developmental Disorders, 24,* 247–257.

Ozonoff, S., Iosif, A. M., Baguio, F., Cook, I. C., Hill, M. M., Hutman, T., . . . Steinfeld, M. B. (2010). A prospective study of the emergence of early behavioral signs of autism. *Journal of the American Academy of Child and Adolescent Psychiatry, 49*(3), 256–266.

Perry, A., Condillac, R. A., Freeman, N. L., Dunn-Geier, J., & Belair, J. (2005). Multisite study of the Childhood Autism Rating Scale (CARS) in five clinical groups of young children. *Journal of Autism and Developmental Disorders, 35*(5), 625–634.

Pierce, K., Courchesne, E., & Bacon, E. (2016). To screen or not to screen universally for autism is not the question: Why the task force got it wrong. *Journal of Pediatrics, 176,* 182–194.

Price, S. K., & Handrick, S. L. (2009). A culturally relevant and responsive approach to screening for perinatal depression. *Research on Social Work Practice, 19*(6), 705–714.

Radecki, L., Sand-Loud, N., O'Connor, K. G., Sharp, S., & Olson, L. M. (2011). Trends in the use of standardized tools for developmental screening in early childhood: 2002–2009. *Pediatrics, 128*(1), 14–19.

Reel, K. H., Lecavalier, L., Butter, E., & Mulick, J. A. (2012). Diagnostic utility of the Pervasive Developmental Disorder Behavior Inventory. *Research in Autism Spectrum Disorders, 6*(1), 458–465.

Rellini, E., Tortolani, D., Trillo, S., Carbone, S., & Montecchi, F. (2004). Childhood Autism Rating Scale (CARS) and Autism Behavior Checklist (ABC) correspondence and conflicts with DSM-IV criteria in diagnosis of autism. *Journal of Autism and Developmental Disorders, 34*(6), 703–708.

Rescorla, L., Kim, A. Y., & Oh, K. J. (2015). Screening for ASD with the Korean CBCL/1½–5. *Journal of Autism and Developmental Disorders, 45,* 4039–4050.

Reznick, J. S., Baranek, G. T., Reavis, S., Watson, L. R., & Crais, E. R. (2007). A parent-report instrument for identifying one-year-olds at risk for an eventual diagnosis of autism: The First Year Inventory. *Journal of Autism and Developmental Disorders, 37,* 1691–1710.

Robins, D. L., Casagrande, K., Barton, M., Chen, C. M. A., Dumont-Mathieu, T., & Fein, D. (2014). Validation of the Modified Checklist for Autism in Toddlers, Revised with follow-up (M-CHAT-R/F). *Pediatrics, 133*(1), 37–45.

Robins, D. L., Fein, D., Barton, M. L., & Green, J. A. (2001). The Modified Checklist for Autism in Toddlers: An initial study investigating the early detection of autism and pervasive developmental disorders. *Journal of Autism and Developmental Disorders, 31*(2), 131–144.

Rogers, S. J. (2004). Developmental regression in autism spectrum disorders. *Mental Retardation and Developmental Disabilities Research Reviews, 10,* 139–143.

Rogers, S. J., Estes, A., Lord, C., Vismara, L., Winter, J., Fitzpatrick, A., . . . Dawson, G. (2012). Effects of a brief Early Start Denver Model (ESDM)-based parent intervention on toddlers at risk for autism spectrum disorders: A randomized controlled trial. *Journal of the American Academy of Child and Adolescent Psychiatry, 51*(10), 1052–1065.

Rutter, M., Bailey, A., & Lord, C. (2003). *The Social Communication Questionnaire.* Los Angeles: Western Psychological Services.

Samadi, S. A., & McConkey, R. (2011). Autism in developing countries: Lessons from Iran. *Autism Research and Treatment, 2011,* Article ID 145359.

Schopler, E., Reichler, R. J., & Renner, B. R. (1988). *CARS: The childhood autism rating scale.* Los Angeles: Western Psychological Services.

Schrader, E., Delehanty, A. D., Casler, A., Petrie, E., Rivera, A., Harrison, K., . . . Wetherby, A. M. (2020). Integrating a new online autism screening tool in primary care to lower the age of referral. *Clinical Pediatrics, 59*(3), 305–309.

Siegel, B. (2013). Pervasive Developmental Disorders Screening Test (PDDST). *Encyclopedia of Autism Spectrum Disorders,* 2211–2215.

Sigman, M., & McGovern, C. (2005). Improvement in cognitive and language skills from preschool to adolescence in autism. *Journal of Autism and Developmental Disorders, 35*(1), 15–23.

Siu, A. L., & the U.S. Preventive Services Task Force. (2016). Screening for autism spectrum disorder in young children: U.S. Preventive Services Task Force Recommendation Statement. *JAMA, 315*(7), 691–696.

Smith, N. J., Sheldrick, R. C., & Perrin, E. C. (2012). An abbreviated screening instrument for autism spectrum disorders. *Infant Mental Health Journal, 34*(2), 149–155.

Soto, S., Linas, K., Jacobstein, D., Biel, M., Migdal, T., & Anthony, B. J. (2015). A review of cultural adaptations of screening tools for autism spectrum disorders. *Autism, 19*(6), 646–661.

Squires, J., & Bricker, D. (2009). *Ages and Stages Questionnaires, third edition (ASQ-3): A parent-completed child-monitoring system.* Baltimore: Brookes.

Stenberg, N., Bresnahan, M., Gunnes, N., Hirtz, D., Hornig, M., Lie, K. K., . . . Stotenberg, C. (2014). Identifying children with autism spectrum disorder at 18 months in a general population sample. *Pediatric and Perinatal Epidemiology, 28*(3), 255–262.

Stone, W. L., Coonrod, E. E., & Ousley, O. Y. (2000). Brief report: Screening Tool for Autism in Two-Year-Olds (STAT): Development and preliminary data. *Journal of Autism and Developmental Disorders, 30*(6), 607–612.

Stone, W. L., Coonrod, E. E., Turner, L. M., & Pozdol, S. L. (2004). Psychometric properties of the STAT for early autism screening. *Journal of Autism and Developmental Disorders, 34*(6), 691–701.

Stone, W. L., McMahon, C. R., & Henderson, L. M. (2008). Use of the Screening Tool for Autism in Two-Year-Olds (STAT) for children under 24 months. *Autism, 12*(5), 557–573.

Stone, W. L., & Ousley, O. Y. (1997). *STAT Manual: Screening tool for autism in two-year-olds.* Unpublished manuscript, Vanderbilt University.

Sturner, R., Howard, B., Bergmann, P., Morrel, T., Andon, L., Marks, D., . . . Landa, R. (2016). Autism screening with online decision support by primary care pediatricians aided by M-CHAT/F. *Pediatrics, 138*(3), 1–11.

Sturner, R., Howard, B., Bergmann, P., Stewart, L., & Afarian, T. E. (2017). Comparison of autism screening in younger and older toddlers. *Journal of Autism and Developmental Disorders, 47*(3), 3180–3188.

Swinkels, S. H. N., Dietz, C., van Daalen, E., Kerkhof, I. H. G. M., van Engeland, H., & Buitelaar, J. K. (2006). Screening for autistic spectrum in children aged 14 to 15 months: I. The development of the Early Screening of Autistic Traits Questionnaire (ESAT). *Journal of Autism and Developmental Disorders, 36*, 723–732.

Szatmari, P., Georgiades, S., Duku, E., Bennett, T. A., Bryson, S., Fombonne, E., . . . Thompson, A. (2015). Developmental trajectories of symptom severity and adaptive functioning in an inception cohort of preschool children with autism spectrum disorder. *JAMA Psychiatry, 72*(3), 276–283.

Thabtah, F., & Peebles, D. (2020). A new machine learning model based on induction of rules for autism detection. *Health Informatics Journal, 26*(1), 264–286.

Turner, L. M., & Stone, W. L. (2007). Variability in outcome for children with an ASD diagnosis at age 2. *Journal of Child Psychology and Psychiatry, 48*(8), 793–802.

Turner-Brown, L. M., Baranek, G. T., Reznick, J. S., Watson, L. R., & Crais, E. R. (2012). The First Year Inventory: A longitudinal follow-up of 12-month-old to 3-year-old children. *Autism, 17*(5), 527–540.

Veenstra-VanderWeele, J., & McGuire, K. (2016). Rigid, inflexible approach results in no recommendation for autism screening. *American Medical Association, 73*(4), 327–328.

Volkmar, F., Cook, E. H., Pomeroy, J., Realmuto, G., Tanguay, P., & the Work Group on Quality Issues. (1999). Practice parameters for the assessment and treatment of children, adolescents, and adults with autism and other pervasive developmental disorders. *Journal of the American Academy of Child and Adolescent Psychiatry, 38*(12), 32S–54S.

Volkmar, F., Siegel, M., Woodbury-Smith, M., King, B., McCracken, J., State, M., & American Academy of Child and Adolescent Psychiatry Committee on Quality Issues. (2014). *Journal of the American Academy of Child and Adolescent Psychiatry, 53*(2), 237–257.

Wadden, N. P. K., Bryson, S. E., & Rodger, R. S. (1991). A closer look at the Autism Behavior Checklist: Discriminant validity and factor structure. *Journal of Autism and Developmental Disorders, 21*(4), 529–541.

Watson, L. R., Baranek, G. T., Crais, E. R., Reznick, J. S., Dykstra, J., & Perryman, T. (2007). The First Year Inventory: Retrospective parent responses to a questionnaire designed to identify one-year-olds at risk for autism. *Journal of Autism and Developmental Disorders, 37,* 49–61.

Wetherby, A. M., Brosnan-Maddox, S., Peace, V., & Newton, L. (2008). Validation of the Infant–Toddler Checklist as a broadband screener for autism spectrum disorders from 9 to 24 months of age. *Autism, 12*(5), 487–511.

Wetherby, A. M., & Prizant, B. M. (2002). *Communication and symbolic behavior scales: Developmental profile, 1st normed.* Baltimore: Brookes.

Wetherby, A. M., Woods, J., Allen, L., Cleary, J. Dickinson, H., & Lord, C. (2004). Early indicators of autism spectrum disorders in the second year of life. *Journal of Autism and Developmental Disorders, 34*(5), 473–493.

Wiggins, L. D., Bakeman, R., Adamson, L. B., & Robins, D. L. (2007). The utility of the Social Communication Questionnaire in screening for autism in children referred for early intervention. *Focus on Autism and Other Developmental Disabilities, 22*(1), 33–38.

Young, R. L. (2007). *Autism detection in early childhood (ADEC) manual.* Camberwell, Australia: ACER Press.

Zuckerman, K. E., Sinche, B., Cobian, M., Cervantes, M., Mejia, A., Becker, T., & Nicolaidis, C. (2014). Conceptualization of autism in the Latino community and its relationship with early diagnosis. *Journal of Developmental and Behavioral Pediatrics, 35*(8), 522–533.

Zwaigenbaum, L., Bryson, S., Rogers, T., Roberts, W., Brian, J., & Szatman, P. (2005). Behavioral manifestations of autism in the first year of life. *International Journal of Developmental Neuroscience, 23*(2–3), 143–152.

CHAPTER 3

• • • • • • •

Psychological Development
of Toddlers with Autism Spectrum Disorder

Suzanne L. Macari, Kelly K. Powell, Megan Lyons,
Celine A. Saulnier, Angelina Vernetti,
and Katarzyna Chawarska

It is increasingly apparent that infants with autism spectrum disorder (ASD), due to early-emerging differences in attention, perception, and cognition underpinned by neurobehavioral and neurobiological variations (Chawarska, Macari, & Shic, 2013; Elison et al., 2013; Jones & Klin, 2013; Jones et al., 2016; Hazlett et al., 2017; Shen et al., 2013; Shic, Macari, & Chawarska, 2014; Wolff et al., 2012), begin to experience the world differently during the first year of life. Likely driven by iterative processes of developmental disruption, by the first birthday, many infants with ASD exhibit overt behavioral differences compared to their peers (Barbaro & Dissanayake, 2013; Bryson et al., 2007; Filliter et al., 2015; Macari et al., 2012; Mitchell et al., 2006; Ozonoff et al., 2010; Rozga et al., 2011; Wan et al., 2013; Zwaigenbaum et al., 2005; Chawarska et al., Chapter 5, this volume; Sifre et al., Chapter 6, this volume). Several questions immediately arise. How do these differences that later culminate in an ASD diagnosis affect the broader psychological development of infants and toddlers? Are there domains outside the core features of the disorder that become part of this cascade of cumulative atypicalities? In this chapter, we focus on areas of early development that appear to be impacted by or to co-occur with the emerging syndrome of ASD. These areas include emotion-related behaviors such as attachment, temperament, and emotional expressivity, as well as early cognitive, language, and adaptive behavior development. These early processes impact the developing brain and thus wield influence over heterogeneous developmental trajectories (see Sifre et al., Chapter 6, this volume). Although experience plays a vital role in specialization of various brain regions (Johnson, 2001), divergence in development can depend highly on initial differences in neuromodulator systems associated with temperament (Lewis, 2005). Furthermore, subcortical neural processes involved in emotion interact with cortical systems in important ways, such as affecting interregional coordination as well as contributing to synaptic pruning and shaping over time (Lewis, 2005).

Studying toddlers with ASD is key to a deeper understanding of the natural history of ASD prior to implementation of intervention and before secondary symptoms and comorbid disorders affect its expression. We review here research focusing on various aspects of psychological development of very young children with ASD in late infancy.

Emotional Development

Given the importance of emotion in shaping social and cognitive development, this topic has gained increased attention in studies of young children with ASD. We begin with attachment, the primary emotional relationship formed between infant and caregiver in the first weeks and months of life. Whether or not children with autism form attachments is no longer the question, but rather, what are the fine-grained differences in these relationships and what child factors influence them? Temperament more broadly and its emotional aspects have also enjoyed renewed interest in the field. Temperament in ASD has been largely examined via parental report, though more recent studies have investigated emotion at behavioral and physiological levels utilizing standardized induction probes in order to elicit emotions in a targeted manner. These areas of inquiry point to the critical role of emotions in shaping highly heterogeneous phenotypes as well as their role in the emergence of comorbid symptoms in older children with ASD.

Attachment

The affective bond between a child and a primary caregiving figure (Ainsworth, Blehar, Waters, & Wall, 1978) has been a frequent topic of study in children with ASD. A young child's behavior during lab-based separation and reunion episodes, or the Strange Situation paradigm, is thought to reflect the history of dyadic interaction and may predict aspects of later functioning. Secure attachment is characterized by greater exploration of the physical environment when accompanied by the caregiver compared to a stranger, as well as by distress and proximity-seeking behaviors in response to separation and reunion episodes, respectively. Although ASD affects the ability to relate socially, studies of toddler- and preschool-age children with ASD utilizing the Strange Situation paradigm have not indicated an absence of proximity-seeking and other behaviors that are emblematic of a secure attachment (Capps, Sigman, & Mundy, 1994; Dissanayake & Crossley,

1996; Naber et al., 2007; Rogers, Ozonoff, & Maslin-Cole, 1993; Waterhouse & Fein, 1998; Willemsen-Swinkels, Bakermans-Kranenburg, Buitelaar, van IJzendoorn, & van Engeland, 2000). However, rates of secure attachment classification are somewhat lower in young children with ASD than in typically developing (TD) or developmentally delayed (DD) groups. According to a meta-analysis of studies involving preschoolers with ASD (Rutgers, Bakermans-Kranenburg, van IJzendoorn, & Berckelaer-Onnes, 2004), 53% of the children displayed a secure attachment. Similarly, a review of studies of children with ASD from a wider age range suggests that approximately 47% are securely attached (Teague, Gray, Tonge, & Newman, 2017), compared with around 60% of TD children (Ainsworth et al., 1978), with an overrepresentation of insecure and disorganized attachment styles in ASD not unlike mental age-matched children with other delays (Naber et al., 2007). However, when matched on adaptive behavior and rated by parents, quality of attachment in preschoolers with ASD was reportedly lower, with more conflict and less closeness (Teague, Newman, Tonge, & Gray, 2018).

Several factors likely contribute to variability across studies, which report secure attachment classification ranging from 40 to 60% of children with ASD (Teague et al., 2017). Moderators of attachment in preschoolers and toddlers include autism symptom severity and mental ability, with both greater severity of social impairments and severity of intellectual disability associated with less secure emotional attachment types and fewer prosocial behaviors during the reunion (Grzadzinski, Luyster, Spencer, & Lord, 2014; Naber et al., 2007). Parental sensitivity and caregivers' own internal models of attachment have also been found to play a role in samples of older children with ASD (Oppenheim, Koren-Karie, Dolev, & Yirmiya, 2012; Seskin et al., 2010). In addition, many studies have used Ainsworth and colleagues' four-category classification system (Ainsworth & Bell, 1970; Ainsworth et al., 1978; Main & Solomon, 1990), while assessment with alternative methods often yields different findings. Studies utilizing the Richters attachment security rating (Richters, Waters, & Vaughn, 1988), the Brief Attachment Screening Questionnaire (Bakermans-Kranenburg, van IJzendoorn, & Juffer, 2003), or a count of prosocial behaviors (Grzadzinski et al., 2014) have revealed significantly lower quality of attachment in 2-year-olds with ASD compared to typical controls and toddlers with non-ASD developmental delays (Rutgers et al., 2007; van IJzendoorn et al., 2007; but see Naber et al., 2007). Other atypical attachment behaviors include increased contact resistance and fewer contact-seeking behaviors (Rogers et al., 1993). Since dimensional measures reveal greater ASD-specific attachment vulnerabilities, discrepancies across results may be attributable in part to measurement issues. Thus, although many young children with ASD are capable of forming secure attachments with their primary caregivers, subtle differences in quality are apparent even in those who are securely attached.

A fundamental contradiction emerges when attempting to reconcile the finding that many children with ASD, a syndrome defined by core deficits in social motivation and reciprocity, exhibit a secure attachment. If attachment underlies basic human sociability and if autism represents the derailment of sociability (Vivanti & Nuske, 2017), the phenomenon of secure attachment in children with ASD is indeed a conundrum. Three lines of reasoning have been set forth: (1) attachment is a biobehavioral system that is highly conserved (Dissanayake & Crossley, 1996); (2) intact attachment behavior in young children with ASD is driven by systems separate from those underlying social affiliation (Chevallier, Kohls, Troiani, Brodkin, & Schultz, 2012); or (3) apparent preserved attachment in ASD is a methodological artifact of experimental paradigms such as the Strange Situation (Hobson, 2019; Moles, Kieffer, & D'Amato, 2004). Vivanti and Nuske (2017) propose a nuanced resolution of this apparent contradiction, with the suggestion that ASD symptoms do have an impact on attachment, but an effect that is perhaps less evident under the threatening and more extreme circumstances provided by the Strange Situation. Instead, ASD symptoms influence the drive to engage socially in a more sustained way in daily life under nonthreatening conditions.

Temperament

Temperament is defined as neurobiologically based individual differences in reactivity and regulation in the domains of attention, motor activity, and emotion that emerge beginning in early infancy (Goldsmith et al., 1987; Rothbart & Bates, 1998; Rothbart & Derryberry, 1981). Viewed as potentially underlying later personality, early temperament has traditionally been studied in relation to healthy and atypical outcomes (Caspi, Henry, McGee, Moffitt, & Silva, 1995; Chess, Thomas, Rutter, & Birch, 1963), with longitudinal links to social competence and peer relationships (Sanson, Hemphill, & Smart, 2004), as well as anxiety, social withdrawal, and externalizing behaviors at early school age (Booth-LaForce & Oxford, 2008; Pérez-Edgar et al., 2011; Rubin, Burgess, Dwyer, & Hastings, 2003).

Temperament in very young children with ASD has been the focus of several recent reports. Clinic-referred 2-year-olds with ASD exhibited temperamental differences across domains compared with TD and DD peers, with the most striking vulnerabilities within the domain of Effortful Control (EC; Macari, Koller, Campbell, & Chawarska, 2017). Toddlers with ASD had difficulties transitioning between activities when prompted and inhibiting actions when directed; were less likely to enjoy and maintain attention to low-intensity activities; and demonstrated less awareness of subtle environmental stimuli compared to both TD and ability-matched delayed peers. Diminished excitement about upcoming pleasant activities (Positive Anticipation) was an ASD-specific vulnerability that drove lower

Surgency domain scores in this group compared to controls. Some temperamental vulnerabilities in ASD were shared with toddlers with developmental delays, including lower soothability (recovering from extreme emotions) and diminished attention focusing.

Similar results have been reported for infants with ASD followed prospectively from birth in familial high-risk cohorts, with group differences emerging as early as 6 months of age (see Chawarska et al., Chapter 5, this volume). Parents reported lower levels of Surgency (positive affect and activity level) in a large cohort of 6-month-old infants who were later diagnosed with ASD (Paterson et al., 2019) as well as in another study in which parents reported lower activity levels in their infants (del Rosario, Gillespie-Lynch, Johnson, Sigman, & Hutman, 2013; but see Clifford, Hudry, Elsabbagh, Charman, & Johnson, 2013, who reported higher Surgency in 7-month-old infants later diagnosed with ASD). Lower Surgency as well as lower EC characterized infants with ASD at 12 months (Clifford et al., 2013; Paterson et al., 2019), as did higher Negative Affectivity (Paterson et al., 2019) and distress (Zwaigenbaum et al., 2005). By 24 months, high-risk toddlers with ASD exhibited more sadness and less cuddliness than low-risk peers; less enjoyment of quiet activities than their high-risk and low-risk TD peers; more shyness and lower soothability than high-risk and low-risk controls (Clifford et al., 2013); reduced ability to shift attention in response to social cues; lower inhibitory control; and less positive anticipation than high-risk and low-risk peers (Garon et al., 2009; Zwaigenbaum et al., 2005). Another study noted significant declines in adaptability and approach behaviors and increases in activity level over the first 3 years in high-risk siblings with ASD compared to other high-risk siblings (del Rosario et al., 2013).

Temperamental vulnerabilities in toddlers with ASD begin early in life and involve attentional and behavioral control as well as affective reactivity. As in nonclinical populations (Putnam, Gartstein, & Rothbart, 2006), individual differences in many temperamental traits were highly stable in children with ASD from the toddler years to preschool age (Macari et al., 2017). Temperamental traits in 2-year-old toddlers with ASD were independent of concurrent severity of social impairments and levels of cognitive functioning (Macari et al., 2017), indicating independent contributions of temperament on the developing ASD phenotype. Furthermore, changes in parent-rated temperament within the EC domain contributed uniquely to social outcomes in the children with ASD, over and above the effects of initial verbal and nonverbal ability, severity of autism symptoms, and adaptive social and communication behavior. Greater severity of autism symptoms at outcome was predicted by minimal improvement in the awareness of and reactivity to low-intensity environmental stimuli (Perceptual Sensitivity) from age 2 to age 3½.

Conversely, improvements in the ability to inhibit behavior (Inhibitory Control) when instructed and increases in the enjoyment of low-key activities (Low-Intensity Pleasure) were both related to better social adaptive skills 1–2 years later. In a large sample of infants at high and low risk (Garon et al., 2016), both Positive Affectivity at 12 months and EC at 24 months were negatively correlated with severity of ASD symptoms at 36 months. However, the relationship between 12-month positive affect and severity of symptoms was completely mediated by 24-month EC in the structural equation model. Thus, positive emotion exerts its effect on severity of symptoms through its connection with EC. Furthermore, the temperamental features that differentiated high-risk infants without ASD from those with ASD were higher positive affect at 12 months and higher EC at 24 months (Garon et al., 2016).

Thus, early temperamental features, reflecting behavioral styles or inherent capacities that promote learning, may influence development in the social domain. For example, attention regulation is advantageous for acquiring skills such as expressive language (Salley, Panneton, & Colombo, 2013) and for monitoring the activities of others, the key to observational learning (Shic, Bradshaw, Klin, Scassellati, & Chawarska, 2011). Attention to social information in late infancy is related to later verbal skills and severity of autism symptoms (Campbell, Shic, Macari, & Chawarska, 2014). Individual differences in the development of attention to faces in the middle part of infancy, in particular, in peak look duration, are related to later executive control in infants at high risk for ASD (Hendry et al., 2018). Similarly, improvement in attentional and behavioral regulation from the second to third year appears to herald more positive social outcomes (Macari et al., 2017), possibly by fostering a focus on details about people or by increased tolerance of normative low-key activities that require well-regulated attention. Given the established links between early temperamental characteristics and later behavioral and affective outcomes in other populations, vulnerabilities in the Effortful Control and Negative Emotionality domains in toddlers with ASD may likewise signal risk for developing attentional, affective, and behavioral symptoms that impede learning and adaptation over and above their social and cognitive disability. Given the ubiquity of comorbid conditions in older children with ASD, particularly attention-deficit/hyperactivity disorder (ADHD) and anxiety (Simonoff et al., 2008), examination of temperamental features as early predictors of such problems may be particularly useful.

Emotional Expressivity and Emotional Experience

Central to some theories of temperament are the emotional aspects of behavior (Goldsmith & Campos, 1982). Emotions play an integral role in learning and communication and in early social and adaptive development (Izard, Fine, Mostrow, Trentacosta, & Campbell, 2002). They are organizers of everyday functioning, serving to motivate arousal as well as to maintain and terminate behavior (Emde, Gaensbauer, & Harmon, 1981).

Emotional expressivity is the external expression of subjective experience and can be quantified by parent report or by ratings of intensity and valence of facial, vocal, and bodily expressions during induction probes. Emotional experience refers to the physiological response of the sympathetic nervous system during induction probes, and can be quantified by a number of measures such as heart rate variability, respiration, and changes in electrodermal activity.

Relatively little is known about emotional expressivity in very young children with autism. Although studies of parent-reported temperament suggest that young children with ASD exhibit more frequent negative emotions and attenuated positive emotions compared to their peers (Adamek et al., 2011; Capps et al., 1994; Clifford et al., 2013; Garon et al., 2009; Macari et al., 2017; Zwaigenbaum et al., 2005), observational studies have reported a range of findings. These studies vary in context, structure, communicative partner, age of children, composition of comparison groups, measurement metric, and so forth, all of which are critical to the results. In social contexts, for example, during interactions with an adult, young children with ASD exhibited reduced positive emotion (Joseph & Tager-Flusberg, 1997; Snow, Hertzig, & Shapiro, 1987; Yirmiya, Kasari, Sigman, & Mundy, 1989), but even this might not be observed in every situation. For example, in requesting contexts, there were no differences in positive affect between TD children and those with ASD (Kasari, Sigman, Mundy, & Yirmiya, 1990).

Emotion induction paradigms involve the presentation of stimuli in a standardized manner to evoke specific emotions. The Laboratory Temperament Assessment Battery (Goldsmith & Rothbart, 1999) is a widely utilized measure that enables elicitation of fear, anger, and joy, and has been used for decades to study development of emotion during infancy and childhood in the general population. Probes from this measure or other similar measures have been employed in a small number of studies of children with ASD to study fear as well as frustration. One study of preschoolers with ASD noted no differences from younger language-matched TD controls in facial or bodily negativity in response to frustrating probes (Jahromi, Meek, & Ober-Reynolds, 2012). In another study, which included a small number of preschool-age children with ASD and children with fragile X syndrome in response to a stranger, facial fear but not escape behavior was more intense in the ASD group compared to TD children and children with fragile X syndrome (Scherr, Hogan, Hatton, & Roberts, 2017).

To address some of the gaps in knowledge, Macari and colleagues (2018) utilized structured induction techniques adapted from the Laboratory Temperament Assessment Battery (Lab-TAB; Goldsmith & Rothbart, 1999) to assess emotional expressivity in the basic affect systems of anger, joy, and fear (Sroufe, 1979) in toddlers with ASD. Stimuli were ecologically valid (e.g., being buckled into a car seat, watching a display of bubbles, being approached by a mechanical spider toy) but minimally social in order to avoid confounding emotional reactions with the social deficits in children with ASD. Participants included 99 very young children with and without ASD (mean age 21 months); two control groups consisted of age-matched TD toddlers and DD toddlers, the latter of whom were also non-verbal and verbal ability-matched. Intensity of emotional expressivity via facial and vocal channels was rated by blinded coders offline. During these essentially nonsocial standardized probes, toddlers with ASD expressed significantly more intense anger during frustrating events compared to DD controls and expressed marginally more intense anger than TD toddlers. When facing novel, potentially threatening situations, the toddlers with ASD expressed less intense fear than both groups of peers. While this increased anger response to goal blockage may challenge the developing emotion regulation system, the diminished fear response suggests atypical appraisal of threat and potential risk for future safety concerns. Intensity of fear and anger expression was independent from severity of autism symptoms (Autism Diagnostic Observation Schedule-2; Lord et al., 2012), suggesting that affective and social areas of vulnerability are dissociable and reciprocally shape ASD phenotypes from infancy onward. Intensity of joy, however, was similar across all three groups, indicating that the capacity to express positive emotions in response to playful, largely nonsocial triggers is intact in very young children with ASD.

In order to better understand these results and to determine the physiological underpinnings of the observed emotional responses, Vernetti and colleagues (2020) recorded electrodermal activity (EDA) during these induction probes in a subset of toddlers with ASD ($n = 42$) and age-matched TD toddlers ($n = 32$) (mean age 22 months). EDA registers a nonvalenced response of the sympathetic nervous system via eccrine glands that release perspiration and thus change the electrical charge of the skin during stressful or exciting events. Patterns of EDA changes from baseline during each probe were similar to the results at the behavioral level from our prior work (Macari et al., 2018). In response to probes aimed to elicit anger, toddlers with ASD exhibited an increase in physiological arousal indexed by electrodermal activity compared to baseline. Although the magnitude of the arousal response was higher than that of TD toddlers, it did not reach statistical significance. During fear-inducing probes, TD toddlers exhibited significantly increased physiological arousal compared to baseline, but this phenomenon was not observed in toddlers with ASD. Further analyses showed that toddlers with ASD exhibited a significantly attenuated physiological response to fear-inducing probes compared to TD controls. Finally, when exposed to playful stimuli, only the ASD group showed a significant decrease in arousal from baseline, reflecting a relaxation response in this group. Changes in physiological arousal during these playful situations also differed significantly between the ASD and TD groups. Together, these findings indicate a typical but somewhat enhanced physiological response to restraint and goal blockage, an attenuated response to threatening stimuli, and a lower, more pronounced physiological response to playful events in toddlers with ASD. Importantly, the intensity of physiological responses was substantially correlated with the intensity of behavioral emotional expressivity in situations eliciting anger or fear, which provides evidence of congruency between behavioral and physiological responses to nonsocial, negatively valenced emotional challenges in the early stages of ASD. In other words, the intensity of emotional expressivity observed via facial and vocal channels in toddlers with ASD mirrors the internal experience in toddlers with ASD (Vernetti et al., 2020). Finally, the physiological responses during the anger, fear, or joy conditions were not significantly correlated with severity of autism symptoms.

Thus, both behavioral and physiological evidence indicates neither a broad negative emotionality bias nor subdued positive emotions in toddlers with ASD upon exposure to largely nonsocial emotion-inducing triggers. The discovery that toddlers with ASD exhibited a muted behavioral and physiological response to novel, intrusive stimuli is important, as it suggests atypical appraisal of threatening elements in the environment and provides motivation for examining its underlying cognitive and neurodevelopmental mechanisms. The fact that neither fear nor anger measured at the behavioral or physiological level was associated with severity of autism symptoms suggests that in very young children, the dimension of emotion may contribute independently to shaping complex and heterogeneous autism phenotypes.

The findings also provide motivation for an investigation into the development of positive emotionality in ASD and its links with core social communicative impairments in ASD. As variability in joyful expression is associated with severity of autism symptoms, it may be a source of heterogeneity in the phenotype. Moreover, the expectation that a child with ASD typically presents with either muted affect or affect marked by a high degree of negativity may lower the detection rate among children who appear to be more affectively engaged, especially around activities that aim to elicit positive emotions. This work on emotional expression adds a much-needed facet to our knowledge of emotional development in young children with ASD and may be consequential for identifying precursors to later comorbid affective problems which are so common in children and adolescents with ASD.

Cognition and Language

Cognitive and Language Profiles

Heterogeneity in the phenotype of young children with ASD is particularly evident in cognitive and language profiles. While 25–30% of individuals with ASD are minimally verbal or nonverbal, the majority acquire spoken language (Anderson et al., 2007; Tager-Flusberg & Kasari, 2013). Estimates suggest that the prevalence of intellectual disability/global developmental delay in preschoolers with ASD is around 50% (Christensen et al., 2016; Delehanty, Stronach, Guthrie, Slate, & Wetherby, 2018). Assessment of cognitive and verbal abilities in children with autism is increasingly important given DSM-5's (American Psychiatric Association, 2013) requirement to specify these alongside the diagnosis (e.g., ASD with or without accompanying intellectual and/or language impairment).

Research examining verbal and nonverbal developmental skills in toddlers with ASD reveals a trend for higher nonverbal compared to verbal abilities (Barbaro & Dissanayake, 2012; Chawarska, Klin, Paul, Macari, & Volkmar, 2009; Chawarska, Macari, & Shic, 2012; Kim, Macari, Koller, & Chawarska, 2015; Landa & Garrett-Mayer, 2006; Macari et al., 2012; Mayes & Calhoun, 2003; Paul, Chawarska, Cicchetti, & Volkmar, 2008). This profile has been observed as early as 12 months of age (Barbaro & Dissanayake, 2012; Macari et al., 2012) and narrows with time (Chawarska et al., 2009; Kim et al., 2015; Landa & Garrett-Mayer, 2006; Mayes & Calhoun, 2003; Paul et al., 2008), though the age at which the gap closes appears to vary across samples and ranges from around 2 years to school age. The degree of verbal–nonverbal discrepancy may depend on overall IQ, but the literature on the nature of this relationship is mixed. In one study of preschool and school-age children, the profile was less prominent in preschoolers with greater overall cognitive impairments (Joseph, Tager-Flusberg, & Lord, 2002). In contrast, in a large study of toddlers within a narrow age range and averaging 22 months, a verbal–nonverbal discrepancy was seen more often in subgroups of toddlers with lower overall IQs than in those with higher IQs (Kim et al., 2015). A similar pattern of greater cross-domain discrepancy in lower-IQ compared to higher-IQ preschoolers was reported (Torras-Maña, Gómez-Morales, González-Gimeno, Fornieles-Deu, & Brun-Gasca, 2016), with longer persistence of this pattern into the school years compared with children possessing IQs > 80 (Mayes & Calhoun, 2003). Subgroups of toddlers with a more substantial verbal–nonverbal split continued to lag behind their more able peers a year later in adaptive communication as well as verbal and nonverbal DQ, though gains were observed in many children (Kim et al., 2015).

Executive Function

Executive function (EF) is the mechanism that coordinates and integrates the processes of several neural systems in the service of regulating and controlling behavior. Like the temperament construct EC, it denotes the deliberate control of attention and behavior. Various component cognitive processes are considered part of this executive system, including inhibition, working memory, and set shifting (Weibe et al., 2011; Garon, Bryson, & Smith,

2008; Best & Miller, 2010). Although they are historically grounded in different literatures, the constructs of EF and EC overlap greatly and are related to self-regulation (Zhou, Chen, & Main, 2012). Because of their separate origins, each is aligned with different methods of measurement: effortful control is primarily ascertained using a parent report such as the Rothbart temperament scales (Early Childhood Behavior Questionnaire; Putnam et al., 2006; Childhood Behavior Questionnaire; Rothbart, Ahadi, Hershey, & Fisher, 2001), and executive functions are more commonly assessed via lab-based tasks such as those measuring working memory, inhibition, rule learning, and set shifting. Because the prefrontal cortex mediates executive functions, these abilities show a protracted developmental trajectory in childhood, beginning in late infancy with notable skill acquisition during the preschool period, and continued development into early adulthood.

Executive dysfunction in individuals with ASD has been widely investigated, with evidence of several areas of impairment in school-age children, adolescents, and adults with ASD, including planning, flexibility, working memory, and response inhibition (for reviews, see Hill, 2004; Kenworthy, Yerys, Anthony, & Wallace, 2008; O'Hearn, Asato, Ordaz, & Luna, 2008). However, studies suggest that although specific EF deficits exist in preschool-age children with ASD at around the age of 5 years (McEvoy, Rogers, & Pennington, 1993; Dawson, Meltzoff, Osterling, & Rinaldi, 1998), cohorts of children with ASD at 3 and 4 years of age do not demonstrate such impairments. When matched with DD and TD controls on mental age, young children with ASD did not differ across a variety of executive functioning tasks, including traditional task A-not-B that taps into both inhibitory control and working memory, as well as cognitive flexibility tasks such as Spatial Reversal (Dawson et al., 2002; Yerys, Hepburn, Pennington, & Rogers, 2007). At age 4, children with ASD either match or outperform their DD and TD peers on a range of lab-based EF tasks (Griffith, Pennington, Wehner, & Rogers, 1999), although variability in task implementation and metrics as well as matching procedures may play a role in these results.

Studies of the emergence of executive functioning in high-risk populations are few. St. John and colleagues (2016) examined executive functioning, measured by the A-not-B paradigm in a cohort of high-risk siblings at 12 and 24 months of age as compared to low-risk controls, identifying vulnerabilities in both the working memory and response inhibition components of the task in the high-risk cohort (with and without ASD) at 24 months but not at 12 months. Findings indicate slower development of both working memory and inhibition in infants at high risk for ASD, with both affected and unaffected siblings performing comparably. Such a pattern of results may be suggestive of early EF vulnerabilities as an endophenotype.

EF task performance observed in a lab setting, though providing the methodological advantage of being standardized, may not necessarily index the application of such skills in everyday life. In other words, the ecological validity of lab-based EF tasks has been called into question (Liss et al., 2001). One approach that may better approximate the use of EF in daily life is eliciting such information from parents via measures such as the BRIEF (Behavioral Rating Inventory of Executive Functioning; Gioia, Isquith, Guy, & Kenworthy, 2000).

As the social demands of daily life involve organizing "a stream of constantly evolving information" (Gilotty, Kenworthy, Sirian, Black, & Wagner, 2002, p. 242), it appears likely that social functioning owes much to intact EF skills such as organizing actions based on prior knowledge, flexibility, inhibitory control, working memory, and so on. The links between "everyday" EF measured by the BRIEF and social skills and impairments have been examined in a small number of studies of youth with ASD (Gilotty et al., 2002; Leung, Vogan, Powell, Anagnostou, & Taylor, 2016). Gilotty and colleagues reported strong negative correlations between the Vineland Adaptive Behavior Scales Socialization score and both the Initiation and Working Memory scales of the BRIEF, as well as both composite scores Behavioral Regulation Index (BRI) and Metacognition Index (MI) in youth and adolescents with ASD. Similarly, a recent study by Leung et al. (2016) found that social abilities indexed by the SRS in youth and teens with ASD were strongly related to the composite scores on the BRIEF, and the relationship between metacognitive skills (MI) and social skills was unique to the ASD group, while BRI was related to social ability in both ASDs and control children. As the BRIEF exists only in school-age and preschool versions, it is not clear how adaptive social skills and EF abilities may be related in toddlers.

Language and Communication

Although timing and patterns of language acquisition among young children with ASD vary considerably, concerns in this domain are often the first that parents note (Chawarska, Klin, Paul, & Volkmar, 2007; De Giacomo & Fombonne, 1998; Goin-Kochel & Myers, 2005; Hess & Landa, 2012; Wetherby et al., 2004). For high-risk siblings of children with autism being followed prospectively from birth (see Chawarska et al., Chapter 5, this volume), concerns about language and communication arise as early as 9–12 months (Sacrey et al., 2015; Ozonoff et al., 2009). During this stage of infancy, a variety of precursors to spoken language are emerging in typically developing infants, followed rapidly by progressively more sophisticated communication and comprehension abilities that provide the foundation for later language acquisition. Efforts to discover early behavioral markers of ASD have resulted in the investigation of preverbal and nonverbal communication in toddlers with ASD. Prelinguistic vocalizations, including whining and crying, preverbal sounds such as vocal play and babbling, and nonverbal communication including deictic (e.g., pointing, showing) and conventional (e.g., waving "bye," nodding head "yes") gestures have all been reported to be atypical in young children developing ASD.

Vocalizations

Among the findings in this area is that very young children with ASD express fewer vocalizations (Plumb & Wetherby, 2013), exhibit atypical cries (i.e., higher fundamental frequency, atypical pause length; English, Tenenbaum, Levine, Lester, & Sheinkopf, 2019; Esposito & Venuti, 2010; Esposito, Nakazawa, Venuti, & Bornstein, 2013), and have a low rate of canonical babbling (Patten et al., 2014) compared to their peers. As in older children with ASD, toddlers exhibit atypical suprasegmental features of speech, including phonation (Sheinkopf, Mundy, Oller, & Steffins, 2000), intonation (Schoen, Paul, & Chawarska, 2011), pitch (Schoen et al., 2011; Santos et al., 2013), and formant (Santos et al., 2013). Furthermore, many infants later diagnosed with ASD show early impairments in comprehension of speech, beginning with a reduction in response to their names compared to low-risk peers by 9–12 months of age (Nadig et al., 2007; Miller et al., 2017) and continuing receptive language deficits into toddlerhood (Luyster, Kadlec, Carter, & Tager-Flusberg, 2008).

Gestures

Atypical development of nonverbal communication such as gesture has long been recognized as a hallmark of ASD (DSM-5; American Psychiatric Association, 2013). Unlike their peers with delays in language, young children with ASD do not appear to compensate for their lagging expressive abilities with gestures. In several studies, toddlers with ASD produced fewer deictic gestures such as pointing, showing, and giving compared to TD and DD toddlers (Özçalışkan, Adamson, & Dimitrova, 2016; Barbaro & Dissanayake, 2013; Clifford, Young, & Williamson, 2007; Li et al., 2011; Shumway & Wetherby, 2009; Werner & Dawson, 2005). Not all studies, however, report differences in such gestures compared to toddlers with other delays (Wetherby et al., 2004; Clifford et al., 2007; Dimitrova, Özçalışkan, & Adamson, 2016). The use of conventional gestures has also been observed significantly less frequently in young children with ASD than in TD and DD controls during play with their mothers (Mastrogiuseppi, Capirci, Cuva, & Venuti, 2015). It is important to note that studies have reported not only a reduced frequency of gestures on average but also a reduced proportion of toddlers with ASD displaying specific gestures in the second year (Barbaro & Dissanayake, 2013).

Differences in the production of gestures are evident from as early as the first year and persist throughout 36 months of age, but across studies, results vary by chronological age and specific communicative functions (for a review, see Manwaring, Stevens, Mowdood, & Lackey, 2018). For example, a gesture such as pointing can be used for imperative purposes ("I want that"), declarative purposes ("look at that"), as well as other purposes. The imperative function of gestural communication appears to be less affected in toddlers with ASD compared to the declarative function, but even this varies with age and specific type of gesture such as reaching or pointing (Clifford et al., 2007; Özçalışkan et al., 2016; Werner & Dawson, 2005). Conclusions about specificity of gesture deficits to ASD compared to toddlers with other delays can depend on all of these factors plus the composition of DD groups and the choice of matching criteria (Manwaring et al., 2018). Early utilization of gestures during the first year facilitates the development of language in typically developing children (Rowe & Goldin-Meadow, 2009; Watt, Wetherby, & Shumway, 2006) and is correlated with concurrent language abilities and later language functioning in children with ASD (Luyster et al., 2008; Gordon & Watson, 2015; Manwaring, Mead, Swineford, & Thurm, 2017) and without ASD (Iverson & Goldin-Meadow, 2005). These associations may not hold over longer periods of follow-up, however (e.g., 9 years; Luyster, Qiu, Lopez, & Lord, 2007b). In terms of developmental sequence of gestures and spoken language, though delayed in ASD, it follows a similar progression as that of TD infants; one notable exception is that pointing often emerges after rather than before first words (Talbott et al., 2018). Similar to TD toddlers, combining gestures with words precedes the expression of two-word utterances in toddlers with ASD. These findings support the use of intervention methods that are guided by principles of typical development (Talbott et al., 2018; see Pizzano and Kasari, Chapter 4, this volume; Green, Chapter 8, this volume).

Rate of Intentional Communication

Long before the emergence of speech, prelinguistic vocalizations, preverbal sounds, and gestures all provide the means to communicate. Intentional communication (IC) involves the deliberate exchange of information between people (Flavell, 1968); it is inherently social in nature and requires a sender and a receiver of a verbal or nonverbal message (MacKay, 1972). During the first year of life, IC occurs through vocalizations (e.g., babbling, vocal utterances) and deictic gestures (e.g., pointing and showing) for a number of communicative functions such as requesting, commenting, protesting, and sharing interest (Crais, Douglas, & Campbell, 2004; Bruner, 1981; Carpenter, Nagell, & Tomasello, 1998). Some of the most striking differences between toddlers with and without ASD involve the rate of intentional communication and the context in which communication occurs. Overall communication rates are lower for toddlers with ASD compared to both TD and DD controls (Wetherby et al., 2004): this is particularly true for communication in which vocalizations or gestures are paired with each other or with eye contact (Shumway & Wetherby, 2009). The majority of communicative acts of young children with autism serve the purpose of behavioral regulation of a partner (Seibert, Hogan, & Mundy, 1982; Wetherby et al., 2004), such as requesting to achieve a desired object or action (Charman et al., 1997), rather than for purposes of sharing attention (Lord, 1995; Wetherby et al., 2004; Shumway & Wetherby, 2009). These differences in profiles of communicative functions distinguish young children with ASD from those with other developmental disorders (Mundy, Sigman, & Kasari, 1990; Lord, 1995; Charman et al., 1997; Wetherby, Prizant, & Hutchinson, 1998; Dawson et al., 2004).

Lexical Development

Expressive language ability has long been known to be an important prognostic indicator of long-term outcomes for individuals with ASD (Lord & Ventner, 1992; see Miller and Ozonoff, Chapter 7, this volume). Recent estimates indicate that approximately 70% of children with ASD acquire spoken language (i.e., the ability to produce more than 20–30 words) (Tager-Flusberg & Kasari, 2013). Despite this growing proportion of verbal children, toddlers with ASD often acquire first words later than their typically developing peers and exhibit weaknesses in receptive and expressive language (Luyster, Lopez, & Lord, 2007a; Ellis Weismer, Lord, & Esler, 2010). Typically developing infants begin producing words at 12 months on average (Fenson et al., 1994), but the mean age at which first words emerge in children with ASD is around the second birthday (Mayo, Chlebowski, Fein, & Eigsti, 2013). Indeed, delayed first words and phrases are the most common primary concern reported by parents of children with ASD (Wetherby et al., 2004).

In typical development, early social-cognitive skills (e.g., joint attention, imitation, gesture use, etc.) are important precursors to the development of vocabulary and other language milestones (Bruner & Sherwood, 1983; Watt et al., 2006). Play, most notably functional and symbolic play, is associated with later language outcome (Ungerer & Sigman, 1984). Similar results have been identified in young children with ASD: joint attention, imitation, and play act as concurrent and longitudinal predictors of language (Carpenter, Pennington, & Rogers, 2002; Charman et al., 2003; Dawson et al., 2004; Kasari, Gulsrud, Freeman, Paparella, & Hellemann, 2012; Mundy, Sigman, Ungerer, & Sherman, 1987; Sigman & McGovern, 2005; Ungerer & Sigman, 1984; Vivanti, Dissanayake, Zierhut, Rogers, & Victorian ASELCC Team, 2013; Yoder & Stone, 2006). Luyster and colleagues (2008) reported that, as observed in TD toddlers, nonverbal cognitive ability and gestures were the strongest correlates of expressive language in a sample of toddlers with ASD. They also documented a predictive relationship between concurrent imitation and expressive language, whereas response to joint attention predicted concurrent receptive language abilities. Furthermore, parent report and direct standardized assessments showed strong agreement, particularly with respect to expressive language (Luyster et al., 2008).

Toddlers with ASD may use a higher proportion of nouns than children with Down syndrome (Tager-Flusberg et al., 1990). Kover and Ellis Weismer (2014) closely examined the lexical characteristics of expressive vocabulary in toddlers with ASD as reported by parents utilizing the extended statistical learning theory of vocabulary delay in late talkers. The specific lexical characteristics examined included neighborhood density (i.e., number of other words in the input that sound like a given word), word frequency, and word length. In typical development, there is evidence that nouns from dense neighborhoods are acquired first, as well as words higher in frequency, and words that are shorter in length (Starkel, Armbruster, & Hogan, 2006). Kover and Ellis Weismer (2014) found that low neighborhood density was the best predictor of vocabulary size for toddlers without ASD, whereas word length may instead play a primary role in vocabulary acquisition for toddlers with ASD.

Receptive–Expressive Language Profiles

A language profile historically considered to characterize very young children with ASD involves lower receptive versus expressive language (Cohen & Volkmar, 1997; Hudry et al., 2010). However, this receptive–expressive language split is only observed when specific developmental measures are utilized, such as the Mullen Scales of Early Learning (Mullen, 1995; Ellis Weismer et al., 2010; Luyster et al., 2008), the MacArthur CDI (Hudry et al., 2010; Luyster et al., 2007a; Charman et al., 2003), or the Preschool Language Scale, Third or Fourth Edition (Hudry et al., 2010; Volden et al., 2011). The split appears to be reversed (i.e., lower expressive than receptive language) when assessments such as the Preschool Language Scale, Fifth Edition (Nevill et al., 2019) or the Vineland Adaptive Behavior Scales (Luyster et al., 2008; Ellis Weismer et al., 2010) are used. In a meta-analysis involving 4,067 children in 74 studies, no significant disparity between receptive and expressive ability was observed, for either younger children (ages 1–5) or older children (ages 6–19) regardless of cognitive ability, developmental level, language skills, or source of language data (parents, clinicians, specific measures; Kwok, Brown, Smyth, & Cardy, 2015). Although this receptive < expressive language profile may be present in some children with ASD when assessing with certain measures, it does not appear to be a universal phenomenon.

Neurological Underpinnings of Atypical Language

Several studies have used functional magnetic resonance imaging (fMRI) during natural sleep to investigate the underlying mechanisms of atypical language development in very young children with ASD. In the first of these studies, brain activation to forward and backward speech was examined in toddlers with ASD who were compared to both a chronological-age-matched group of children and to a younger, mental-age-matched group of children (Redcay & Courchesne, 2008). The toddlers with ASD exhibited both delays and atypical patterns of brain activity compared to the chronological-age-matched controls, with enhanced responses in right frontal regions instead of left frontal regions. When compared to the mental-age-matched children, those with ASD showed reduced activity in left frontal networks, areas known to be involved in speech processing. The enhanced activity in right and medial frontal areas was significantly and positively correlated in the ASD group with receptive language scores. Thus, toddlers with ASD exhibited both a delayed and a deviant pattern of brain response to speech, with greater recruitment of right-hemisphere frontal regions during perception of speech. In line with these initial findings, the same diminished response to speech in the left temporal cortex was reported in a much larger group of toddlers with ASD (Eyler et al., 2012). This occurred once again alongside an enhanced response in the right hemisphere. These differences in lateralization of language-related areas were most pronounced in the oldest children in the sample (3- to 4-year-olds). In contrast, typically developing children showed expected left-lateralized activation, which was stable with age.

Extending this work, Lombardo and colleagues (2015) investigated brain activation in the same cohort of toddlers with respect to their later language outcomes. Children with average ("good") language outcomes, defined by average Mullen Verbal scores at ages 3–4, were more likely to display patterns of cortical response to speech stimulation in the second year that were similar to that of their TD and language-delayed peers, including superior temporal regions. In contrast, those with below-average ("poor") language scores on the Mullen at early preschool age exhibited very little activation in these speech-related areas in toddlerhood.

Synchronization between areas involved in language processing is another area of investigation, with weaker interhemispheric synchronization in the inferior frontal gyrus (IFG) and superior temporal gyrus (STG) in toddlers with ASD in comparison to TD and language-delayed toddlers (Dinstein et al., 2011). The strength of IFG synchronization was positively correlated with language abilities and negatively related to autism severity in the ASD group. Taken together, these results are suggestive of a possible underlying mechanism for atypical language development that is specific to young children with ASD.

ASD affects language development on multiple levels. Although poor vocal production is one of the most common presenting symptoms of toddlers who will be diagnosed with ASD, many more aspects of language as well as communication are impacted. Quality of vocalizations and cries, sensitivity to and comprehension of speech, and production of gestures are all diminished or atypical in various ways. Whether these features differ from children with other developmental and language delays depends heavily on several factors including the composition of the comparison groups, matching criteria, age, and consideration of the specific type of function of given communicative acts. Lexical development appears to proceed on a delayed schedule in young children with ASD and, in some respects, in an atypical fashion. The long-standing view that receptive language level is lower than expressive language in children with ASD may be measure-dependent and does not necessarily hold for all children on the spectrum. Neuroimaging studies are beginning to illuminate potential mechanisms of language impairments in ASD, with reported differences in lateralization of speech processing and weaker interhemispheric synchronization in putative cortical language areas during sleep. Furthermore, these studies underscore the importance of stratification by later language ability level.

Adaptive Functioning

Adaptive behavior is defined as the application of abilities that foster personal independence and social sufficiency (Cicchetti & Sparrow, 1990). Compared with ability-matched or IQ-matched controls, children with autism have historically been found to function at an overall lower level of adaptive behavior (Lord & Schopler, 1989). However, recent research has shown that the profile of adaptive skills can vary by IQ in that children with intact cognition tend to show significant delays in adaptive behavior compared to their cognitive abilities and age, whereas children with cognitive impairment tend to have adaptive skills that are on par with or exceed their mental age (Fenton et al., 2003; Perry, Flanagan, Geier, & Freeman, 2009; Kanne et al., 2011). Moreover, the gap between cognitive and adaptive skills has been found to be larger in older versus younger individuals without cognitive impairment (e.g., Klin et al., 2007; Kanne et al., 2011). Research on older children, adolescents, and adults with ASD has shown that specific deficits in adaptive socialization skills surpass impairments in other adaptive areas (Volkmar, Carter, Sparrow, & Cicchetti, 1993). However, research on toddlers with ASD varies as to what type of adaptive skills are most significantly delayed during these very young ages. For instance, one study on 2-year-old toddlers with ASD found below-average scores on the Communication, Socialization, and Daily Living Skills domains of the Vineland Adaptive Behavior Scales, Second Edition, but the Communication domain was found to be the lowest overall score (Ray-Subramanian, Huai, & Weismer, 2011). Another study comparing toddlers with ASD to chronological age- and verbal/nonverbal age-matched controls with developmental delays found lower scores in the ASD group in the Socialization and Receptive Communication domains only (Ventola, Saulnier, Steinberg, Chawarska, & Klin, 2014), whereas in yet another study, adaptive delays were only evident in the Receptive Communication and Daily Living Skills domains (Paul, Loomis, & Chawarska, 2014).

The gap between higher cognitive and lower adaptive skills has also been observed in preschool-age children (e.g., Stone, Ousley, Hepburn, Hogan, & Brown, 1999; Ventola et al., 2014; Paul et al., 2014), but until recently it has been unclear as to how early this gap emerges. In a sample of high-risk toddlers who developed ASD, Vineland Socialization scores were lower compared to DD peers at 12, 18, and 24 months, and discrepancies were already observed between cognitive abilities and adaptive socialization skills by the second year of life (Saulnier, Caravella, Klin, & Chawarska, 2013). In a study following infants at high and low risk for ASD, Estes and colleagues (2015) found significantly lower adaptive motor skills in infants later diagnosed with ASD compared to low-risk infants as early as 6 months of age, but they did not observe a gap between cognitive and adaptive skills until 24 months. Salomone and colleagues (2018) followed high-risk infants with and without ASD from 7 months to 7 years and found a similar emerging gap between cognitive and adaptive socialization skills in the ASD sample that began by age 2, and a significant lag in adaptive daily living skills was evident by age 7. In a more recent longitudinal study following high- and low-risk infants, the gap between nonverbal cognition and adaptive socialization and daily living skills was observed to increase between 12 and 36 months in both high-risk toddlers who were diagnosed with ASD at outcome and in those with the broader autism phenotype, or autism symptomatology falling below a diagnostic threshold (Bradshaw, Gillespie, Klaiman, Klin, & Saulnier, 2019. This suggests that the mere presence of autism symptoms was associated with derailment in adaptive development early on.

When individual items of the Vineland Socialization domain were examined, the behaviors differentiating toddlers with ASD from age- and verbal/nonverbal ability-matched toddlers with non-ASD developmental delays were nearly exclusively social abilities that emerge in the first several months of life in typical infants (Ventola et al., 2014). However, these findings were by retrospective report and not prospectively observed and assessed, leaving open the question as to whether these skills are acquired and then lost or whether they are never fully developed.

The lag between adaptive skills and overall cognitive ability in ASD suggests that, even as early as toddlerhood, children have the capacity to acquire a large repertoire of conceptual skills but fall behind in translating these skills to real-life contexts. Although they often continue to acquire conceptual skills throughout childhood and beyond, their adaptive development does not keep pace. Consequently, evidence increasingly suggests that adaptive deficits are strongly associated with poor adolescent and adult outcome, even when cognition and language are intact (e.g., Howlin, Goode, Hutton, & Rutter, 2004; Howlin, Moss, Savage, & Rutter, 2013; Howlin, Savage, Moss, Tempier, & Rutter, 2014; Farley et al., 2009; Meyer, Powell, Butera, Klinger, & Klinger, 2018). This calls for direct and intensive intervention targeting adaptive skills acquisition and application from diagnosis throughout the lifespan, as it cannot be assumed that individuals with and at risk for ASD will naturally and independently apply a behavior in their repertoire when life demands it.

Summary and Conclusions

With a growing number of studies focusing on characteristics beyond the core features of the syndrome, the picture of more general psychological development of young children with ASD is beginning to come into sharper focus. The topic of emotions in toddlers with ASD, including attachment, temperament, and emotional expressivity, has been of greater interest in recent years, perhaps owing to the recognition of emotion's central role in many aspects of daily life and its relevance to later comorbidities that affect a large proportion of older children with the disorder. As the Interagency Autism Coordinating Committee (IACC, 2017) has designated research on co-occurring mental health conditions as among its priorities, covering them in two separate objectives, this increased inquiry is timely. Research on early verbal ability in toddlers with ASD has continued to focus on gestures, early vocal expression, rates of communication, and lexical development, with an emphasis on fine-grained consideration of specific behaviors and specific communicative functions. Adaptive behavior has been another area of interest in which researchers have devoted more attention to more specific subdomains, profiles across domains, and younger children.

In recent years, the field has expanded its focus from core features of autism to investigate broader issues in the psychological development of very young children with ASD. The studies reviewed here show a burgeoning interest in dimensions that shed light on noncore facets of the ASD phenotype, which are potentially relevant to the heterogeneity of syndrome expression. Even during the earliest stages of the disorder, heterogeneity is evident along a number of dimensions. Although a recent study (Chaste et al., 2015) demonstrated that reducing phenotypic heterogeneity based on clinical features only modestly improved genetic homogeneity, the pursuit of subgrouping individuals based on variables beyond clinical assessment scores may yet aid in identifying more uniform groups of children for the purposes of stratification biomarker identification (Loth et al., 2017; McPartland, 2016), critical to predicting an individual's response to a specific type of treatment. Evaluation of these associated features may also provide insight into the likelihood of future affective and behavioral difficulties and the comorbid disorders that affect many older children, adolescents, and adults with autism.

ACKNOWLEDGMENTS

We gratefully acknowledge the support of the National Institute of Child Health and Human Development (Grant P01 HD003008), the National Institute of Mental Health (Grants U54 MH066594, P50 MH081756, P50 MH115716, R01 MH111652, R01 MH100182, DOD W81XWH-12-ARP-IDA, R01 MH087554, R21 MH102572, R21 MH103550, R03 MH092617, R03 MH086732, and R03 MH092618), the FAR Fund, the V & L Marx Foundation, the Yale Child Study Center Junior Faculty Fund, and the Associates of the Child Study Center. We thank Kohrissa Joseph, Nicole Powell, and Chaela Nutor for their assistance in the preparation of this chapter.

REFERENCES

Adamek, L., Nichols, S., Tetenbaum, S. P., Bregman, J., Ponzio, C. A., & Carr, E. G. (2011). Individual temperament and problem behavior in children with autism spectrum disorders. *Focus on Autism and Other Developmental Disabilities, 26*(3), 173–183.

Ainsworth, M. D. S., & Bell, S. M. (1970). Attachment, exploration, and separation— illustrated by behavior of one-year-olds in a Strange Situation. *Child Development, 41,* 49–67.

Ainsworth, M. D. S., Blehar, M. C., Waters, E., & Wall, S. (1978). *Patterns of attachment: A psychological study of the Strange Situation.* New York: Routledge.

American Psychiatric Association. (2013). *Diagnostic and statistical manual of mental disorders* (5th ed.). Arlington, VA: Author.

Anderson, D. K., Lord, C., Risi, S., DiLavore, P. S., Shulman, C., Thurm, A., . . . Pickles, A. (2007). Patterns of growth in verbal abilities among children with autism spectrum disorder. *Journal of Consulting and Clinical Psychology, 75*(4), 594.

Bakermans-Kranenburg, M. J., van IJzendoorn, M. H., & Juffer, F. (2003). Less is more: Meta-analyses of sensitivity and attachment interventions in early childhood. *Psychological Bulletin, 129*(2), 195–215.

Barbaro, J., & Dissanayake, C. (2012). Developmental profiles of infants and toddlers with autism spectrum disorders identified prospectively in a community-based setting. *Journal of Autism and Developmental Disorders, 42*(9), 1939–1948.

Barbaro, J., & Dissanayake, C. (2013). Early markers of autism spectrum disorders in infants and toddlers prospectively identified in the Social Attention and Communication Study. *Autism, 17*(1), 64–86.

Best, J. R., & Miller, P. H. (2010). A developmental perspective on executive function. *Child Development, 81,* 1641–1660.

Booth-LaForce, C., & Oxford, M. L. (2008). Trajectories of social withdrawal from grades 1 to 6: Prediction from early parenting, attachment, and temperament. *Developmental Psychology, 44*(5), 1298.

Bradshaw, J., Gillespie, S., Klaiman, C., Klin, A., & Saulnier, C. (2019). Early emergence of discrepancy in adaptive behavior and cognitive skills in toddlers with autism spectrum disorder. *Autism, 23*(6), 1485–1496.

Bruner, J. (1981). The social context of language acquisition. *Language and Communication, 1,* 155–178.

Bruner, J., & Sherwood, V. (1983). Thought, language and intersection in infancy. In J. D. Call, E. Galenson, & R. L. Tyson (Eds.), *Frontiers of infant psychiatry* (pp. 38–52). New York: Basic Books.

Bryson, S. E., Zwaigenbaum, L., Brian, J., Roberts, W., Szatmari, P., Rombough, V., & McDermott, C. (2007). A prospective case series of high-risk infants who developed autism. *Journal of Autism and Developmental Disorders, 37*(1), 12–24.

Campbell, D., Shic, F., Macari, S., & Chawarska, K. (2014). Gaze patterns in response to dyadic bids at 2 years predict functioning at 3 years in autism spectrum disorders: A subtyping analysis. *Journal of Autism and Developmental Disorders, 44*(2), 431–442.

Capps, L., Sigman, M., & Mundy, P. (1994). Attachment security in children with autism. *Development and Psychopathology, 6*(2), 249–261.

Carpenter, M., Nagell, K., & Tomasello, M. (1998). Social cognition, joint attention, and communicative competence from 9 to 15 months of age. *Monographs of the Society for Research in Child Development, 63*(4, Serial No. 255), i–174.

Carpenter, M., Pennington, B., & Rogers, S. (2002). Interrelations among social-cognitive skills in young children with autism. *Journal of Autism and Developmental Disorders, 32,* 91–106.

Caspi, A., Henry, B., McGee, R. O., Moffitt, T. E., & Silva, P. A. (1995). Temperamental origins of child and adolescent behavior problems: From age three to age fifteen. *Child Development, 66*(1), 55–68.

Charman, T., Baron-Cohen, S., Swettenham, J., Baird, G., Drew, A., & Cox, A. (2003). Predicting language outcome in infants with autism and pervasive developmental disorder. *International Journal of Language and Communication Disorders, 38*(3), 265–285.

Charman, T., Swettenham, J., Baron-Cohen, S., Cox, A., Baird, G., & Drew, A. (1997). Infants with autism: An investigation of empathy, pretend play, joint attention, and imitation. *Developmental Psychology, 33,* 781–789.

Chaste, P., Klei, L., Sanders, S. J., Hus, V., Murtha, M. T., Lowe, J. K., . . . Geschwind, D. (2015). A genome-wide association study of autism using the Simons Simplex Collection: Does reducing phenotypic heterogeneity in autism increase genetic homogeneity? *Biological Psychiatry, 77*(9), 775–784.

Chawarska, K., Klin, A., Paul, R., Macari, S., & Volkmar, F. (2009). A prospective study of toddlers with ASD: Short-term diagnostic and cognitive outcomes. *Journal of Child Psychology and Psychiatry, 50*(10), 1235–1245.

Chawarska, K., Klin, A., Paul, R., & Volkmar, F. (2007). Autism spectrum disorder in the second year: Stability and change in syndrome expression. *Journal of Child Psychology and Psychiatry, 48*(2), 128–138.

Chawarska, K., Macari, S., & Shic, F. (2012). Context modulates attention to social scenes in toddlers with autism. *Journal of Child Psychology and Psychiatry, 53*(8), 903–913.

Chawarska, K., Macari, S., & Shic, F. (2013). Decreased spontaneous attention to social scenes in 6-month-old infants later diagnosed with autism spectrum disorders. *Biological Psychiatry, 74*(3), 195–203.

Chess, S., Thomas, A., Rutter, M., & Birch, H. G. (1963). Interaction of temperament and environment in the production of behavioral disturbances in children. *American Journal of Psychiatry, 120*(2), 142–148.

Chevallier, C., Kohls, G., Troiani, V., Brodkin, E. S., & Schultz, R. T. (2012). The social motivation theory of autism. *Trends in Cognitive Sciences, 16*(4), 231–239.

Christensen, D. L., Bilder, D. A., Zahorodny, W., Pettygrove, S., Durkin, M. S., Fitzgerald, R. T., & Yeargin-Allsopp, M. (2016). Prevalence and characteristics of autism spectrum disorder among 4-year-old children in the autism and developmental disabilities monitoring network. *Journal of Developmental and Behavioral Pediatrics, 37*(1), 1–8.

Cicchetti, D. V., & Sparrow, S. S. (1990). Assessment of adaptive behavior in young children. In J. H. Johnson & J. Goldman (Eds.), *Developmental assessment in clinical child psychology: A handbook* (Vol. 163, pp. 173–196). New York: Pergamon Press.

Clifford, S. M., Hudry, K., Elsabbagh, M., Charman, T., & Johnson, M. H. (2013). Temperament in the first 2 years of life in infants at high-risk for autism spectrum disorders. *Journal of Autism and Developmental Disorders, 43*(3), 673–686.

Clifford, S., Young, R., & Williamson, P. (2007). Assessing the early characteristics of autistic disorder using video analysis. *Journal of Autism and Developmental Disorders, 37*(2), 301–313.

Cohen, D., & Volkmar, F. (1997). Autism and pervasive developmental disorders. *Child and Adolescent Psychiatry, 10*(4), 282–285.

Crais, E., Douglas, D., & Campbell, C. (2004). The intersection of the development of gestures and intentionality. *Journal of Speech, Language, and Hearing Research, 47,* 678–694.

Dawson, G., Meltzoff, A. N., Osterling, J., & Rinaldi, J. (1998). Neuropsychological correlates of early symptoms of autism. *Child Development, 69*(5), 1276–1285.

Dawson, G., Toth, K., Abbott, R., Osterling, J., Munson, J., Estes, A., & Liaw, J. (2004). Early social attention impairments in autism: Social orienting, joint attention, and attention to distress. *Developmental Psychology, 40,* 271–283.

Dawson, G., Webb, S., Schellenberg, G. D., Dager, S., Friedman, S., Aylward, E., & Richards, T. (2002). Defining the broader phenotype of autism: Genetic, brain, and behavioral perspectives. *Development and Psychopathology, 14*(3), 581–611.

De Giacomo, A., & Fombonne, E. (1998). Parental recognition of developmental abnormalities in autism. *European Child and Adolescent Psychiatry, 7*(3), 131–136.

del Rosario, M. D., Gillespie-Lynch, K., Johnson, S., Sigman, M., & Hutman, T. (2013). Parent-reported temperament trajectories among infant siblings of children with autism. *Journal of Autism and Developmental Disorders, 44*(2), 381–393.

Delehanty, A. D., Stronach, S., Guthrie, W., Slate, E., & Wetherby, A. M. (2018). Verbal and nonverbal outcomes of toddlers with and without autism spectrum disorder, language delay, and global developmental delay. *Autism and Developmental Language Impairments, 3,* 1–19.

Dimitrova, N., Özçalışkan, Ş., & Adamson, L. B. (2016). Parents' translations of child gesture facilitate word learning in children with autism, Down syndrome and typical development. *Journal of Autism and Developmental Disorders, 46*(1), 221–231.

Dinstein, I., Pierce, K., Eyler, L., Solso, S., Malach, R., Behrmann, M., & Courchesne, E. (2011). Disrupted neural synchronization in toddlers with autism. *Neuron, 70*(6), 1218–1225.

Dissanayake, C., & Crossley, S. A. (1996). Proximity and sociable behaviours in autism: Evidence for attachment. *Journal of Child Psychology and Psychiatry, 37*(2), 149–156.

Elis Weismer, S., Lord, C., & Esler, A. (2010). Early language patterns of toddlers on the autism spectrum compared to toddlers with developmental delay. *Journal of Autism and Developmental Disorders, 40,* 1259–1273.

Elison, J. T., Wolff, J. J., Heimer, D. C., Paterson, S. J., Gu, H., Hazlett, H. C., . . . IBIS Network. (2013). Frontolimbic neural circuitry at 6 months predicts individual differences in joint attention at 9 months. *Developmental Science, 16*(2), 186–197.

Emde, R. N., Gaensbauer, T., & Harmon, R. J. (1981). Using our emotions: Some principles for appraising emotional development and intervention. In *Developmental disabilities* (pp. 409–424). Dordrecht, the Netherlands: Springer.

English, M. S., Tenenbaum, E. J., Levine, T. P., Lester, B. M., & Sheinkopf, S. J. (2019). Perception of cry characteristics in 1-month-old infants later diagnosed with autism spectrum disorder. *Journal of Autism and Developmental Disorders, 49*(3), 834–844.

Esposito, G., Nakazawa, J., Venuti, P., & Bornstein, M. H. (2013). Componential deconstruction of infant distress vocalizations via tree-based models: A study of cry in autism spectrum disorder and typical development. *Research in Developmental Disabilities, 34*(9), 2717–2724.

Esposito, G., & Venuti, P. (2010). Developmental changes in the fundamental frequency (f0) of infants' cries: A study of children with autism spectrum disorder. *Early Child Development and Care, 180*(8), 1093–1102.

Estes, A., Zwaigenbaum, L., Gu, H., John, T. S., Paterson, S., Elison, J. T., . . . Kostopoulos, P. (2015). Behavioral, cognitive, and adaptive development in infants with autism spectrum disorder in the first 2 years of life. *Journal of Neurodevelopmental Disorders, 7*(1), 24.

Eyler, L. T., Pierce, K., & Courchesne, E. (2012). A failure of left temporal cortex to specialize for language is an early emerging and fundamental property of autism. *Brain, 135*(3), 949–960.

Farley, M. A., McMahon, W. M., Fombonne, E., Jenson, W. R., Miller, J., Gardner, M., . . . Coon, H. (2009). Twenty-year outcome for individuals with autism and average or near-average cognitive abilities. *Autism Research, 2*(2), 109–118.

Fenson, L., Dale, P. S., Reznick, J. S., Bates, E., Thal, D. J., Pethick, S. J., . . . Stiles, J. (1994). Variability in early communicative development. *Monographs of the Society for Research in Child Development, 59,* 1–185.

Fenton, G., D'ardia, C., Valente, D., Del Vecchio, I., Fabrizi, A., & Bernabei, P. (2003). Vineland Adaptive Behavior Profiles in children with autism and moderate to severe developmental delay. *Autism, 7*(3), 269–287.

Filliter, J. H., Longard, J., Lawrence, M. A., Zwaigenbaum, L., Brian, J., Garon, N., . . . Bryson, S. E. (2015). Positive affect in infant siblings of children diagnosed with autism spectrum disorder. *Journal of Abnormal Child Psychology, 43*(3), 567–575.

Flavell, J. H. (1968). *The development of role-taking and communication skills in children.* Oxford, UK: Wiley.

Garon, N., Bryson, S. E., & Smith, I. M. (2008). Executive function in preschoolers: A review using an integrative framework. *Psychological Bulletin, 134*(1), 31–60.

Garon, N., Bryson, S. E., Zwaigenbaum, L., Smith, I. M., Brian, J., Roberts, W., & Szatmari, P. (2009). Temperament and its relationship to autistic symptoms in a high-risk infant sib cohort. *Journal of Abnormal Child Psychology, 37*(1), 59–78.

Garon, N., Zwaigenbaum, L., Bryson, S., Smith, I. M., Brian, J., Roncadin, C., . . . Roberts, W. (2016). Temperament and its association with autism symptoms in a high-risk population. *Journal of Abnormal Child Psychology, 44*(4), 757–769.

Gilotty, L., Kenworthy, L., Sirian, L., Black, D. O., & Wagner, A. E. (2002). Adaptive skills and executive function in autism spectrum disorders. *Child Neuropsychology, 8*(4), 241–248.

Gioia, G. A., Isquith, P. K., Guy, S. C., & Kenworthy, L. (2000). Test review behavior rating inventory of executive function. *Child Neuropsychology, 6*(3), 235–238.

Goin-Kochel, R. P., & Myers, B. J. (2005). Parental report of early autistic symptoms: Differences in ages of detection and frequencies of characteristics among three autism-spectrum disorders. *Journal on Developmental Disabilities, 11*(2), 21–39.

Goldsmith, H. H., Buss, A. H., Plomin, R., Rothbart, M. K., Thomas, A., Chess, S., . . . McCall, R. B. (1987). Roundtable: What is temperament?: Four approaches. *Child Development, 58*(2), 505–529.

Goldsmith, H. H., & Campos, J. J. (1982). Toward a theory of infant temperament. In *The development of attachment and affiliative systems* (pp. 161–193). Boston: Springer.

Goldsmith, H. H., & Rothbart, M. K. (1999). The laboratory temperament assessment battery. *Locomotor Version, 3.1.*

Gordon, R., & Watson, L. (2015). Brief report: Gestures in children at risk for autism spectrum disorders. *Journal of Autism and Developmental Disorders, 45,* 2267–2273.

Griffith, E. M., Pennington, B. F., Wehner, E. A., & Rogers, S. J. (1999). Executive functions in young children with autism. *Child Development, 70*(4), 817–832.

Grzadzinski, R. L., Luyster, R., Spencer, A. G., & Lord, C. (2014). Attachment in young children with autism spectrum disorders: An examination of separation and reunion behaviors with both mothers and fathers. *Autism, 18*(2), 85–96.

Hazlett, H. C., Gu, H., Munsell, B. C., Kim, S. H., Styner, M., Wolff, J. J., . . . Statistical Analysis (2017). Early brain development in infants at high risk for autism spectrum disorder. *Nature, 542*(7641), 348–351.

Hendry, A., Jones, E. J., Bedford, R., Gliga, T., Charman, T., & Johnson, M. H. (2018). Developmental change in look durations predicts later effortful control in toddlers at familial risk for ASD. *Journal of Neurodevelopmental Disorders, 10*(1), 3.

Hess, C. R., & Landa, R. J. (2012). Predictive and concurrent validity of parent concern about young children at risk for autism. *Journal of Autism and Developmental Disorders, 42*(4), 575–584.

Hill, E. L. (2004). Executive dysfunction in autism. *Trends in Cognitive Sciences, 8*(1), 26–32.

Hobson, R. P. (2019). *Autism and the development of mind.* New York: Routledge.

Howlin, P., Goode, S., Hutton, J., & Rutter, M. (2004). Adult outcome for children with autism. *Journal of Child Psychology and Psychiatry, 45*(2), 212–229.

Howlin, P., Moss, P., Savage, S., & Rutter, M. (2013). Social outcomes in mid- to later adulthood among individuals diagnosed with autism and average nonverbal IQ as children. *Journal of the American Academy of Child and Adolescent Psychiatry, 52*(6), 572–581.

Howlin, P., Savage, S., Moss, P., Tempier, A., & Rutter, M. (2014). Cognitive and language skills in adults with autism: A 40-year follow-up. *Journal of Child Psychology and Psychiatry, 55*(1), 49–58.

Hudry, K., Leadbitter, K., Temple, K., Slonims, V., McConachie, H., Aldred, C., . . . Pact Consortium. (2010). Preschoolers with autism show greater impairment in receptive compared with expressive language abilities. *International Journal of Language and Communication Disorders, 45*(6), 681–690.

Interagency Autism Coordinating Committee (IACC). (2017). 2016–2017 Interagency Autism Coordinating Committee Strategic Plan for Autism Spectrum Disorder. Retrieved from the author at *https://iacc.hhs.gov/publications/strategic-plan/2017.*

Iverson, J., & Goldin-Meadow, S. (2005). Gesture paves the way for language development. *Psychological Science, 16,* 367–371.

Izard, C. E., Fine, S., Mostow, A., Trentacosta, C., & Campbell, J. (2002). Emotion processes in normal and abnormal development and preventive intervention. *Development and Psychopathology, 14*(4), 761–787.

Jahromi, L. B., Meek, S. E., & Ober-Reynolds, S. (2012). Emotion regulation in the context of frustration in children with high functioning autism and their typical peers. *Journal of Child Psychology and Psychiatry, 53*(12), 1250–1258.

Johnson, M. H. (2001). Functional brain development in humans. *Nature Reviews Neuroscience, 2*(7), 475.

Jones, E. J., Venema, K., Earl, R., Lowy, R., Barnes, K., Estes, A., . . . Webb, S. J. (2016). Reduced engagement with social stimuli in 6-month-old infants with later autism spectrum disorder: A longitudinal prospective study of infants at high familial risk. *Journal of Neurodevelopmental Disorders, 8*(1), 7.

Jones, W., & Klin, A. (2013). Attention to eyes is present but in decline in 2–6-month-old infants later diagnosed with autism. *Nature, 504*(7480), 427–431.

Joseph, R. M., & Tager-Flusberg, H. (1997). An investigation of attention and affect in children with autism and Down syndrome. *Journal of Autism and Developmental Disorders, 27*(4), 385–396.

Joseph, R. M., Tager-Flusberg, H., & Lord, C. (2002). Cognitive profiles and social-communicative functioning in children with autism spectrum disorder. *Journal of Child Psychology and Psychiatry, 43*(6), 807–821.

Kanne, S. M., Gerber, A. J., Quirmbach, L. M., Sparrow, S. S., Cicchetti, D. V., & Saulnier, C. A. (2011). The role of adaptive behavior in autism spectrum disorders: Implications for functional outcome. *Journal of Autism and Developmental Disorders, 41*(8), 1007–1018.

Kasari, C., Gulsrud, A., Freeman, S., Paparella, T., & Hellemann, G. (2012). Longitudinal follow-up of children with autism receiving targeted interventions on joint attention and play. *Journal of the American Academy of Child and Adolescent Psychiatry, 51*(5), 487–495.

Kasari, C., Sigman, M., Mundy, P., & Yirmiya, N. (1990). Affective sharing in the context of joint attention interactions of normal, autistic, and mentally retarded children. *Journal of Autism and Developmental Disorders, 20*(1), 87–100.

Kenworthy, L., Yerys, B. E., Anthony, L. G., & Wallace, G. L. (2008). Understanding executive control in autism spectrum disorders in the lab and in the real world. *Neuropsychology Review, 18*(4), 320–338.

Kim, S. H., Macari, S., Koller, J., & Chawarska, K. (2015). Examining the phenotypic heterogeneity of early autism spectrum disorder: Subtypes and short-term outcomes. *Journal of Child Psychology and Psychiatry, 57*(1), 93–102.

Klin, A., Saulnier, C. A., Sparrow, S. S., Cicchetti, D. V., Volkmar, F. R., & Lord, C. (2007). Social and communication abilities and disabilities in higher functioning individuals with autism spectrum disorders: The Vineland and the ADOS. *Journal of Autism and Developmental Disorders, 37*(4), 748–759.

Kover, S., & Eliis Weismer, S. (2014). Lexical characteristics of expressive vocabulary in toddlers with autism spectrum disorder. *Journal of Speech, Language, and Hearing Research, 57,* 1428–1441.

Kwok, E. Y., Brown, H. M., Smyth, R. E., & Cardy, J. O. (2015). Meta-analysis of receptive and expressive language skills in autism spectrum disorder. *Research in Autism Spectrum Disorders, 9,* 202–222.

Landa, R., & Garrett-Mayer, E. (2006). Development in infants with autism spectrum disorders: A prospective study. *Journal of Child Psychology and Psychiatry, 47*(6), 629–638.

Leung, R. C., Vogan, V. M., Powell, T. L., Anagnostou, E., & Taylor, M. J. (2016). The role of executive functions in social impairment in autism spectrum disorder. *Child Neuropsychology, 22*(3), 336–344.

Lewis, M. D. (2005). Self-organizing individual differences in brain development. *Developmental Review, 25*(3–4), 252–277.

Li, Y.-M., Jing, J., Jin, Y., Zou, X.-B., Igarashi, K., & Chan, R. C. (2011). Visual attention, emotional and behavioral responses to facial expression in young children with autism. *Psychologia, 54*(3), 156–165.

Liss, M., Fein, D., Allen, D., Dunn, M., Feinstein, C., Morris, R., . . . Rapin, I. (2001). Executive functioning in high-functioning children with autism. *Journal of Child Psychology and Psychiatry and Allied Disciplines, 42*(2), 261–270.

Lombardo, M., Pierce, K., Eyler, L., Carter Barnes, C., Ahrens-Barbeau, C., Solso, S., . . . Courchesne, E. (2015). Different functional neural substrates for good and poor language outcome in autism. *Neuron, 86*(2), 567–577.

Lord, C. (1995). Follow-up of two-year-olds referred for possible autism. *Journal of Child Psychology and Psychiatry, 36*(8), 1365–1382.

Lord, C., Rutter, M., DiLavore, P., Risi, S., Gotham, K., & Bishop, S. (2012). *Autism diagnostic observation schedule, 2nd edition (ADOS-2).* Los Angeles: Western Psychological Corporation.

Lord, C., & Schopler, E. (1989). The role of age at assessment, developmental level, and test in the stability of intelligence scores in young autistic children. *Journal of Autism and Developmental Disorders, 19*(4), 483–499.

Lord, C., & Ventner, A. (1992). Outcome and follow-up studies of high-functioning autistic individuals. In E. Schopler & G. Mesibov (Eds.), *High-functioning individuals with autism* (pp. 187–199). New York: Plenum Press.

Loth, E., Charman, T., Mason, L., Tillmann, J., Jones, E. J., Wooldridge, C., . . . Banaschewski, T. (2017). The EU-AIMS Longitudinal European Autism Project (LEAP): Design and methodologies to identify and validate stratification biomarkers for autism spectrum disorders. *Molecular Autism, 8*(1), 24.

Luyster, R. J., Kadlec, M. B., Carter, A., & Tager-Flusberg, H. (2008). Language assessment and development in toddlers with autism spectrum disorders. *Journal of Autism and Developmental Disorders, 38*(8), 1426–1438.

Luyster, R., Lopez, K., & Lord, C. (2007a). Characterizing communicative development in children referred for autism spectrum disorders using the MacArthur–Bates Communicative Development Inventory (CDI). *Journal of Child Language, 34*(3), 623–654.

Luyster, R., Qiu, S., Lopez, K., & Lord, C. (2007b). Predicting outcomes of children referred for autism using the MacArthur–Bates Communicative Development Inventory. *Journal of Speech, Language, and Hearing Research, 50*, 667–681.

Macari, S. L., Campbell, D., Gengoux, G. W., Saulnier, C. A., Klin, A. J., & Chawarska, K. (2012). Predicting developmental status from 12 to 24 months in infants at risk for autism spectrum disorder: A preliminary report. *Journal of Autism and Developmental Disorders, 42*(12), 2636–2647.

Macari, S., DiNicola, L., Kane-Grade, F., Prince, E., Vernetti, A., Powell, K., . . . Chawarska, K. (2018). Emotional expressivity in toddlers with autism spectrum disorder. *Journal of the American Academy of Child and Adolescent Psychiatry, 57*(11), 828–836.

Macari, S. L., Koller, J., Campbell, D. J., & Chawarska, K. (2017). Temperamental markers in toddlers with autism spectrum disorder. *Journal of Child Psychology and Psychiatry, 58*(7), 819–828.

MacKay, D. M. (1972). Formal analysis of communicative processes. In R. A. Hinde, *Non-verbal communication.* Cambridge, UK: Cambridge University Press.

Main, M., & Solomon, J. (1990). Procedures for identifying infants as disorganized/disoriented during the Ainsworth Strange Situation. *Attachment in the Preschool Years: Theory, Research, and Intervention, 1,* 121–160.

Manwaring, S., Mead, D., Swineford, L., & Thurm, A. (2017). Modeling gesture use and early language development in autism spectrum disorder. *International Journal of Language and Communication Disorder, 52,* 637–651.

Manwaring, S. S., Stevens, A. L., Mowdood, A., & Lackey, M. (2018). A scoping review of deictic gesture use in toddlers with or at-risk for autism spectrum disorder. *Autism and Developmental Language Impairments, 3,* 1–27.

Mastrogiuseppe, M., Capirci, O., Cuva, S., & Venuti, P. (2015). Gestural communication in children with autism spectrum disorders during mother–child interaction. *Autism, 19*(4), 469–481.

Mayes, S. D., & Calhoun, S. L. (2003). Analysis of WISC-III, Stanford–Binet: IV, and academic achievement test scores in children with autism. *Journal of Autism and Developmental Disorders, 33*(3), 329–341.

Mayo, J., Chlebowski, C., Fein, D. A., & Eigsti, I. M. (2013). Age of first words predicts cognitive ability and adaptive skills in children with ASD. *Journal of Autism and Developmental Disorders, 43*(2), 253–264.

McEvoy, R. E., Rogers, S. J., & Pennington, B. F. (1993). Executive function and social communication deficits in young autistic children. *Journal of Child Psychology and Psychiatry, 34*(4), 563–578.

McPartland, J. C. (2016). Considerations in biomarker development for neurodevelopmental disorders. *Current Opinion in Neurology, 29*(2), 118.

Meyer, A. T., Powell, P. S., Butera, N., Klinger, M. R., & Klinger, L. G. (2018). Brief report: Developmental trajectories of adaptive behavior in children and adolescents with ASD. *Journal of Autism and Developmental Disorders, 48*(8), 2870–2878.

Miller, M., Iosif, A. M., Hill, M., Young, G. S., Schwichtenberg, A. J., & Ozonoff, S. (2017). Response to name in infants developing autism spectrum disorder: A prospective study. *Journal of Pediatrics, 183,* 141–146.

Mitchell, S., Brian, J., Zwaigenbaum, L., Roberts, W., Szatmari, P., Smith, I., & Bryson, S. (2006). Early language and communication development of infants later diagnosed with autism spectrum disorder. *Journal of Developmental and Behavioral Pediatrics, 27*(Suppl. 2), S69–S78.

Moles, A., Kieffer, A. L., & D'Amato, F. R. (2004). Deficit in attachment behavior in mice lacking the μ-opioid receptor gene. *Science, 304*(5679), 1983–1986.

Mullen, E. (1995). *Mullen Scales of Early Learning: AGS edition.* Circle Pines, MN: American Guidance Serivce.

Mundy, P., Sigman, M., & Kasari, C. (1990). A longitudinal study of joint attention and language development in autistic children. *Journal of Autism and Developmental Disorders, 20,* 115–128.

Mundy, P., Sigman, M., Ungerer, J., & Sherman, T. (1987). Nonverbal communication and play correlates of language development in autistic children. *Journal of Autism and Developmental Disorders, 17*(3), 349–364.

Naber, F. B., Swinkels, S. H., Buitelaar, J. K., Bakermans-Kranenburg, M. J., van IJzendoorn, M. H., Dietz, C., . . . van Engeland, H. (2007). Attachment in toddlers with autism and other developmental disorders. *Journal of Autism and Developmental Disorders, 37*(6), 1123–1138.

Nadig, A. S., Ozonoff, S., Young, G. S., Rozga, A., Sigman, M., & Rogers, S. J. (2007). A prospective study of response to name in infants at risk for autism. *Archives of Pediatrics and Adolescent Medicine, 161*(4), 378–383.

Nevill, R., Hedley, D., Uljarević, M., Sahin, E., Zadek, J., Butter, E., & Mulick, J. A. (2019). Language profiles in young children with autism spectrum disorder: A community sample using multiple assessment instruments. *Autism, 23*(1), 141–153.

O'Hearn, K., Asato, M., Ordaz, S., & Luna, B. (2008). Neurodevelopment and executive function in autism. *Development and Psychopathology, 20*(4), 1103–1132.

Oppenheim, D., Koren-Karie, N., Dolev, S., & Yirmiya, N. (2012). Maternal sensitivity mediates the link between maternal insightfulness/resolution and child–mother attachment: The case of children with autism spectrum disorder. *Attachment and Human Development, 14*(6), 567–584.

Özçalışkan, Ş, Adamson, L. B., & Dimitrova, N. (2016). Early deictic but not other gestures predict later vocabulary in both typical development and autism. *Autism, 20*(6), 754–763.

Ozonoff, S., Iosif, A. M., Baguio, F., Cook, I. C., Hill, M. M., Hutman, T., . . . Young, G. S. (2010). A prospective study of the emergence of early behavioral signs of autism. *Journal of the American Academy of Child and Adolescent Psychiatry, 49*(3), 256–266.

Ozonoff, S., Young, G. S., Steinfeld, M. B., Hill, M. M., Cook, I., Hutman, T., . . . Sigman, M. (2009). How early do parent concerns predict later autism diagnosis? *Journal of Developmental and Behavioral Pediatrics, 30*(5), 367–375.

Paterson, S. J., Wolff, J. J., Elison, J. T., Winder-Patel, B., Zwaigenbaum, L., Estes, A., . . . Hazlett, H. C. (2019). The importance of temperament for understanding early manifestations of Autism Spectrum Disorder in high-risk infants. *Journal of Autism and Developmental Disorders, 49*(7), 2849–2863.

Patten, E., Belardi, K., Baranek, G. T., Watson, L. R., Labban, J. D., & Oller, D. K. (2014). Vocal patterns in infants with autism spectrum disorder: Canonical babbling status and vocalization frequency. *Journal of Autism and Developmental Disorders, 44*(10), 2413–2428.

Paul, R., Chawarska, K., Cicchetti, D., & Volkmar, F. (2008). Language outcomes of toddlers with autism spectrum disorders: A two year follow-up. *Autism Research, 1*(2), 97–107.

Paul, R., Loomis, R., & Chawarska, K. (2014). Adaptive behavior in toddlers under two with autism spectrum disorders. *Journal of Autism and Developmental Disorders, 44*(2), 264–270.

Pérez-Edgar, K., Reeb-Sutherland, B. C., McDermott, J. M., White, L. K., Henderson, H. A., Degnan, K. A., . . . Fox, N. A. (2011). Attention biases to threat link behavioral inhibition to social withdrawal over time in very young children. *Journal of Abnormal Child Psychology, 39*(6), 885–895.

Perry, A., Flanagan, H. E., Geier, J. D., & Freeman, N. L. (2009). Brief report: The Vineland Adaptive Behavior Scales in young children with autism spectrum disorders at different cognitive levels. *Journal of Autism and Developmental Disorders, 39*(7), 1066–1078.

Plumb, A. M., & Wetherby, A. M. (2013). Vocalization development in toddlers with autism spectrum disorder. *Journal of Speech, Language, and Hearing Research, 56*(2), 721–734.

Putnam, S. P., Gartstein, M. A., & Rothbart, M. K. (2006). Measurement of fine-grained aspects of toddler temperament: The Early Childhood Behavior Questionnaire. *Infant Behavior and Development, 29*(3), 386–401.

Ray-Subramanian, C. E., Huai, N., & Weismer, S. E. (2011). Brief report: Adaptive behavior and cognitive skills for toddlers on the autism spectrum. *Journal of Autism and Developmental Disorders, 41*(5), 679–684.

Redcay, E., & Courchesne, E. (2008). Deviant functional magnetic resonance imaging patterns of brain activity to speech in 2–3-year-old children with autism spectrum disorder. *Biological Psychiatry, 64*(7), 589–598.

Richters, J. E., Waters, E., & Vaughn, B. E. (1988). Empirical classification of infant–mother relationships from interactive behavior and crying during reunion. *Child Development, 59*(2), 512–522.

Rogers, S. J., Ozonoff, S., & Maslin-Cole, C. (1993). Developmental aspects of attachment behavior in young children with pervasive developmental disorders. *Journal of the American Academy of Child and Adolescent Psychiatry, 32*(6), 1274–1282.

Rothbart, M. K., Ahadi, S. A., Hershey, K. L., & Fisher, P. (2001). Investigations of temperament at three to seven years: The Children's Behavior Questionnaire. *Child Development, 72*(5), 1394–1408.

Rothbart, M. K., & Bates, J. E. (1998). Temperament. In W. Damon (Series Ed.) & N. Eisenberg (Vol. Ed.), *Handbook of child psychology: Vol. 3, Social, emotional, and personality development* (5th ed., pp. 105–176). New York: Wiley.

Rothbart, M. K., & Derryberry, D. (1981). Development of individual differences in temperament. In M. E. Lamb & A. L. Brown (Eds.), *Advances in developmental psychology* (Vol. 1, pp. 37–86). Hillsdale, NJ: Erlbaum.

Rowe, M. L., & Goldin-Meadow, S. (2009). Early gesture selectively predicts later language learning. *Developmental Science, 12,* 182–187.

Rozga, A., Hutman, T., Young, G. S., Rogers, S. J., Ozonoff, S., Dapretto, M., & Sigman, M. (2011). Behavioral profiles of affected and unaffected siblings of children with autism: Contribution of measures of mother–infant interaction and nonverbal communication. *Journal of Autism and Developmental Disorders, 41*(3), 287–301.

Rubin, K. H., Burgess, K. B., Dwyer, K. M., & Hastings, P. D. (2003). Predicting preschoolers' externalizing behaviors from toddler temperament, conflict, and maternal negativity. *Developmental Psychology, 39*(1), 164.

Rutgers, A. H., Bakermans-Kranenburg, M. J., van IJzendoorn, M. H., & Berckelaer-Onnes, I. A. (2004). Autism and attachment: A meta-analytic review. *Journal of Child Psychology and Psychiatry, 45*(6), 1123–1134.

Rutgers, A. H., van IJzendoorn, M. H., Bakermans-Kranenburg, M. J., Swinkels, S. H., van Daalen, E., Dietz, C., . . . van Engeland, H. (2007). Autism, attachment and parenting: A comparison of children with autism spectrum disorder, mental retardation, language disorder, and non-clinical children. *Journal of Abnormal Child Psychology, 35*(5), 859–870.

Sacrey, L. A. R., Zwaigenbaum, L., Bryson, S., Brian, J., Smith, I. M., Roberts, W., . . . Vaillancourt, T. (2015). Can parents' concerns predict autism spectrum disorder?: A prospective study of high-risk siblings from 6 to 36 months of age. *Journal of the American Academy of Child and Adolescent Psychiatry, 54*(6), 470–478.

Salley, B., Panneton, R. K., & Colombo, J. (2013). Separable attentional predictors of language outcome. *Infancy, 18*(4), 462–489.

Salomone, E., Shephard, E., Milosavljevic, B., Johnson, M. H., Charman, T., & BASIS Team. (2018). Adaptive behaviour and cognitive skills: Stability and change from 7 months to 7 years in siblings at high familial risk of autism spectrum disorder. *Journal of Autism and Developmental Disorders, 48*(9), 2901–2911.

Sanson, A., Hemphill, S. A., & Smart, D. (2004). Connections between temperament and social development: A review. *Social Development, 13*(1), 142–170.

Santos, J. F., Brosh, N., Falk, T. H., Zwaigenbaum, L., Bryson, S. E., Roberts, W., . . . Brian, J. A. (2013). *Very early detection of autism spectrum disorders based on acoustic analysis of pre-verbal vocalizations of 18-month old toddlers.* Paper presented at the 2013 IEEE International Conference on Acoustics, Speech and Signal Processing.

Saulnier, C. A., Caravella, K. E., Klin, A., & Chawarska, K. (2013). *Differences in adaptive socialization skills in ASD vs. non-ASD developmental delays in the first two years of life.* Paper presented at the International Meeting for Autism Research (IMFAR), Seattle, WA.

Scherr, J. F., Hogan, A. L., Hatton, D., & Roberts, J. E. (2017). Stranger fear and early risk for social anxiety in preschoolers with fragile X syndrome contrasted to autism spectrum disorder. *Journal of Autism and Developmental Disorders, 47*(12), 3741–3755.

Schoen, E., Paul, R., & Chawarska, K. (2011). Phonology and vocal behavior in toddlers with autism spectrum disorders. *Autism Research, 4*(3), 177–188.

Seibert, J. M., Hogan, A. E., & Mundy, P. C. (1982). Assessing interactional competencies: The early social-communication scales. *Infant Mental Health Journal, 3*(4), 244–258.

Seskin, L., Feliciano, E., Tippy, G., Yedloutschnig, R., Sossin, K. M., & Yasik, A. (2010). Attachment and autism: Parental attachment representations and relational behaviors in the parent–child dyad. *Journal of Abnormal Child Psychology, 38*(7), 949–960.

Sheinkopf, S. J., Mundy, P., Oller, D. K., & Steffens, M. (2000). Vocal atypicalities of preverbal autistic children. *Journal of Autism and Developmental Disorders, 30*(4), 345–354.

Shen, M. D., Nordahl, C. W., Young, G. S., Wootton-Gorges, S. L., Lee, A., Liston, S. E., . . . Amaral, D. G. (2013). Early brain enlargement and elevated extra-axial fluid in infants who develop autism spectrum disorder. *Brain, 136*(9), 2825–2835.

Shic, F., Bradshaw, J., Klin, A., Scassellati, B., & Chawarska, K. (2011). Limited activity monitoring in toddlers with autism spectrum disorder. *Brain Research, 1380*, 246–254.

Shic, F., Macari, S., & Chawarska, K. (2014). Speech disturbs face scanning in 6-month-old infants who develop autism spectrum disorder. *Biological Psychiatry, 75*(3), 231–237.

Shumway, S., & Wetherby, A. M. (2009). Communicative acts of children with autism spectrum disorders in the second year of life. *Journal of Speech, Language and Hearing Research, 52*(5), 1139–1156.

Sigman, M., & McGovern, C. (2005). Improvement in cognitive and language skills from preschool to adolescence in autism. *Journal of Autism and Developmental Disorders, 35*, 15–23.

Simonoff, E., Pickles, A., Charman, T., Chandler, S., Loucas, T., & Baird, G. (2008). Psychiatric disorders in children with autism spectrum disorders: Prevalence, comorbidity, and associated factors in a population-derived sample. *Journal of the American Academy of Child and Adolescent Psychiatry, 47*(8), 921–929.

Snow, M. E., Hertzig, M. E., & Shapiro, T. (1987). Expression of emotion in young autistic children. *Journal of the American Academy of Child and Adolescent Psychiatry, 26*(6), 836–838.

Sroufe, L. A. (1979). The ontogenesis of emotion. In J. D. Osofsky (Ed.), *Handbook of infant development* (pp. 462–516). New York: Wiley.

Starkel, H. L., Armbruster, J., & Hogan., T.P. (2006). Differentiating phonotactic probability and neighborhood density in adult word learning. *Journal of Speech, Language, and Hearing Research, 49,* 1175–1192.

St.John, T. , Estes, A. M., Dager, S. R., Kostopoulos, P., Wolff, J. J., Pandey, J., . . . Piven, J. (2016). Emerging executive functioning and motor development in infants at high and low risk for autism spectrum disorder. *Frontiers in Psychology, 7,* 1–12.

Stone, W. L., Ousley, O. Y., Hepburn, S. L., Hogan, K. L., & Brown, C. S. (1999). Patterns of adaptive behavior in very young children with autism. *American Journal on Mental Retardation, 104*(2), 187–199.

Tager-Flusberg, H., Calkins, S., Nolin, T., Baumberger, T., Anderson, M., & Chadwick-Dias, A. (1990). A longitudinal study of language acquisition in autistic and Down syndrome children. *Journal of Autism and Developmental Disorder, 20,* 1–21.

Tager-Flusberg, H., & Kasari, C. (2013). Minimally verbal school-aged children with autism spectrum disorder: The neglected end of the spectrum. *Autism Research, 6*(6), 468–478.

Talbott, M. R., Young, G. S., Munson, J., Estes, A., Vismara, L. A., & Rogers, S. J. (2018). The developmental sequence and relations between gesture and spoken language in toddlers with autism spectrum disorder. *Child Development.* [Epub ahead of print]

Teague, S. J., Gray, K. M., Tonge, B. J., & Newman, L. K. (2017). Attachment in children with autism spectrum disorder: A systematic review. *Research in Autism Spectrum Disorders, 35,* 35–50.

Teague, S. J., Newman, L. K., Tonge, B. J., & Gray, K. M. (2018). Caregiver mental health, parenting practices, and perceptions of child attachment in children with autism spectrum disorder. *Journal of Autism and Developmental Disorders, 48*(8), 2642–2652.

Torras-Mañá, M., Gómez-Morales, A., González-Gimeno, I., Fornieles-Deu, A., & Brun-Gasca, C. (2016). Assessment of cognition and language in the early diagnosis of autism spectrum disorder: Usefulness of the Bayley Scales of Infant and Toddler Development. *Journal of Intellectual Disability Research, 60*(5), 502–511.

Ungerer, J., & Sigman, M. (1984). The relation of play and sensorimotor behavior to language in the second year. *Child Development, 55,* 1448–1455.

van IJzendoorn, M. H., Rutgers, A. H., Bakermans-Kranenburg, M. J., Swinkels, S. H., van Daalen, E., Dietz, C., . . . van Engeland, H. (2007). Parental sensitivity and attachment in children with autism spectrum disorder: Comparison with children with mental retardation, with language delays, and with typical development. *Child Development, 78*(2), 597–608.

Ventola, P., Saulnier, C. A., Steinberg, E., Chawarska, K., & Klin, A. (2014). Early-emerging social adaptive skills in toddlers with autism spectrum disorders: An item analysis. *Journal of Autism and Developmental Disorders, 44*(2), 283–293.

Vernetti, A., Shic, F., Boccanfuso, L., Macari, S., Kane-Grade, F., Milgramm, A., . . . Chawarska, K. (2020). *Atypical physiological arousal to emotion inducing probes in toddlers with autism spectrum disorder.* Manuscript under review.

Vivanti, G., Dissanayake, C., Zierhut, C., Rogers, S. J., & Victorian ASELCC Team. (2013). Brief report: Predictors of outcomes in the Early Start Denver Model delivered in a group setting. *Journal of Autism and Developmental Disorders, 43*(7), 1717–1724.

Vivanti, G., & Nuske, H. J. (2017). Autism, attachment, and social learning: Three challenges and a way forward. *Behavioural Brain Research, 325,* 251–259.

Volden, J., Smith, I. M., Szatmari, P., Bryson, S., Fombonne, E., Mirenda, P., . . . Thompson, A. (2011). Using the Preschool Language Scale, Fourth Edition to characterize language in preschoolers with autism spectrum disorders. *American Journal of Speech-Language Pathology, 20*(3), 200–208.

Volkmar, F. R., Carter, A., Sparrow, S. S., & Cicchetti, D. V. (1993). Quantifying social development in autism. *Journal of the American Academy of Child and Adolescent Psychiatry, 32*(3), 627–632.

Wan, M. W., Green, J., Elsabbagh, M., Johnson, M., Charman, T., Plummer, F., & BASIS Team. (2013). Quality of interaction between at-risk infants and caregiver at 12–15 months is associated with 3-year autism outcome. *Journal of Child Psychology and Psychiatry, 54*(7), 763–771.

Waterhouse, L., & Fein, D. (1998). Autism and the evolution of human social skills. In F. R. Volkmar (Ed.), *Autism and pervasive developmental disorders* (pp. 242–267). New York: Cambridge University Press.

Watt, N., Wetherby, A., & Shumway, S. (2006). Prelinguistic predictors of language outcome at 3 years of age. *Journal of Speech, Language and Hearing Research, 49*(6), 1224–1237.

Weibe, S. A., Sheffield, T., Nelson, J. M., Clark, C. A., Chevalier, N., & Espy, K. A. (2011). The structure of executive function in 3-year-olds. *Journal of Experimental Child Psychology, 108*(3), 436–452.

Werner, E., & Dawson, G. (2005). Validation of the phenomenon of autistic regression using home videotapes. *Archives of General Psychiatry, 62*(8), 889–895.

Wetherby, A. M., Prizant, B. M., & Hutchinson, T. A. (1998). Communicative, social/affective, and symbolic profiles of young children with autism and pervasive developmental disorders. *American Journal of Speech-Language Pathology, 7*(2), 79–91.

Wetherby, A., Woods, J., Allen, L., Cleary, J., Dickinson, H., & Lord, C. (2004). Early indicators of autism spectrum disorders in the second year of life. *Journal of Autism and Developmental Disorders, 34*(5), 473–493.

Willemsen-Swinkels, S. H., Bakermans-Kranenburg, M. J., Buitelaar, J. K., van IJzendoorn, M. H., & van Engeland, H. (2000). Insecure and disorganised attachment in children with a pervasive developmental disorder: Relationship with social interaction and heart rate. *Journal of Child Psychology and Psychiatry and Allied Disciplines, 41*(6), 759–767.

Wolff, J. J., Gu, H., Gerig, G., Elison, J. T., Styner, M., Gouttard, S., . . . Evans, A. C. (2012). Differences in white matter fiber tract development present from 6 to 24 months in infants with autism. *American Journal of Psychiatry, 169*(6), 589–600.

Yerys, B. E., Hepburn, S. L., Pennington, B. F., & Rogers, S. J. (2007). Executive function in preschoolers with autism: Evidence consistent with a secondary deficit. *Journal of Autism and Developmental Disorders, 37*(6), 1068–1079.

Yirmiya, N., Kasari, C., Sigman, M., & Mundy, P. (1989). Facial expressions of affect in autistic, mentally retarded and normal children. *Journal of Child Psychology and Psychiatry, 30*(5), 725–735.

Yoder, P., & Stone, W. L. (2006). Randomized comparison of two communication interventions for preschoolers with autism spectrum disorders. *Journal of Consulting and Clinical Psychology, 74*(3), 426–435.

Zhou, Q., Chen, S. H., & Main, A. (2012). Commonalities and differences in the research on children's effortful control and executive function: A call for an integrated model of self-regulation. *Child Development Perspectives, 6*(2), 112–121.

Zwaigenbaum, L., Bryson, S., Rogers, T., Roberts, W., Brian, J., & Szatmari, P. (2005). Behavioral manifestations of autism in the first year of life. *International Journal of Developmental Neuroscience, 23*(2–3), 143–152.

CHAPTER 4

• • • • • • • •

Early Interventions for Young Children with Autism Spectrum Disorder

Maria Pizzano and Connie Kasari

S igns of autism spectrum disorder (ASD) can be detected early in the second year of life. These early signs often center on social communication abilities, such as difficulties with eye contact, responsiveness to others, orienting to name, shared affect, and vocalizations (Landa, Holman, & Garrett-Mayer, 2007; American Psychiatric Association, 2013). However, young children showing these early signs also exhibit great heterogeneity, challenging clinicians in making a definitive diagnosis of ASD. One push for earlier and earlier diagnoses of ASD is the strong belief in the benefits of early intervention. In this chapter, we review evidence for the benefits of early interventions aimed at young children with ASD and the goals for future improvements in our current intervention models and research designs.

Targets of Early Interventions

The focus of early interventions is often on the core impairments unique to children with ASD, but it may also include more general goals aimed at addressing delays in development. Intervention goals may be focused (e.g., concentrated on specific skills such as joint attention and play skills) or comprehensive (e.g., targeted on any and all areas of development). Targeted and comprehensive models are implemented and studied in different ways as described below.

The two core developmental impairments necessary for a diagnosis of ASD are social communication and restricted and repetitive behaviors. Social communication refers to communication used for the purpose of sharing information with a social partner. In early childhood, social communication requires appropriate initiation and response to social partners, back-and-forth conversation with sharing of interests, adjustment of behavior for social contexts, and shared relationships with peers. Social communication integrates verbal and nonverbal language, and those with ASD may have difficulty understanding and using eye contact, body language, and gestures in social exchanges. For very young children, the earliest signs may be nonverbal, as gestures and gaze patterns are precursors to children using verbal language (Bruner, 1985; Tomasello & Farrar, 1986). These nonverbal behaviors may include eye contact, pointing, and reaching, with the function of these behaviors used to share an experience with another person or to request help. These abilities are important foundational skills with downstream effects on language abilities and social cognition such as theory of mind (Charman et al., 2000; Mundy, Sigman, & Kasari, 1990).

The second core impairment of ASD—restricted, repetitive behaviors, interests, or activities—can manifest as inflexibility, stereotyped movements, intense and fixated interests, and over- or underreaction to sensory information. These behaviors can impact learning and social interaction and often worsen over the early years of life. Many interventions take aim directly on these core impairments, while others address the impairments in more general ways.

Although language is no longer considered a core deficit of children with ASD, nearly all children with ASD also demonstrate early-language delays (American Psychiatric Association, 2013). Language is a powerful predictor of children's outcomes and is critical to developing independence later in life (Howlin, Mawhood, & Rutter, 2000). Therefore, early interventions for children with ASD often target language skills due to the integral role they play in adaptive functioning, although the methods used to teach language vary among programs. Because at least 30–50% of preverbal preschoolers with ASD will not develop enough functional language to be considered fluent communicators by kindergarten age (Tager-Flusberg & Kasari, 2013), interventions have also focused on developing communication and language skills through alternative and augmentative means (such as picture exchange systems to communicate and speech-generating devices).

Evidence for Early Interventions

Early interventions are indicated for any child showing developmental delays or differences such as in the case of children with ASD. In 2001, the National Research Council Committee on Educational Interventions for Children with Autism reviewed existing intervention literature to recommend that more studies use rigorous group comparisons, individualized treatment plans, appropriate measures, parental involvement, and targets of spontaneous language (National Research Council, 2001). Perhaps because of the unique developmental impairments noted in children with ASD, or because of the increasing numbers of identified children (now 1 in

54 children; Maenner et al., 2020), the numbers of distinct, named intervention models specifically for ASD have proliferated over the last decade. However, the majority of these programs have been undertested, or not tested at all, using rigorous scientific methods. As a result, many of the evidence-based reviews of early intervention have found significant deficiencies in our ability to claim strong evidence of early intervention models for children with ASD (Kasari & Smith, 2016; Smith & Iadarola, 2015; Wong et al., 2015).

Below we address empirical evidence for interventions for children ages 2–5 that are comprehensive (aimed at improving all areas of development) and those that are more targeted (such as on social communication skills). (See Table 4.1 on pp. 140–149.) For intervention during the prodromal stage of ASD, see Chapter 8. In this chapter, we describe studies that focus on group-based research designs. Most studies reviewed will use randomization (similar to flipping a coin) to assign children to groups that can be compared. Randomization ensures that the "deck is not stacked" to find the positive effects of one intervention over another. This procedure is critically important in protecting the outcome from bias. Children will have an equal opportunity to receive one intervention or another (or standard care), so that the effects of the intervention can be fairly evaluated (Sibbald & Roland, 1998; Jüni, Altman, & Egger, 2001). While an intervention may have several behavioral targets, the effect of the intervention is judged by a predetermined primary outcome measure (as well as at times secondary, indirect outcomes of the intervention; Bakhai, Chhabra, & Wang, 2006).

In this review, we have not included an evaluation of the hundreds of studies that have manipulated a single strategy (e.g., discrete trial teaching of one joint attention skill) or a singular goal in intervention (e.g., decrease in mouthing toys), as these have been reviewed in previous papers (Odom et al., 2003; White et al., 2011; Wong et al., 2015), with noted limitations in determining the effectiveness of early interventions based on the quality of the research (Kasari & Smith, 2016). These studies often use single-case study designs, with repeated measurement of a single subject serving as their own control to compare data collected before and after an intervention is applied. These studies can help provide insight into potentially beneficial new practices (Horner et al., 2005). However, single-case designs have limited usefulness in providing evidence for the efficacy of early interventions, given their limitations in determining moderators of outcomes, comparison of approaches, and long-term change (Kasari & Smith, 2016).

Comprehensive Early Interventions

Comprehensive early intervention programs include considerations of both dose (how many hours of intervention per week and for how long) and targets of intervention that focus on multiple areas, including cognition, social communication, language, adaptive behaviors, motor development, and challenging or problem behaviors (including repetitive behaviors and restricted interests). In a previous review, interventions for preschool-age children delivered for at least 20 hours per week were shown to effectively improve the developmental outcomes of children with ASD (Virués-Ortega, 2010).

It is widely believed that children with ASD require comprehensive interventions (National Research Council, 2001). The vast heterogeneity among children means that some children will need greater focus on some areas than others, but nearly all children benefit from a comprehensive examination of developmental skills and behavioral challenges. How to select or build a comprehensive program for a child is a matter of some debate. For example, some programs are marketed as all-inclusive comprehensive packages (e.g., the discrete trial teaching approach or the Early Start Denver Model). Some argue that building a comprehensive model of intervention using evidence-based, targeted modules can better personalize interventions for individual children (Chorpita & Weisz, 2009; Kasari & Smith, 2016). Below we review comprehensive intervention packages, as well as modular, targeted interventions.

The most common comprehensive intervention package in the field of ASD is referred to as *early intensive behavioral intervention (EIBI)* and draws largely from the work pioneered by Ivar Lovaas. Lovaas used a method of intervention referred to as discrete trial teaching (DTT). This method is based on the science of applied behavior analysis (ABA) and uses the repeated delivery of a stimulus–response–consequence to the child to teach specific skills. Discrete trials are based in Skinner's operant conditioning theory and include methods of shaping, chaining, discrimination training, and establishing contingencies. While ABA refers to an umbrella of strategies used to individualize instruction based on principles of behavior theory, DTT is probably the most common, and widely accepted, ABA method.

Lovaas's research study of EIBI greatly influenced the early intervention field (Lovaas, 1987). In the original paper, treatment was implemented by therapists individually with a child for up to 40 hours or only 10 hours per week in the child's home. The study included three nonrandomized groups of children with ASD all under 46 months. The intensive treatment group of 19 children was assigned to 40 hours per week of 1:1 home-based intervention consisting primarily of discrete trials to teach new skills. The low-dosage comparison group of 19 children was assigned to the same intervention program but for just 10 hours per week, and the second comparison group of 21 was given early intervention services also at 10 hours per week but sampled from community services. The intervention lasted a total of 3 years, representing a significant investment of time and resources.

Results showed that of the 19 children in the intensive treatment group, 9 entered general education classrooms in the first grade and had cognitive scores in the average normative range. Differences in measured cognitive scores averaged nearly 30 points between the low- and high-dose groups. Whereas 10% of the original intensive group were placed in classes for intellectual disability, 53% of the control group was placed in classes for intellectual disability. A follow-up of the landmark 1987 study showed that 6 years later, the intensive treatment group maintained their level of functioning and had significantly higher scores on IQ and adaptive functioning than the low-dose comparison group (McEachin, Smith, & Lovaas, 1993).

Subsequent studies continued to refine, replicate, and elucidate nuances of Lovaas's program. Despite decades of research, just two studies have been published using rigorous scientific methods that include randomization of participants into intervention groups. Smith, Groen, and Wynn (2000) randomly assigned 28 children 18–42 months old to intensive (30 hours per week) treatment or low-intensity (5 hours per week) parent training based on developmental quotient (DQ)-matched pairs. DQ describes the ratio of a subject's developmental age and chronological age to provide a view of overall development. The intensive treatment was based on Lovaas's original intervention manual. The intensive group had significant gains on cognitive scores, visual–spatial skills, language, and academic skills but did not outperform the parent group on adaptive skills and maladaptive behaviors. Moreover, the results were driven by children with pervasive developmental disorder not otherwise specified (PDD-NOS), in other words, children with the least impairment (American Psychiatric Association, 2000). Children with more severe delays made little progress in either group. A subsequent 2005 randomized controlled trial (RCT) of 24 children randomized to an intensive 37-hour weekly clinic-directed EIBI group did no better than a parent-directed EIBI group of similar intensity, the same curriculum, and the same therapists, with the only difference in groups being fewer supervision hours. As there were no group differences, the data were presented as pre–post data on a single group; therefore, data from the randomized trial were not reported (Sallows & Graupner, 2005). For both groups combined, approximately 48% of the children made rapid progress, so that 4 years later they had achieved average intelligence and were in general education classrooms, much as was found through Lovaas's original study data (Lovaas, 1987).

Other attempts to deliver EIBI using less intense workforce demands include the development of an app for parents to use in implementation of EIBI. The TOBY (Therapy Outcomes by You) app is designed to support parents in implementing ABA at home. In a trial of 80 families over a 6-month period, the TOBY app was randomly assigned to families that were receiving treatment in the community (Whitehouse et al., 2017). Parents were asked to use the TOBY app for 20 minutes per day. No significant differences were found on the primary outcome of the Autism Treatment Evaluation Checklist or on the expressive and receptive subscales of the Mullen Scales of Early Learning (MSEL; Mullen, 1995). The TOBY group did outperform at the 3-month midpoint and 6-month exit time points on secondary outcomes of the nonverbal and fine motor skills measured by the MSEL and parent-reported words understood as measured by the MacArthur–Bates Communication Development Inventory (MBCDI; Fenson et al., 1991). Of note, parents used the app for the required time during the first 3 months but then significantly decreased use over the next 3 months, raising questions about the sustainability, acceptability, and usability of the intervention app.

These tests of the efficacy of EIBI are not a strong endorsement of DTT used alone as an effective early intervention model. There appears to be some gain for children who are the least impaired, but it is unclear what is driving these effects. It may be that a minimum dose level is needed to make significant gains (e.g., 20 hours per week), but it is unclear whether DTT as a method of intervention drives these effects since DTT has not been rigorously compared to another method, nor has dose been rigorously compared. Despite these findings, there is strong belief in the community that EIBI, and specifically DTT, is the most (and only?) effective early intervention approach.

Despite community perceptions, researchers note that there are issues with interpreting current research studies with common concerns about inconsistent methods, in particular nonrandomization, unclear content, variations in delivery, and lack of attention to core deficits (Kasari et al., 2005; Smith & Iadarola, 2015). Nonrigorously tested studies can find replicated IQ advantages, but in contrast to Lovaas (1987), participants' autism classification remains unchanged due to minimal change in ASD symptoms and social skills (Sheinkopf & Siegel, 1998; Cohen, Amerine-Dickens, & Smith, 2006; Reed, Osborne, & Corness, 2007; Zachor, Ben-Itzchak, Rabinovich, & Lahat, 2007). At low intensities (< 15 hours per week) or at an intensity equal to that of many in the community, EIBI does not necessarily result in significant gains over interventions that combine many different approaches (often referred to as eclectic models), again raising the question of whether dose is a more important factor versus the intervention approach (Eldevik, Eikeseth, Jahr, & Smith, 2006; Howard, Sparkman, Cohen, Green, & Stanislaw, 2005; Magiati, Charman, & Howlin, 2007). Further criticisms of EIBI are limited generalizability after intervention ceases and diminished group differences by follow-up (Kovshoff, Hastings, & Remington, 2011).

ABA alternatives to the DTT model are those that alter the traditional DTT approach with naturalistic, developmental methods, particularly important with younger children (infants and toddlers). In 2015, several interventions were developed independently by separate research groups but grouped together to recognize some common elements that differentiated them from the more traditional ABA methods of DTT. The new group of interventions is called *naturalistic developmental behavioral interventions (NDBIs)*; Schreibman et al., 2015). NDBI refers to interventions that are implemented in natural contexts, are more child versus adult centered, and use natural reinforcements and learning opportunities but are similar to other ABA methods in using a number of behavioral strategies to teach children with ASD developmentally anchored skills in an appropriate sequence. The goal of these interventions is to reduce prompt dependence, promote motivating exchanges, ensure generalization of skills, and teach meaningful and relevant language. Several NDBIs were derived primarily from principles of ABA (e.g., pivotal response training [PRT], enhanced milieu training [EMT], and others from developmental principles, including joint attention, symbolic play, engagement, and regulation [JASPER] and social communication/emotion regulation/transactional support [SCERTS]), but all models use a mixture of strategies combining developmental and behavioral theories. NDBIs include the *Early Start Denver Model (ESDM)*; PRT; early achievements (EA); JASPER; reciprocal imitation training (RIT); improving parents as communication teachers (Project ImPACT); EMT; and SCERTS. Although some of these interventions are derived from comprehensive packages (e.g., SCERTS, PRT), most are research tested as targeted interventions. Below we describe research-tested comprehensive NDBI models that were evaluated as a comprehensive intervention package over several hours per day or week and delivered by therapists, the ESDM and EA.

A comprehensive intervention model that focuses on integrating ABA and developmental principles within natural, everyday contexts is the ESDM. Intervention is delivered at home at high intensity, approximately 20 hours per week, but it emphasizes generalization across contexts. In one of the first RCTs of a comprehensive intervention for children under 30 months, ESDM was compared to treatment as usual (TAU). Dose was reported as comparable between the two groups but not tightly controlled. Results from 2 years of the intervention yielded significant gains in overall DQ as measured by the MSEL and all adaptive domains, except socialization, as measured by the Vineland Adaptive Behavior Scales (VABS; Sparrow, Cicchetti, & Balla, 2005) versus the TAU group (Dawson et al., 2010). There were no group differences in autism severity as measured by the Autism Diagnostic Observation Schedule (ADOS; Lord, Rutter, DiLavore, & Risi, 2008) and in repetitive behaviors as measured by the Repetitive Behavior Scale (RBS; Bodfish, Symons, & Lewis, 1998). A follow-up 2 years after intervention concluded that the ESDM group maintained the gains made in the intervention period, although differences between the groups had diminished (Estes et al., 2015). Of note here is that the ESDM comprehensive model applied to younger children with ASD yielded similar outcomes in DQ gains to the Smith et al. (2000) randomized trial of DTT with preschool-age children (about 16–20 DQ points). Again, a question remains as to whether dose alone (rather than approach) may be important to changes in DQ in early childhood, particularly since core deficits of ASD (repetitive behavior and socialization) were unaffected by the 2-year intervention. It will be important to establish the extent to which any of the intervention packages improve the outcomes of core deficits in autism (social communication and restricted and repetitive behaviors) since DQ is not considered a core deficit of ASD.

A multisite replication of the original ESDM intervention study (Dawson et al., 2010) was rigorously tested with close attention to fidelity at each of the three sites, independent outcome assessments on a standardized measure of language, and data analyses by an independent group. Thus, the data from this study were carefully examined, and results indicated that the study did not replicate the earlier findings on DQ; rather, it found a complicated site by treatment interaction effect on a combined measure of language not used in the original study (replication used a combined language measure from the MSEL; Rogers et al., 2019). The site interaction effect, as noted by the authors, is difficult to interpret. Several factors may have contributed to the limited replication. One was that the community group had 42% attrition over the course of the 27-month-long intervention period versus 18% attrition in the ESDM group, leading to questions about the validity of the control group comparisons. Another was the possibility that the available interventions for the community control group had significantly improved over the last 10 years, thus lessening the differences between groups.

Another early intervention model that consists of multiple hours per day and is delivered by therapists in clinic-based classrooms is the *early achievements (EA)* intervention. In this intervention study, toddlers received two different versions of group-based, therapist-mediated intervention, largely based on a pivotal response training (PRT) approach to intervention (see below), for 10 hours per week for 6 months with a 6-month follow-up. The study tested the effect of adding in treatment components aimed at core impairments in social communication. One version of the intervention added in teaching joint attention, imitation, and shared affect, while the other did not. A randomized controlled trial of 50 toddlers found that there was a significant treatment effect for imitation with eye contact that generalized and was maintained at follow-up, but no differences were found in initiations of joint attention (IJA) or shared positive affect (Landa, Holman, O'Neill, & Stuart, 2011). Indeed, joint attention initiations appear to be a significant impairment in young children's development and one that is particularly difficult to improve in interventions.

Comprehensive Models Are Difficult to Compare

Despite the fact that comprehensive intervention models are desirable, they are difficult to evaluate for multiple reasons (Kasari et al., 2005). Besides being expensive to test in research studies (e.g., staff costs to execute many hours per week for months or years), there has been overall general improvement in community-delivered early intervention. Because control groups consist of students receiving interventions that have improved over time, replication studies may not find the same results as reported earlier. Such lack of difference suggests that, on the one hand, our community interventions have improved significantly and, on the other hand, our experimental interventions may not be potent enough to rise above the current treatment as usual.

Take, for example, a model of intervention developed in the 1960s, *Treatment and Education of Autistic and Related Communication Handicapped Children (TEACCH)*. TEACCH has core tenets that include structured environments, organization of time, use of special interests as rewards and communication opportunities, and emphasis on visual supports to communicate. The goal of TEACCH is to use individualized approaches to the generalized curriculum to adapt work systems, teaching tasks, and routines, based on the learning style of children with ASD. However, TEACCH was never tested as a stand-alone model. Today TEACCH core ingredients have ubiquitous influence in nearly every model of intervention. In fact, in a quasi-experimental comparison of three early intervention models (a preschool classroom based on the TEACCH model versus one based in learning experiences, an alternative program for preschoolers and parents [LEAP], an inclusion model of early intervention [Strain & Bovey, 2011], versus a general, quality, eclectic special education model), no differences were found on any child outcome measures (Boyd et al., 2014). All children seemed to benefit from early intervention generally; it may be that each model had more similarities than differences in approach, speaking to the general improvement and blending of early interventions over time.

Another reason comprehensive interventions are difficult to compare is that, to date, none of the models has determined the active ingredients of why the intervention might provide benefit (Kasari et al., 2005; Kasari & Smith, 2016). Particular strategies or targets have not been distilled in ways to determine the active ingredient in a comprehensive model. The one potential element to date has been dose, where interventions of similar dose appear to provide comparable benefit on the same outcome (e.g., 20 hours of DTT or ESDM per week on DQ outcomes compared to lower dose comparison, TAU groups).

We also have limited information on who benefits the most from any particular intervention model. Studies that have tested moderators (variables that might be associated with better or worse outcomes) have found that children who begin with the most skills prior to intervention and children who are the youngest make the most progress. We don't know how other factors about children or families may fit better with intervention models allowing us to better personalize interventions to particular children.

An Alternative Approach to Testing Comprehensive Models

As we do not know the active ingredients of comprehensive models, an alternative is to distill intervention components into smaller, focused interventions, testing the resulting module on targeted outcomes and/or subgroups of individuals. Indeed, several models designed to be "comprehensive" have actually tested their "model" over brief periods of time and for only certain outcomes or only certain subpopulations of individuals. Examples include studies based on PRT or SCERTS that are tested by training parents to implement the intervention with their children.

Therefore, another approach has been to design an intervention to be modular from the beginning. These modules are typically targeted toward particular child skills (e.g., social communication), with effectiveness of the intervention determined by testing outcomes that are theoretically related and often proximal to the intervention focus (e.g., tests of social communication). A modular approach has several advantages over existing comprehensive models. In particular, when a tested module is shown to be efficacious on a targeted behavior or set of behaviors, combining different modules to create a comprehensive program for a child lends itself to greater personalization of intervention, an approach we have advocated for in previous publications (Kasari et al., 2005; Kasari & Smith, 2013, 2016). In other words, modules are combined into an intervention program that targets skills deficits or behavioral excesses particular to the child, thus creating an individualized, person-centered intervention program. Below we describe studies that test a distilled, briefer version of a comprehensive program and studies that were designed as modular, or targeted, from the beginning.

Focused Interventions

Some focused interventions were developed as brief versions of comprehensive models delivered by therapists. While several models of intervention have been developed as comprehensive packages, the developers have tested the intervention model in a targeted or focused fashion only, or they have narrowed the intervention to teach in a more focused manner especially when teaching parents. For example, the *Autism 1–2–3* intervention aims to teach language using EIBI principles (primarily DTT). The intervention applies a developmental sequence with physical and verbal prompting to teach social communication requesting skills in a discrete fashion, and candy is given as reinforcement for correct responses. A pilot investigation randomized 17 participants to either the intervention or a wait-list control. When randomized participants were compared to a wait-list group, parents did not report improvements for the intervention group compared to the control group. However, compared to the control group, those in the Autism 1–2–3 group showed improvements on the ADOS in the areas of vocalization, pointing, and gestures, as well as on the reciprocal interaction subscale (Wong & Kwan, 2010). Because of small group sizes, results warrant further investigation with larger samples before making definitive conclusions.

Another ABA model uses Skinner's Verbal Behavior method coupled with music therapy to target communication. In this study, 22 children were randomly assigned to music plus verbal behavior, speech therapy plus verbal behavior, or no training (Lim & Draper, 2011). Both active treatment conditions improved child speech with no difference between music and speech, but music plus ABA resulted in more echoed language. In a subsequent RCT, 23 children received either 4 months of family-centered music therapy (FCMT) in addition to their early intervention program or their early intervention program alone (Thompson, McFerran, & Gold, 2014). The music therapy did not show any additional benefit to language skills or social responsiveness but did improve social engagement in the home and in the community. Thus, there may be some benefit to adding music therapy into treatment as usual, but further studies are indicated.

Other focused models derived from comprehensive interventions evolved from different theoretical frameworks, often as a contrast to issues identified with EIBI methods such as poor generalization (Schreibman et al., 2015). PRT is one model that modified Lovaas's approach to DTT by altering the basic approach to reflect shared control between adult and child, use of natural reinforcers, and targeting of pivotal behaviors that were viewed as addressing motivational issues in learning of children with ASD. PRT can be used to address a number of intervention goals and to build a comprehensive model. Indeed, several NDBIs use PRT methods as the foundation of their intervention approach, such as reciprocal imitation training, Project ImPACT, ESDM, Social ABCs, and EA. Many of these models test the intervention by targeting social communication or language skills specifically (thus, more targeted than comprehensive) and mediate the intervention through parents (described below). One model, *reciprocal imitation training (RIT)*, mediates the intervention through therapists and focuses on imitation specifically. RIT aims to teach object and gesture imitation with naturalistic techniques. In two very small randomized trials (both with fewer than 30 participants), the experimental RIT group made significant improvements over a TAU control group in elicited and spontaneous imitation (Ingersoll & Dvortcsak, 2010) and joint attention, and in social–emotional functioning (Ingersoll, 2012). These results replicated earlier single-subject studies of RIT (Ingersoll & Gergans, 2007; Ingersoll, Lewis, & Kroman, 2007).

Specifically Targeted Interventions

Some interventions were developed to be targeted or focused interventions, and not derived from a comprehensive program. A common target for these interventions is improving communication and language skills. While studies report on therapist-mediated versions of the model, they have also developed parent-mediated versions of the same models (discussed below).

Enhanced milieu treatment (EMT) and responsive education and prelinguistic milieu training (RPMT) share certain behaviorally based methods in teaching expressive language skills, one by targeting verbal language specifically (EMT) and the other by targeting prelinguistic gestures (joint attention and requesting) as a means to improve expressive language (RPMT). EMT emphasizes environmental arrangement, responsive interaction, specific language modeling and expansions, and milieu teaching prompts. Milieu teaching prompts are composed of modeling, verbal prompts, time delay, and incidental teaching. Similar to PRT, it was developed primarily via single-subject designs. Such single-subject evidence shows that EMT increases language complexity and the social function of language (Hancock & Kaiser, 2002). Two randomized trials have been reported with children with developmental disabilities and toddlers with language delays, but not autism. Kaiser and Roberts (2013) reported comparisons of EMT as implemented by a therapist versus EMT implemented by a therapist plus a parent. Although the parent was able to use EMT strategies effectively, and conceivably was able to continue the intervention beyond the therapy sessions, there were no group differences on child language measures (Kaiser & Roberts, 2013). For toddlers with language delays, a primarily caregiver-mediated EMT intervention led to improved receptive language over treatment as usual, but not expressive language (Roberts & Kaiser, 2015). A follow-up of this intervention 12 months post-intervention did not find maintained effects (Hampton, Kaiser, & Roberts, 2017). EMT when combined with JASPER (see below) has shown effectiveness for older children with autism (5- to 8-year-old, minimally verbal children; Kasari et al., 2014a); thus, specific ABA-based language prompting methods may be more effective with older than younger children, or when combined with an intervention that also focuses on prelinguistic skills.

RPMT is derived from EMT strategies, using similar responsive and prompting strategies, but focuses on earlier-developing gestural skills that are associated with later expressive language, and more often on samples of children with ASD. In a study of preschoolers with ASD, RPMT has been compared to the Picture Exchange Communication System (PECS) using randomized controlled methods, and similar to the earlier reported PRT versus PECS study (Schreibman & Stahmer, 2014), no group differences were noted. However, there were positive effects for some children. Children who began the study with at least some joint attention initiations made greater gains in generalizing initiation of joint attention, and these gains were due to RPMT (Yoder & Stone, 2006).

An intervention model developed specifically to address core impairments in social communication is *joint attention, symbolic play, engagement, and regulation (JASPER)*. This intervention specifically targets joint engagement, joint attention, and play skills to effect later-developing language and cognitive skills. In the developmental phases of this intervention, children ages 36–48 months were randomized to receive one of three brief interventions added into their existing early intervention program that involved 30 hours of group-based ABA per week. These intervention modules were either (1) a targeted joint attention intervention (JA) or (2) a symbolic play intervention (SP) or (3) the existing early intervention program alone (control; Kasari, Freeman, & Paparella, 2006). The JA and SP interventions were delivered by clinicians 5 days a week for 30 minutes each day for 5–6 weeks on average. Both groups improved significantly over the control group, with the JA group increasing in responding to joint attention (RJA) and initiating joint attention (IJA) skills. The SP group had significantly more diverse types of symbolic play and higher play levels. A follow-up 1 year after the JA and SP interventions showed that gains made during the intervention period continued to increase, with children who received the JA and SP interventions having greater growth in expressive language over time versus the control, more growth in joint attention initiations, and increased durations of joint engagement, with play skills also growing more in the intervention groups versus the control group (Kasari, Paparella, Freeman, & Jahromi, 2008). A 5-year follow-up revealed that 80% of all participants had functional language by age 8–10 years, with play level at the start of the study predicting spoken language at follow-up, diversity of functional play type predicting cognitive scores (IQ), and spoken vocabulary at follow-up associated with initial IJA skills and receiving the early JA or SP treatment compared to the control group (Kasari, Gulsrud, Freeman, Paparella, & Hellemann, 2012). In another examination of these data at the 5-year follow up, the JA group had the sharpest increase in JA looks and showing, and early pointing predicted later spoken language development (Gulsrud, Hellemann, Freeman, & Kasari, 2014). These investigations determined that targeted skills could be taught in a short time (30 minutes daily for 5–6 weeks), with durable and wide-reaching effects. The joint attention gains were found to be higher not only in quantity in the JA and SP groups, but in quality as well, with JA gains having increases in shared positive affect with and without language (Lawton & Kasari,

2012a). Those in the JA group were more likely to acknowledge a novel event and respond with JA (Gulsrud, Kasari, Freeman, & Paparella, 2007). Because there were few differences between the JA and SP conditions, with both superior to the control group, the JA and SP conditions were later combined into the JASPER intervention package. However, several studies built upon this initial JA and SP study, with adaptation mediated mostly by teachers (see below).

Parent-Mediated Models

Given that young children spend most of their time with their family members, a number of early intervention studies have been reported that teach parents to implement an intervention. Some of these are derived from comprehensive models and are distilled to be delivered over brief periods of time (3 to 9 months, one to three times per week). Others are designed to be targeted for parents from the beginning. Although intuitively and theoretically logical, results have proven to be mixed. Almost all studies show they can teach parents strategies with their children (i.e., parents can get to high levels of fidelity in implementing the intervention), but fewer find significant improvements in child behaviors. The reasons for the mixed findings are unclear, but they likely concern how focused the intervention is; how long it may take for these interventions to take hold and have an effect on parent and/or child behavior; and how natural and sustainable they are in the real world. Below we review evidence from randomized controlled parent-mediated models.

Parent-Mediated Interventions Derived from Comprehensive Models

The TEACCH model has been adapted for use by parents. An RCT of *TEACCH for toddlers* with a comparison of 20 families randomized to parent-implemented TEACCH versus a wait list found improvements in developmental and adaptive skills but lacked the power to detect a significant group difference (Welterlin, Turner-Brown, Harris, Mesibov, & Delmolino, 2012). A subsequent RCT of TEACCH for toddlers versus treatment as usual found treatment effects for decreased parent stress and well-being but no treatment effects for global child measures (Turner-Brown, Hume, Boyd, & Kainz, 2019). Evidence for the TEACCH model for improving child outcomes has not been found, but studies are based on very small, and likely underpowered samples.

PRT has been used with therapists and with parents, often in combination. One such randomized comparison where PRT was implemented by both parents and clinicians revealed no group differences on spoken language outcomes between the PRT intervention and an intervention using the PECS (Schreibman & Stahmer, 2014). PECS is an assistive communication system intended to increase communication via picture exchange. This comparison yielded similar findings between treatment approaches for increasing language outcomes. Another RCT compared video delivery of PRT information versus wait list for 34 participants. The PRT parents significantly changed their behavior, and their children's use of functional utterances increased significantly more than those in a wait-list control (Nefdt, Koegel, Singer, & Gerber, 2010).

Project ImPACT was developed in collaboration with parents, teachers, and service providers with the goal of improving the speed of dissemination from research to implementation. It is a parent training program with the goal of helping parents improve their child's social communication skills via play and home routines (Ingersoll & Dvortcsak, 2010; Ingersoll & Wainer, 2013a). Project ImPACT has been assessed primarily through single-case designs and shows some promise in training teachers to coach groups of parents in improving parent strategies to increase a child's spontaneous language (Ingersoll & Wainer, 2013a, 2013b; Ingersoll, Wainer, Berger, & Walton, 2017). A small pilot RCT randomized 28 families to receive either self-directed access to Project ImPACT content via an online website for 6 months with 12 self-directed lessons, or therapist-assisted access to the same website and content with two 30-minute videoconferenced coaching sessions per week (Ingersoll, Wainer, Berger, Pickard, & Bonter, 2016). Results showed that both models improved parent fidelity, parent perceptions, and child language, with only the therapist-assisted children showing improvements on parent-reported social skills via the VABS. Project ImPACT shows some promise, but further study utilizing experimental group designs is warranted, especially as remote access to interventions is particularly important to expand reach for families who have limited access to professionals.

The *parent-delivered ESDM (P-ESDM)* intervention was delivered weekly over 12 weeks and compared to treatment as usual in a group of nearly 100 parent–child dyads. No group differences were found in child or parent outcomes (Rogers et al., 2012). Both groups of parents improved their interactions with their children, and younger age of child and more community intervention hours were positively related to children's improvement. In a second P-ESDM study, the researchers enhanced the model in order to improve on the earlier null findings (Rogers et al., 2019). In this study, 45 parent–child dyads were randomized to receive P-ESDM as before (1.5-hour clinic visit per week for 12 weeks) versus the enhanced version of P-ESDM involving another 1.5-hour visit in the home and other techniques to motivate parents to maintain their engagement in the study. This study found that the enhanced version improved parent fidelity and maintenance in the trial (only 20% attrition) compared to the P-ESDM standard model, which had over 40% attrition by the end of the trial. However, the models had similar, nonsignificant findings on child behavior. These null findings associated with the P-ESDM model may illustrate the difficulty in translating an interventionist-delivered program that is comprehensive and delivered in high doses into a caregiver-implemented low-dose program. This particular model at reduced dose (in both hours per week and duration of intervention) has not shown efficacy.

Another caregiver-implemented intervention also based on a comprehensive model, *social communication/emotion regulation/transactional support (SCERTS)*, was tested in 82 caregivers and toddlers with ASD. The intervention, *early social interaction (ESI)*, was delivered more intensely than the P-ESDM study to children randomized to either individual (ESI) or group parent-implemented training that focused on supporting active engagement in the home setting (Wetherby et al., 2014). ESI parents received home-based instruction 2–3 times per week for 9 months, while those in the group condition met in groups of 4–5 with a therapist in the clinic one time per week for 9 months. Results indicated significant effects of the parent-mediated ESI intervention on children's receptive language and social communication skills.

In a parent-implemented intervention derived from the *DIR/Floortime* comprehensive model, *Play and Language for Autistic Youngsters (PLAY)* teaches parents to promote child progression through developmental levels, from self-regulation and interest in the world to thinking logically. Groups randomized to receive the PLAY intervention versus treatment as usual over 1 year had significantly better social functioning and parent and child interactions but were not different on autism classification or cognitive scores (Solomon, Van Egeren, Mahoney, Huber, & Zimmerman, 2014). Another shorter-term parent-mediated intervention based on DIR/Floortime also reported significantly improved functional outcomes on the DIR/Floortime-created assessment and diminished autism symptoms on the CARS over 3 months (Pajareya & Nopmaneejumruslers, 2011).

Targeted Parent-Mediated Models of Intervention

Models that were designed to be targeted and mediated through parents share similar characteristics. Many of these models provide one to three sessions per week over 3 months and focus on child outcomes of social communication and language.

Preschool Autism Communication Trial (PACT) is a parent-mediated social communication intervention. It aims to improve children's communication by training parents to alter their own communication in favor of nonintrusive communication that matches their child's language development. An initial small RCT showed that PACT yielded significant group effects on autism symptom scores and improved parent–child social interaction versus TAU (Aldred, Green, & Adams, 2004). A subsequent larger randomized, controlled study examined the effectiveness of PACT versus TAU and found a significant group effect favoring the intervention for parental synchrony but not for autism symptoms (Green et al., 2010). Four years postintervention, however, there was a group difference in favor of the PACT intervention in ADOS severity score and child initiations but no group differences on language measures (Pickles et al., 2016).

Another parent-mediated model, *Focused Playtime Intervention (FPI)*, aims to enhance child outcome via increasing responsive parent communication, with intervention goals that include establishing coordinated play. An RCT comparing FPI to a parent advocacy group showed a significant treatment effect for FPI on parent responsiveness but not on child outcomes. There was a significant moderated effect for a subgroup of children; those who began treatment with the lowest expressive language scores made the most progress (Siller, Hutman, & Sigman, 2013). Similarly, when FPI was applied to parents of infants at high risk for developing autism, parents significantly increased responsiveness but were not able to increase child outcomes over the TAU control group (Kasari et al., 2014c).

JASPER (the merging of the original joint attention and play modules in Kasari et al., 2006) was first tested with parents implementing the intervention. The results of parent-mediated JASPER are reported with toddlers and preschoolers. In Kasari, Gulsrud, Wong, Kwon, and Locke (2010), toddlers were randomized to either a caregiver-mediated intervention group with individual interventionist coaches or a wait-list control, with both groups again enrolled in the same intensive early intervention program (30 hours per week of base early intervention). The caregiver-mediated group made significant gains in joint engagement, RJA, and diversity of play, and these gains were maintained at the one-year follow-up. In a subsequent study of toddlers and parents, the caregiver-mediated protocol had significantly greater effects over a comparative parent education intervention on joint engagement that was maintained at follow-up (Kasari, Gulsrud, Paparella, Hellemann, & Berry, 2015). The caregiver-mediated group also saw effects on play and generalization to the child's classroom, while parent education effectively reduced parental stress. Furthermore, the caregiver-mediated group responded more frequently and more successfully to their child's restricted and repetitive behaviors (RRBs; Harrop, Gulsrud, Shih, Hovsepyan, & Kasari, 2017). The same parent-mediated intervention was taught to low-resourced families of preschool-age children with ASD in the community setting and randomly compared to a parent education program taught to caregivers in small groups. Both the parent education and parent-mediated groups made gains in IJA and joint engagement (JE), but the gains of the caregiver-mediated group were significantly greater (Kasari et al., 2014b).

Group-Based Parent-Mediated Interventions

Most parent-mediated interventions are delivered one-on-one with parent and child. However, some group interventions have been reported. In addition to the PRT study noted above (Hardan et al., 2015), *Hanen's More Than Words* is a group-based intervention designed to teach parents to structure everyday routines to be sensitive to their child's development and provide communication opportunities. This intervention is supervised by speech and language professionals and has been tested in a randomized trial of parents of at-risk autism toddlers. Results of this study of 60 parent–child dyads who received the Hanen intervention found no effect on child communication or parental responsivity when compared to TAU (Carter et al., 2011).

PRT has been delivered in a parent training group and compared to a parent psychoeducation group to find that parents who were taught PRT could implement PRT at fidelity. The outcome measure was language, and the study reported that parents were more successful in increasing *prompted* language in their children if they received PRT (Hardan et al., 2015). Most recently, a pilot study randomized 23 families to receive pivotal response intervention for social motivation (PRISM), a modified PRT approach that included additional components designed specifically to target social motivation, or a TAU wait list for 6 months (Vernon et al., 2019). The researchers reported that the treatment group improved significantly in reduced ADOS severity, increased MSEL receptive language and visual reception scores, PLS total score, PPVT score, and Vineland communication score and that the control group did not improve. These effects were examined within each sample and not between samples, so it is not clear if the children receiving PRT were significantly different from children receiving the TAU (the authors indicated that their samples were too small to test between-group differences).

Other group-delivered parent-mediated interventions have focused on increasing parenting strategies, particularly for challenging child behaviors. When comparing *parent education and behavior management (PEBM)* to counseling and parent education (PEAC), the children in the behavior management group significantly improved in adaptive behavior and showed decreased autism symptoms as compared to the counseling group (Tonge, Brereton, Kiomall, Mackinnon, & Rinehart, 2014). Grahame et al. (2015) compared an intervention targeting behavior management to a control group and found that when taught skills to manage their child's restricted and repetitive behavior, parents' self-efficacy increases and children's RRBs decrease. Bearss et al. (2015) compared *parent training* for behavior management to parent education for behavior management, with both groups reporting decreases in problem behavior, but the training group was found to have a significantly greater decrease in problem behavior, improved home behavior, and significantly greater improvement on clinical global impression (CGI) ratings by researchers. Scahill et al. (2016) used the same data and found that when parent training was compared directly to parent education for behavior management, there was a significant group difference in daily living skills favoring the parent training group.

Teacher-Mediated Interventions

A few studies have been reported where an intervention model has been mediated through teachers or paraprofessionals. These studies are reported with varying success. For example, in extensions of ESDM, small pilot studies have been reported with an adaption for preschool programs (Group-based Early Start Denver Model; G-ESDM). This model shows pre–post differences but has not been rigorously tested against a different model or treatment as usual. Children receiving G-ESDM over a year in a clinic-based classroom showed improvements in DQ, adaptive behavior, and socialization. These improvements were greater than those for a non-randomized, community comparison group of children receiving early intervention (Vivanti et al., 2014). However, because the children were not randomly assigned to intervention groups, significant advantage of G-ESDM cannot be reliably concluded. Subsequently, however, a small group of children were randomized to G-ESDM strategies applied to an inclusive classroom, or within an autism-specific classroom. Here improvements were made on the Vineland (VABS) and DQ on the MSEL with no differences found for children in inclusive or autism-specific classrooms (Vivanti et al., 2019). Rigorous tests of G-ESDM have not been published, so the effects of this intervention versus community interventions are unclear.

The model most adapted for classroom use has been the original model of teaching joint attention by Kasari (Kasari et al., 2006), which was later developed into JASPER. In an initial RCT for preschoolers in Norway, 61 students were randomized to receive either the JA component of Kasari et al. (2006) in addition to their preschool program or their preschool program alone. The JA group had greater JA initiations in a treatment effect that generalized to longer periods of engagement with their mothers versus the control (Kaale, Smith, & Sponheim, 2012). In an RCT comparing a wait-list control to teacher-implemented JASPER, teachers used the strategies they were taught and their students used significantly more JA, spending significantly more time in a supported engagement state over the wait-list group (Lawton & Kasari, 2012b). Wong (2013) independently combined JA and SP to teach the interventions based on Kasari et al. (2006) to preschool education teachers. Participants were randomized to receive either JA first and then SP, SP first and then JA, or a wait-list control group for 4 weeks. After 4 weeks, the control group was randomized to receive either one of the two intervention combinations. The initial intervention group teachers were able to learn the strategies, and their students' joint engagement significantly improved over the wait list at 4 weeks. The treatment groups also saw significant JA and play skill improvements, although no differences were found between the two sequences and no differences were found compared to the wait list halfway through the intervention.

Finally, the advancing social communication and play (ASAP) intervention was designed as a classroom-based intervention, with the teaching staff taught how to improve children's social communication and play skills. Seventy-eight classrooms involving 161 children with ASD were randomized to ASAP or business-as-usual comparison classrooms (Boyd et al., 2018). No significant group differences were found for the primary outcomes of children's social communication and play. However, children in the ASAP group showed increased classroom engagement.

None of the above studies implemented JASPER exactly as it was designed, but rather adopted key components as chosen by the investigators. Kaale et al. (2012) stayed closest to the original JA, SP study with similar findings when teachers implemented the intervention as when therapists implemented the study in Kasari et al. (2006). In implementation of JASPER by teachers and paraprofessionals, two studies have been reported. First, teachers in public preschool classrooms successfully implemented the JASPER program at high fidelity to significantly improve joint engagement, joint attention gestures, language, and play over the wait-list control (Chang, Shire, Shih, Gelfand, & Kasari, 2016). In this study, small groups of students were taught in classroom center rotations. Improvements were noted after 3 months and were maintained over a 1-month follow-up. In a study of toddlers who were taught one-on-one by paraprofessional teaching assistants (TAs), the TAs learned JASPER in person and then were supported via remote support. High levels of fidelity were achieved, and significant child effects were found after 3 months of intervention and a 1-month follow-up on child-initiated joint engagement and functional play (Shire et al., 2017). Toddlers receiving JASPER also improved their spoken language at rates higher than the control group. TAs were able to deliver JASPER at high levels of fidelity the next year with a new group of children; these children achieved similar levels of improvement in social communication and language skills as children in the first year where the TAs received more external supports (Shire et al., 2019). These examples of successful implementation of clinic-based JASPER into local and remote classrooms demonstrate a rare example of translation of results and show promise for the train-the-trainer model and remote feedback as a method of diffusing interventions from the clinic to the community.

A multitude of other programs have been developed, sometimes incorporating aspects of different models. Most are reported as pilot RCT studies with very few participants. One such model for a teacher-implemented program is STAR, which includes DTT, PRT, and structured teaching methods (Arick, Krug, Loos, & Falco, 2004). STAR, only examined in one single group pre–post study for preschoolers, was found to improve social interaction and expressive speech (Arick et al., 2003). In an RCT, STAR was examined with older school-age students to find mixed effectiveness on child DQ and was apparently based on teacher fidelity to the program (Mandell et al., 2013). Another teacher-delivered program, the Comprehensive Autism Program (CAP; combining STAR, PRT, and DTT), was evaluated by a study that involved 84 teachers and 320 preschoolers with ASD (Young, Falco, & Hanita, 2016). This study found small effects on child receptive language and teacher-reported social skills. Effects were stronger for those with more severe ASD symptoms. One examination looked at the addition of a computer-assisted instruction program accompanied with in-class activities versus a wait-list control in a large public school district and found that those using the computer program showed improvement in language and cognitive outcomes (Whalen et al., 2010).

Summary

What Do We Know?

The previous review of evidence for early intervention is not exhaustive but covers most of the RCTs published for interventions for children with ASD, ages 2–5. A consistent picture begins to emerge about the state of the science for early interventions. While comprehensive intervention programs are indicated, given the broad developmental needs of children with ASD, current models are limited to positive effects on overall cognition (DQ as measured by the MSEL or similar standardized measures), with unknown or limited effect on core ASD deficits of social communication and restricted interests and repetitive behaviors. Current comprehensive models show some positive effects in randomized trials but are complicated by lack of efficacy on replication trials (Dawson et al., 2010; Rogers et al., 2019; Sallows & Graupner, 2005; Smith et al., 2000). Comprehensive models have yet to explicate the mechanisms (active ingredients) underlying the model and to show who may or may not benefit. Indeed, the focus on non-responders to early interventions has been a topic of recent, as yet unpublished, studies. To date, we cannot refute any of the best practice assumptions made in the National Academy Sciences report of 2001 (see below). It may be that as these recommendations are implemented, we have greater difficulty showing that the experimental early intervention in research studies is superior to the counterfactual. This is certainly not a bad place to be. We need interventions to improve in the community, so that more children can reach their optimal outcome (Georgiades & Kasari, 2018). Yet, we still

(text resumes on page 150)

TABLE 4.1. Preschool Interventions: RCTs for Children with ASD

Authors (date)	Groups	EIBI or NDBI	Tx dur.	Age (mo)	N	Primary target	Measures	Finding
		Comprehensive: Interventionist-delivered						
*Smith, Groen, & Wynn (2000)	EIBI 30 h/wk vs. parent training 5 h/wk	EIBI	2 yr	18–42	28	IQ	S-B, BSID, M-P, REY, VABS, ABC	Significant EIBI effect for cognitive, nonverbal, and language skills, but no other effects
*Sallows & Graupner (2005)	EIBI 37 h/wk vs. parent-directed 30 h/wk	EIBI	4 yr	36	24	IQ	BSID, M-P, REY, VABS, WPPSI, WISC-II, CBCL, ELM	No group differences on measures
*Dawson et al. (2010)	ESDM 20 h/wk vs. TAU approx. 20 h/wk	NDBI-ESDM	2 yr	18–30	48	MSEL, VABS	ADOS, VABS, MSEL, RBS, ADI-R	ESDM group had significant treatment effect on IQ, adaptive behaviors, and autism symptoms
*Estes et al. (2015)	2-year follow-up to Dawson et al. (2010)				39	MSEL, VABS	ADOS, VABS, MSEL, RBS, ADI-R	ESDM group maintained gains and group differences for autism symptoms and adaptive behaviors but not for IQ
Dawson et al. (2012)	Secondary outcome of Dawson et al. (2010)				48	ERP	ADOS, VABS, MSEL, RBS, ADI-R, EEG	ERP of ESDM group was more similar to TD children than to the control group
*Landa et al. (2011)	Class + EA 12.5 h/wk vs. class only 10 h/wk	NDBI	6 mo	21–33	50	IJA	CSBS, behavioral videos, MSEL	Treatment has significant effect for imitation with eye contact that generalized and maintained, but no effect for IJA or positive affect
*Whitehouse et al. (2017)	TOBY plus TAU 1.5 h/wk vs. TAU only	TOBY app for ABA	6 mo	39	80	ATEC	VABS, MSEL, ATEC, MCDI	No group difference on overall outcome but treatment group improves on specific subscales
*Rogers et al. (2019)	ESDM 1:1 20 h/wk + 1 h parent coaching/wk vs. TAU	NDBI-ESDM	2 yr	12–24	118	MSEL EL	MSEL, VABS, ADOS, JA task	Equal group gains, some sites show treatment effect on language; no other group effects; 40% attrition in community group

						Targeted:	Interventionist-delivered	
*Yoder & Stone (2006)	RPMT 1 h/wk vs. PECS 1 h/wk	NDBI	6 mo	18–60	36	IJA	ESCS, PCX, unstructured free play	RPMT group has greater joint attention initiations
*Kasari, Freeman, & Paparella (2006)	JA 2.5 h/wk vs. SP 2.5 h/wk vs. control	NDBI-JASPER	5 wk	36–48	58	ESCS and SPA	ESCS, SPA, PCX, MSEL, REY	JA group has significant gains in RJA and IJA; SP group has significant gains in diversity of play and play levels
*Gulsrud et al. (2007)	Use Kasari et al. (2006) data			33–54	35	JA	Coded probe responses	JA group more likely to acknowledge and respond to novel probe with JA
*Kasari, Paparella, Freeman, & Jahromi (2008)	1-year follow-up to Kasari et al. (2006)			36–48	58	ESCS and SPA	ESCS, SPA, PCX, MSEL, REY	JA and SP have greater growth in expressive language, types of play, and play level
*Lawton & Kasari (2012a)	Use Kasari et al. (2006) data			36–48	58	ESCS	ESCS	Higher JA quality in JA and SP groups
*Kasari et al. (2012)	5-year follow-up to Kasari et al. (2006)			36–48	40	EVT, DAS	ESCS, SPA, EVT, DAS, PCX	80% have functional language; cognition and language predicted by play at baseline, vocabulary predicted by IJA and intervention
*Gulsrud et al. (2014)	5-year follow-up to Kasari et al. (2006)			36–48	40	ESCS, EVT	ESCS, EVT	JA group has most growth in JA looks and showing, early pointing predicts later language
*Wong & Kwan (2010)	Autism 1-2-3 2.5 h/wk vs. WL	ABA	2 wk	17–36	17	ADOS, RFRLRS	ADOS, RFRLRS, SPT, PSI	Individual groups show improvements, but between-group comparisons were not conducted
*Ingersoll (2010)	Pilot of Ingersoll (2012)				21	Imit.	MIS, UIA	Significant treatment effect for elicited and spontaneous imitation
*Ingersoll (2012)	RIT 3 h/week vs. control	NDBI-RIT	10 wk	27–47	27	Imit.	PLS, ESCS, BSID, MIS, UIA	Significant treatment effect for IJA and social–emotional functioning

(continued)

141

TABLE 4.1. (continued)

Authors (date)	Groups	EIBI or NDBI	Tx dur.	Age (mo)	N	Primary target	Measures	Finding
*Lim & Draper (2011)	Music + ABA 15 m/wk vs. speech + ABA 15 m/wk vs. TAU	ABA-VB	2 wk	36–60	22	Verbal lang.	Verbal Production Evaluation Scale	Music and speech helped EL, but music had the most echoed language and speech had the most shared language
Williams, Gray, & Tonge (2012)	Targeted DVD 1.25 h/wk vs. noninstructional DVD 1.25 h/wk	Video	4 wk	48–84	55	Emotion	Emotion recognition and theory of mind tasks	Treatment effect only for the recognition of anger; no other treatment effects
Casenhiser, Shanker, & Stieben (2013)	MEHRIT 2 h/wk vs. TAU 4 h/wk	DSP	12 mo	24–60	51	PLS	PLS, M/CBRS, CASL	Social interactions significantly improve but not language
Casenhiser et al. (2015)	Reanalysis of Casenhiser et al. (2013)					PLS	PLS, BSID, videotapes of play	MEHRIT has significant effects on length of utterances, number of utterances, and speech type
*Kaiser & Roberts (2013)	EMT therapist only vs. EMT parent + therapist 3 additional hr	NDBI-EMT	4 mo	30–54	77	Lang.	Leiter, PPVT, EVT, PLS-4, LS, MCDI, CBCL, PSI	No group differences on language measures, parent group has effect on observational measures and parents are able to use EMT strategies
*Thompson, McFerran, & Gold (2014)	Music therapy + intervention vs. intervention only	EIBI	16 wk	36–60	23	VABS	VABS, SRS, MCDI, engagement	Treatment effect on socialization and improvement in parent–child relationship; no other group effects
*Schreibman & Stahmer (2014)	PRT 10 h/wk vs. PECS 10 h/wk	NDBI-PRT	23 wk	24–48	39	EL	MSEL, MCDI, VABS, E/ROWPVT	No group differences, spoken language improvements in both

Study	Intervention	Type	Duration	Age (mo)	N	Primary measure	Measures	Outcomes
Bremer, Balogh, & Lloyd (2015)	Motor intervention 1 h/wk vs. WL	ABA	12 wk	48	9	Motor skills	PPVT, Movement Battery, VABS, SSIS, videos	Significant effect for object manipulation and motor domain but no effect for global measures
*Roberts & Kaiser (2015)	Caregiver-implemented EMT 2 sessions/wk vs. WL	NDBI-EMT	3 mo	24–42	97	PLS	PLS, PSI, PPVT, MCDI, E/ROWPVT	Significant group effect on receptive language only; parents improve strategy use
*Hampton et al. (2017)	1-year follow-up to Roberts & Kaiser (2015)							No group differences; those with RL/EL delays were persistently delayed at follow-up
Comprehensive: Caregiver-delivered								
Jocelyn et al. (1998)	Daycare + parent ed & bx training 3 h/wk vs. daycare only	ABA	10 wk	24–72	35	IQ, CARS	CARS, TAQ, EIDP	Parent ed had significant gains in child language and caregiver outcomes; no group differences on cognition or ASD symptoms
Rickards et al. (2007)	Home-based + center-based 6.5 h/wk vs. center-based 5 h/wk	ABA	12 mo	36–60	59	IQ	BSID, WPPSI-R, MSEL, VABS, PBCL	No differences on outcomes, but children with the additional home component improved most in high-stress families
*Nefdt et al. (2010)	1 h DVD with 12 chapters vs. WL	NDBI-PRT	—	< 60	27	EL	Videos coded for language and fidelity	Parents significantly improve behaviors and increase child communication
*Pajareya & Nopmaneejumruslers (2011)	DIR 20 h/wk vs. TAU	NDBI-Floortime	3 mo	24–72	32	FEAS	CARS, FEAS, FEDQ	DIR group had significant gains on all measures—functional development, autism symptoms, and emotional development

(continued)

TABLE 4.1. *(continued)*

Authors (date)	Groups	EIBI or NDBI	Tx dur.	Age (mo)	N	Primary target	Measures	Finding
Roberts et al. (2011)	Home-based 1 h/wk vs. center-based 2 h/wk vs. WL	ABA	40 wk	36–60	85	VABS, DBC	PSI, VABS, REY, DBC, BFQL	Center-based has significant effect on social communication and parent perception, but variability in response
*Rogers et al. (2012)	P-ESDM 1 h/wk vs. TAU >4 h/wk	NDBI-ESDM	12 wk	12–24	98	MSEL, ADOS	ADOS, MSEL, VABS, MCDI	No group differences on parent or child outcome measures
*Rogers et al. (2019)	P-ESDM 1.5 h clinic/wk vs. enhanced P-ESDM + 1.5 h/wk home	NDBI-ESDM	12 wk	12–30	45	MSEL DQ, VABS	MSEL, VABS, ADOS, PATH-CC, CBCL	Enhanced group has significant effect on improving parent interaction skill; no treatment effect on child outcomes; parent change related to child gains
*Solomon et al. (2014)	PLAY + special ed 15 h/wk vs. special ed only	NDBI-PLAY	12 mo	36–60	128	None ID'd	ADOS, MSEL, PSI, FEAS, M/CBRS,	Significant group improvements for PLAY group for parent/child interaction and social functioning
*Wetherby et al. (2014)	Individual ESI 2–3 sessions/wk vs. group-ESI 1/wk	NDBI	9 mo	16–20	82	None ID'd	ADOS, VABS, MSEL, CSBS	Individual ESI has group effect on social communication, VABS, and RL
*Turner-Brown et al. (2019)	TEACCH 1.25 h/wk vs. TAU	TEACCH	6 mo	<36	50	ADOS, MSEL	ADOS, MSEL, PIA, PSI, RAND-36	Significant treatment benefit for parent stress and well-being but no effect on global child outcomes
*Ingersoll et al. (2016)	Therapist-assist ImPACT 1 h/wk vs. self-directed ImPACT online	NDBI-ImPACT	6 mo	19–73	28	None ID'd	VABS, MCDI, PSOC, parent intervention	Therapist-assisted group improved in social skills only, both groups improved on other measures

144

					Targeted: Parent-delivered			
Drew et al. (2002)	Parent training 0.5 h/wk vs. TAU	Blend	12 mo	22	24	MDCI	MCDI, PSI	Minimal group differences
*Aldred, Green, & Adams (2004)	PACT 3 h/wk vs. TAU	NDBI-PACT	2 yr	24–72	28	ADOS	ADOS, VABS, MCDI, PSI, PCX	Significant treatment effect on ADOS
*Green et al. (2010)	PACT 1 h/wk vs. TAU	NDBI-PACT	13 mo	24–60	152	ADOS	ADOS, PCX, VABS, PLS, MCDI, CSBSDP	Significant treatment effect for parent synchrony but no effect on ASD severity
*Pickles et al. (2016)	Follow-up to Green et al. (2010)			24–48	121	ADOS	ADOS, DCMA, language composite	Parent synchrony effects did not maintain to follow-up, and group effects vs. TAU are minimal
Oosterling et al. (2010)	FOCUS parent training 8 h/wk vs. TAU	Blend	2 yr	34	75	MCDI, ADOS	ADOS, MCDI, CBCL, Erikson	No group effects on child outcomes
*Kasari et al. (2010)	Caregiver-mediated 2 h/wk vs. WL	NDBI-JASPER	8 wk	21–36	38	JE	PCX	Significant treatment effect for JE, RJA, and play diversity, maintained 1 year later
Gulsrud, Jahromi, & Kasari (2010)	Use Kasari et al. (2010) data			21–36	34	ER	Videotaped PCX	After intervention, children decrease negativity and mothers increase scaffolding
*Carter et al. (2011)	Hanen's 1 session/wk vs. TAU	NDBI-Hanen's	3.5 mo	15–25	62	EL and Parent bx	STAT, VABS, ESCS, dyad play, DPA, FOT	No significant treatment effects on child or parent measures
Schertz et al. (2013)	JAML 3 h/wk vs. TAU	NDBI-JAML	16 wk	< 30	23	JA	Focusing on faces and RJA, MSEL, VABS	Time effects for the intervention but no significant group differences
*Siller, Hutman, & Sigman (2013)	FPI 90 m/wk vs. parent advocacy approx. 20 m/wk	NDBI-FPI	12 wk	33–82	70	EL and Parent bx	MSEL, ADOS, ESCS	Significant group effect for FPI on children's EL at follow-up, strongest when baseline language level is below 12 months at entry

(continued)

TABLE 4.1. (continued)

Authors (date)	Groups	EIBI or NDBI	Tx dur.	Age (mo)	N	Primary target	Measures	Finding
*Tonge et al. (2014)	PEBM 1.25 h/wk vs. parent ed counseling 1.25 h/wk vs. TAU	ABA	20 wk	30–60	105	VABS	VABS, DBC, PEP-R, S-B, REY	PEBM significantly improved in adaptive bx and ASD symptoms vs. others and improved on communication, social, and daily living
*Kasari et al. (2014b)	Caregiver-mediated 2 h/wk vs. caregiver education 2 h/wk	NDBI-JASPER	3 mo	42	112	JE	MSEL, PCX, SPA, ESCS	Significantly greater gains in joint engagement and IJA in CMM are maintained at follow-up
Carr et al. (2016)	Use Kasari et al. (2014b) data					Tx adherence	Treatment attendance and adherence, videos	Intervention gains predicted by treatment attendance; attendance predicted by SES and intervention
*Kasari et al. (2015)	Caregiver-mediated 1 h/wk vs. caregiver education 1 h/wk	NDBI-JASPER	10 wk	21–36	82	JE	Videos coded for JE and play	Significant treatment effect on JE was maintained at follow-up, treatment effects on play, and generalization to the classroom
*Hardan et al. (2015)	Group PRT 1.5 h/wk vs. group parent education 1.5 h/wk	NDBI-PRT	12 wk	24–72	53	Lang. freq.	Video coded for fidelity and lang., MCDI, VABS, SRS, CGI	PRT group has greater improvement in language and parents were able to learn PRT
*Grahame et al. (2015)	MRB 2 h/wk vs. control	ABA	8 wk	36–72	45	RBQ, CGI, parent–child bx	SRS, CGI, VABS, PCX, RBQ-2	MRB intervention significantly improves RRBs into follow-up vs. the control and improves parent self-efficacy
*Bearss et al. (2015)	Parent training 45 m/week vs. parent education 45 m/week	ABA	24 wk	36–72	180	Problem bx	ABC-I, CGI, HSQ-ASD	Significantly greater decrease for parent training group in aberrant behavior and home behavior, and greater CGI improvement

Study	Intervention	NDBI	Duration	Age	N		Measures	Outcomes
*Scahill et al. (2016)	Secondary measure report of Bearss et al. (2015)					VABS	VABS, ADOS, ABC, HSQ-ASD, S-B, MSEL, CGI	Parent training group has moderate improvement in daily living skills versus parent education; no other group differences
Rahman et al. (2016)	PASS 30 m/wk vs. TAU	NDBI-PACT	6 mo	24–108	65	Parent and child dyad	Dyadic Comm. Measure for Autism; VABS	PASS significantly improves parent synchrony and child initiation of communication but no other outcomes
Fletcher-Watson et al. (2016)	App vs. TAU	App	2 mo	<72	54	BOSCC	BOSCC, MSEL, ADOS, MCDI, CSBS	No significant group difference in child or parent outcomes
Ginn et al. (2017)	PCIT 1 h/wk vs. WL	NDBI-PCIT	10 wk	36–72	30	None ID'd	CARS, DAS, PPVT, ECBI, DPICS-III, PSI, SRS, word count	PCIT group significantly improved parenting behaviors; fewer disruptive behaviors and less distress, no other group differences
*Vernon et al. (2019)	PRISM 8 h/wk vs. WL	NDBI-PRT	6 mo	18–56	23	PLS	PLS, ADOS, MSEL, EVT, PPVT, VABS	Significant changes in PRISM not found in WL on ADOS severity, Mullen EL, PLS, and PPVT with no changes on EVT and VABS
				Teacher-delivered				
*Whalen et al. (2010)	TeachTown 20 m/day computer program vs. TAU	NDBI-PRT	9 mo	36–72	47	CARS	CARS, PPVT, EVT	TeachTown group shows significant treatment effect on PPVT, EVT, and cognition
*Lawton & Kasari (2012b)	JASPER 5 h/wk vs. WL	NDBI-JASPER	5 wk	36–60	16	JE, JA, and play	ESCS, class observation, TCX	JASPER teachers use the strategies to improve their students' JE and JA
*Kaale, Smith, & Sponheim (2012)	JA + preschool 3.5 h/wk vs. preschool only	NDBI-JASPER	8 wk	29–60	61	JA	ESCS, PCX, MSEL	JA group has more JA initiation and the effect generalizes to longer JE with caregivers

(continued)

TABLE 4.1. (continued)

Authors (date)	Groups	EIBI or NDBI	Tx dur.	Age (mo)	N	Primary target	Measures	Finding
*Wong (2013)	SP, then JA 1 h/wk vs. JA, then SP 1 h/wk vs. WL	NDBI-JASPER	8 wk	36–72	33	JE, JA, and play	ESCS, SPA, classroom observation, CARS, MSEL	Significantly improve JE; intervention groups have significant gains in JA and play after 8 but not after 4 weeks
Goods et al. (2013)	JASPER 1 h/wk vs. TAU	NDBI-JASPER	12 wk	36–60	15	ESCS and SPA	MSEL, REY, SPA, classroom observation, ESCS	Significant treatment effect on play, initiation of gestures, and time spent unengaged
Ruble et al. (2013)	Face-to-face 4.5 h vs. Web 4.5 h vs. placebo	COMPASS	2 mo	36–108	49	Goal mastery	PET-GAS, DAS	No differences, both groups have significant cognitive gains
*Young, Falco, & Hanita (2016)	CAP vs. BAU classrooms	Mixed-PRT and DTT	8 mo	36–60	302	EL, RL, social skills	VABS, BDI-2, E/ROWPVT, ASIEP-3, SSRS	Small treatment effect on student receptive language and social skills moderated by ASD severity
*Chang et al. (2016)	JASPER 2.5 h/wk vs. WL	NDBI-JASPER	8 wk	36–60	66	JE, JA, and play	MSEL, TCX, ESCS, SPA	Teachers at high fidelity; intervention effect in JE, JA gestures, language, and play skills
*Shire et al. (2017)	JASPER 2.5 h/wk vs. TAU 2.5 h/wk	NDBI-JASPER	10 wk	31	113	JE, JA, and play	MSEL, TCX, SPACE, CGI	Trained to 80% fidelity, and JASPER had significant effects in child-initiated JE, JA, and play
*Vivanti et al. (2019)	G-ESDM in autism-only class vs. G-ESDM in inclusive class	NDBI-ESDM	9 mo	15–32	44	LENA	LENA, M-COSMIC, MSEL, VABS	Improvements across both groups not significantly different

| *Boyd et al. (2018) | ASAP 2 h/mo vs. TAU | NDBI-JASPER based | 4 yr | 36–60 | 161 | JE, JA, play | ADOS, SP | Significant treatment effect on classroom engagement, no group differences on other outcomes |

Note. *Discussed in text; ABA, applied behavior analysis; ABA-VB, Applied Behavior Analysis: Verbal Behavior; ABC, Achenbach Behavior Checklist; *ABC-I, Autism Behavior Checklist–Irritability Subscale; ADI, Autism Diagnostic Interview; ADI-R, Autism Diagnostic Interview—Revised; ADOS, Autism Diagnostic Observation Schedule; ASAP, advancing social communication and play; ASD, autism spectrum disorder; ASIEP-3, Autism Screening Instrument for Educational Planning—Third Edition; ATEC, Autism Treatment Evaluation Checklist; BAU, business as usual; BDI, Battelle Developmental Inventory; BFQL, Beach Family Quality of Life Questionnaire; BOSCC, Brief Observation of Social Communication Change; BSID, Bayley Scales of Infant Development; bx, behavior; CAP, Comprehensive Autism Program; CARS, Childhood Autism Rating Scale; CASL, Comprehensive Assessment of Spoken Language; CBCL, Child Behavior Checklist; CGI, Clinical Global Impressions; Comm., communication; COMPASS, Collaborative Model for Promoting Competence and Success; CSBS, Communication and Symbolic Behavior Scales; CMM, Caregiver-Mediated Modules; CSBS DP, Communication and Symbolic Behavior Scales Developmental Profile; DAS, Differential Ability Scales; DBC, Developmental Behavior Checklist; DCMA, Dyadic Communication Assessment Measure; DIR, Developmental, Individual-Differences, Relationship-Based Model/Floortime; DPA, Developmental Play Assessment; DPICS, Dyadic Parent–Child Interaction Coding System; DQ, developmental quotient; DSP, Developmental Social Pragmatic; DTT, discrete trial teaching; E/ROWPVT, Expressive/Receptive One Word Picture Vocabulary Test; EA, early achievements; ECBI, Eyberg Child Behavior Inventory; EEG, electroencephalogram; EIBI, early intensive behavioral intervention; EIDP, Early Intervention Developmental Profile; EL, expressive language; ELM, Early Learning Measure; EMT, enhanced milieu treatment; ER, emotion regulation; ERP, Event-Related Potential; ESCS, Early Social Communication Scales; ESDM, Early Start Denver Model; ESI, early social interaction; EVT, Expressive Vocabulary Test; FEAS, Functional Emotional Assessment Scale; FEDQ, Functional Emotional Developmental Questionnaire; FOT, fidelity of treatment; FPI, Focused Playtime Intervention; Freq, frequency; G-ESDM, group-based Early Start Denver Model; HSQ-ASQ, Home Situations Questionnaire–Autism Spectrum Disorder; IJA, initiations of joint attention; imit, imitation; imPACT, improving parents as communication teachers; IQ, intelligence quotient; JA, joint attention; JAML, joint attention mediated learning; JASPER, joint attention, symbolic play, engagement, and regulation; JE, joint engagement; LENA, Language Environment Analysis; LS, language sample; M/CBRS, Maternal/Child Behavior Rating Scale; M-COSMIC, Modified Classroom Observation Schedule to Measure Intentional Communication; MCDI, MacArthur Communicative Development Inventory; MEHRIT, Milton and Ethel Harris Research Initiative treatment program; MIS, Motor Imitation Scale; M-P, Merrill-Palmer; MRB, Managing Repetitive Behaviors Programme; MSEL, Mullen Scales of Early Learning; NDBI, Naturalistic Developmental Behavioral Intervention; P-ESDM, parent-delivered Early Start Denver Model; PACT, Preschool Autism Communication Trial; PASS, parent-mediated intervention for autism spectrum disorders in South Asia; PATH-CC, PATH Curriculum Checklist; PBCL, Preschool Behavior Checklist; PCIT, Parent–Child Interaction Therapy; PCX, Parent–Child Interaction; PEBM, parent education and behavior management; PECS, Picture Exchange Communication System; PEP-R, Psychoeducational Profile–Revised; PET-GAS, Psychometrically Equivalence Tested Goal Attainment Scaling; PIA, Parent Interview for Autism; PLAY, Play and Language for Autistic Youngsters; PLS, Preschool Language Scale; PPVT, Peabody Picture Vocabulary Test; PRISM, pivotal response intervention for social motivation; PRT, pivotal response training; PSI, Parenting Stress Index; PSOC, Parent Sense of Competence Scale; RBQ, Repetitive Behavior Questionnaire; RBS, Repetitive Behavior Scales; REY, Reynell; RFRLRS, Ritvo-Freeman Real Life Rating Scale; RIT, reciprocal imitation training; RJA, responding joint attention; RL, receptive language; RPMT, responsive education and prelinguistic milieu training; RRB, restricted and repetitive behavior; S-B, Stanford–Binet; SES, socioeconomic status; SP, symbolic play; SPA, spontaneous play assessment; SPACE, Symbolic Place and Communication Examination; SPT, Symbolic Play Test; SRS, Social Responsiveness Scale; SSIS, Social Skills Improvement System; SSRS, Social Skills Rating System; STAT, Screening Tool for Autism in Two-Year Olds; TAQ, The Activity Questionnaire; TAU, treatment as usual; TCX, Teacher–Child Interaction; TD, typically developing; TEACCH, Treatment and Education of Autistic and Related Communication Handicapped Children; TOBY (Therapy Outcomes by You); tx, treatment; UIA, Unstructured Imitation Assessment; VABS, Vineland Adaptive Behavior Scales; WISC, Weschler Intelligence Scale for Children; WL, wait list; WPPSI, Weschler Preschool and Primary Scale of Intelligence.

149

have room for improvement. Since anywhere from 30 to 50% of children enter school without fluent language and show impairments in core deficits (social communication and restricted, repetitive behaviors) (Anderson et al., 2007), there continues to be room for innovation in interventions.

We argue that innovation is likely to be achieved through use of a modular, personalized approach to early intervention. Indeed, a lot of innovations have already been reported, with significant effects on child outcomes against the backdrop of their usual community intervention. Combining modules or using a module to target an area of deficiency may more readily improve outcomes for individual children. Applying these innovations to the most underrepresented children in research, those with comorbid intellectual disability, with minimal language, or rare genetic syndromes, may improve outcomes for far more children in our community settings which cannot include some children and exclude others.

In addition to effective targeted interventions focused on teaching parents to reduce behavior problems, or those used by therapists to improve core social communication deficits, we are seeing an increase in translational intervention programs. More studies are focused on the implementation practices of community practitioners, with positive outcomes on children (Chang et al., 2016; Kaale et al., 2012; Shire et al., 2017). Train-the-trainer, remote support, and community-partnered research have proven to be effective models for teaching teachers and paraprofessionals to implement clinic-based interventions (Ingersoll, 2012; Shire et al., 2017). We know that staff members can be trained in targeted interventions, can implement these interventions at high fidelity, and can use the strategies they learn to improve their students' engagement, joint attention, and play (Chang et al., 2016; Shire et al., 2017, 2019).

Our confidence in treatment models, however, needs the additional support of studies with far greater methodological rigor and studies that examine for whom the intervention works best, and why the intervention might work. Currently, few studies examine moderators, mediators, and long-term outcomes. For example, we understand that a single intervention will not be effective for all children. Researchers are beginning to study subgroups of underrepresented children, such as those who are slow to develop language or who have comorbid intellectual disabilities (Paparella, Goods, Freeman, & Kasari, 2011). New designs are being applied in order to study responders and nonresponders to particular interventions (Kasari, Sturm, & Shih, 2018). In other work, we are beginning to address the mechanisms underlying why an intervention is effective for certain outcomes. In parent-mediated interventions, parent-mirrored pacing and parent synchronization are associated with the social communication outcomes of children (Gulsrud, Hellemann, Shire, & Kasari, 2016; Pellecchia et al., 2015; Aldred, Green, Emsley, & McConachie, 2012; Bono, Daley, & Sigman, 2004). For more about long-term outcomes of infants at risk for

ASD, see Chapter 7. Long-term treatment outcomes, though sparse, have only been published for a few models, including ESDM, JASPER, PACT, and EIBI. Those in Lovaas's original study, approximately 4.5 years later, who had achieved the best outcomes, maintained average intelligence and adaptive behavior, with the rest of the experimental group also maintaining their gains (McEachin et al., 1993). Five years after the original JA/SP study, functional language was predicted by play level at baseline, cognitive scores were predicted by play diversity at baseline, and vocabulary was predicted by IJA and intervention group membership (Kasari et al., 2012). Pickles et al. (2016) found that 5 years after intervention, there were no group effects of the PACT intervention, with both interventions improving child outcomes over time. While these studies begin to reveal for whom an intervention works, why an intervention works, and how long gains with intervention last, much more research is needed to further inform future effective models of early intervention.

What Is Next?

A review of interventions for preschool children with ASD points to clear gaps, particularly when addressing the 2001 National Research Council goals for intervention. Despite developing interventions that effectively improve core deficits with delivery by interventionists, parents, or teachers, a number of the 2001 goals for intervention for children with ASD and their families remain unaddressed. These gaps should be the focus of future studies and represent the next step in intervention research. Comparing the original National Research Council recommendations to current preschool intervention literature reveals a need for more investigation into (1) personalizing intervention by identifying subcategories within the ASD spectrum, isolating specific strategies of interventions for specific aspects of ASD, and adequately comparing different interventions to combine them into a personalized program; (2) supporting families by effectively training and educating parents; (3) developing interventions that generalize to promote independence and have effects beyond the initial treatment period, with frequent ongoing measurement; and (4) developing more precise measurement of outcome.

Personalization of Intervention

Heterogeneity is a well-established aspect of ASD that affects intervention outcome but remains inadequately addressed in intervention development (Howlin, Magiati, & Charman, 2009; Fernell & Gillberg, 2010). Community providers recognize heterogeneity in intervention planning and response and do not choose just one intervention but rather use a combination of evidence-based and non-evidence-based interventions in ways they were not designed to be combined (Stahmer, Collings, & Palinkas, 2005). Across all evidence-based approaches, 50% of children make substantial gains, while 50% make variable or limited progress (Stahmer, Schreibman, & Cunningham, 2011). Individual differences within ASD have been characterized based on personality, neurocognitive profile, symptom severity, cognitive scores, verbal ability, joint attention skills, and peer engagement, but these characterizations are not yet systematically organized (Tager-Flusberg & Joseph, 2003; Schwartzman, Wood, & Kapp, 2016; Georgiades et al., 2013; Sherer & Schreibman, 2005; Anderson et al., 2007; Shih, Patterson, & Kasari, 2016). In particular, having few spoken words, low social motivation, and less joint attention initiation is linked to a decreased response to intervention, independent of IQ scores (Kasari et al., 2008; Bopp, Mirenda, & Zumbo, 2009). Further, despite minimal verbal language being a known predictor of treatment response, there is heterogeneity within the minimally verbal subgroup, and few interventions have been designed to address this heterogeneity and response to intervention (Tager-Flusberg & Kasari, 2013).

The heterogeneity of the ASD phenotype leads to large heterogeneity in response to intervention, with some children responding quickly and others responding more slowly to an intervention. Investigations as to what characteristics may predict or be related to response to an intervention are just beginning but show promise in the hopes of creating more personalized interventions. For example, Sherer and Schreibman (2005) found that response to PRT may be related to higher levels of toy play and lower levels of avoidance. A follow-up found that improving toy play can lead to an improved PRT response (Schreibman, Stahmer, Barlett, & Dufek, 2009). These types of studies are essential to understanding how all individuals with ASD can best succeed and become responders.

There are some promising approaches to experimentally evaluating the best method for targeting a child's individual needs, however. Sequential Multiple Assignment Randomized Trials (SMART designs) offer the opportunity to test sequences of intervention that are adaptive based on child response. In this design, a child is initially randomized to receive one of two treatments and is then assessed for response to intervention midway through the study. Based on response status (responder or nonresponder), the child is then re-randomized to one of multiple interventions. The goal in this type of design is to determine not just what intervention may be most effective, but what intervention may be most effective for whom—and in which order. Kasari et al. (2014a) used a SMART design to look at the impact of adding an alternative and augmentative communication (AAC) device to JASPER intervention by comparing groups initially randomized to JASPER alone or JASPER plus and AAC with the option of staying the course, intensifying treatment, or adding AAC upon the second randomization. Results indicated that those who started with an AAC made the most improvements in socially communicative utterances and spontaneous comments.

Personalized medicine is a growing trend in the biological sciences and medical field and has only recently been applied to mental health disorders and ASD (Almirall & Chronis-Tuscano, 2016). Bringing together components of interventions or modular programs according to child characteristics has been examined for conduct disorder, anxiety, and depression and is needed to address the varied needs and responses of ASD (Hawes, Dadds, Brennan, Rhodes, & Cauchi, 2013; Almirall, Compton, Gunlicks-Stoessel, Duan, & Murphy, 2012; Dawson, Lavori, Luby, Ryan, & Geller, 2007). While limited preliminary work has been done for personalized clinic-based, therapist-delivered interventions, there is no established and systematic adaptive approach and no known attempts to personalize parent-mediated programs. Testing separately developed modular interventions together presents a realistic scenario of how these clinic-developed, evidence-based approaches can be combined by community service providers.

Family Support

Interviews with parents of children with ASD reveal that parent quality of life is heavily dependent on the child's service situation, the family's financial burden, and parental physical health (Kuhlthau et al., 2014). Depressive symptoms in parents are higher when their child has fewer social communication skills, more ASD symptomology present, and in particular more behavioral problems (Baker-Ericzén, Brookman-Frazee, & Stahmer, 2005; Barker et al., 2011; Zablotsky, Anderson, & Law, 2013). The rate of depression in parents of a child with ASD is estimated to be 20%, over two times the percentage in parents whose child does not have ASD (8%), and about three times the national average (6%) (Cohrs & Leslie, 2017). Parents of children with ASD also have anxiety that may decrease over time, but parent depression is stable or may even increase (Barker et al., 2011). National Resource Council guidelines have concluded that parents are vital to their child's education and should be provided additional support for their increased stress (National Research Council, 2001). However, the lowest level of implementation of the National Resource Council's guidelines occurs in the area of family support (Tincani, Cucchiarra, Thurman, Snyder, & McCarthy, 2013). Previous studies have shown that a high level of parent stress is associated with unsuccessful child interactions and diminished treatment outcomes (Kasari & Sigman, 1997; Osborne, McHugh, Saunders, & Reed, 2008). Parent support and parent-mediated interventions have shown mixed effectiveness when it comes to improving both child and parent outcomes (e.g., Patterson, Smith, & Mirenda, 2012;

Oono, Honey, & McConachie, 2013). Optimal child outcomes depend on optimal parent mental health and parent knowledge. Future parent education and training programs need to ensure that both parent and child outcomes are central to the intervention.

Generalization

Generalization is infrequently included as an outcome measure for ASD interventions and therefore has been noted as a challenge in early intervention (Smith & Iadarola, 2015). Generalization refers to applying a skill or an idea in a context other than the specific context in which it was learned. A few studies have included measures of generalization to find that JA skills may generalize to other people, other settings, and over time, but measures of generalization and maintenance are still not standard components of research designs (Kaale, Fagerland, Martinsen, & Smith, 2014; Kasari et al., 2008, 2015). Parents are particularly powerful in solidifying learned skills as they are present in all contexts of a child's daily experience. Parents can consistently use teaching strategies to create continued learning opportunities and ensure that their child's skills are maintained after intervention support ends (e.g., Kaiser, Hancock, & Nietfeld, 2000; Kasari et al., 2015). Establishing generalization across natural contexts and daily activities is needed to investigate the efficacy of parent-mediated interventions.

Choice of Outcome Measure

Choice of outcome is essential for measurement of an intervention's effectiveness. Outcomes of intervention are generally cognitive functioning, or ASD symptomatology. These measures are weakly related to social communication, a core deficit of ASD, and may be poorly suited to the duration and targets of ASD intervention (Kasari, 2002; Kasari & Smith, 2016). Global assessments cannot detect small, meaningful change, and in the case of ASD, appropriate measurement of small and meaningful change is essential to recording gains in areas of core deficits. Small but meaningful changes in joint attention skills have been linked to meaningful gains in verbal language (Kasari et al., 2012). Despite the inability of global measures of functioning to capture core deficits of ASD and changes in core deficits, they persist as primary outcome measures. Additionally, parent and self-report questionnaires are frequently used as main sources for outcome measurement (Lord et al., 2005). A literature review for interventions reveals that there are few agreed-upon assessments standardized to measure change in core deficits of ASD (Anagnostou et al., 2015). There also remains a need for more nuanced measures of adaptive functioning, as this outcome has relevance across the lifespan.

Preschool interventions for children with ASD have proliferated, but there are still gaps in the literature that remain. Autism intervention research, having established the effectiveness of early individualized programs, needs to begin to compare programs, focus on parent and child outcomes at the same time, and develop personalized courses of intervention.

ACKNOWLEDGMENTS

We acknowledge funding from the National Institutes of Health to Connie Kasari (Grants R01HD073975, P50HD055784, and 5R01HD090138-04) from National Institute of Child Health and Human Development (Grant 5P50HD055784-13), and from the Health, Resources and Services Administration (Grant UA3MC11055).

REFERENCES

Aldred, C., Green, J., & Adams, C. (2004). A new social communication intervention for children with autism: Pilot randomised controlled treatment study suggesting effectiveness. *Journal of Child Psychology and Psychiatry, 45*(8), 1420–1430.

Aldred, C., Green, J., Emsley, R., & McConachie, H. (2012). Brief report: Mediation of treatment effect in a communication intervention for pre-school children with autism. *Journal of Autism and Developmental Disorders, 42*(3), 447–454.

Almirall, D., & Chronis-Tuscano, A. (2016). Adaptive interventions in child and adolescent mental health. *Journal of Clinical Child and Adolescent Psychology, 45*(4), 383–395.

Almirall, D., Compton, S. N., Gunlicks-Stoessel, M., Duan, N., & Murphy, S. A. (2012). Designing a pilot sequential multiple assignment randomized trial for developing an adaptive treatment strategy. *Statistics in Medicine, 31*(17), 1887–1902.

American Psychiatric Association. (2000). *Diagnostic and statistical manual of mental disorders* (4th ed., text rev.). Washington, DC: Author.

American Psychiatric Association. (2013). *Diagnostic and statistical manual of mental disorders* (5th ed.). Arlington, VA: Author.

Anagnostou, E., Jones, N., Huerta, M., Halladay, A. K., Wang, P., Scahill, L., . . . Sullivan, K. (2015). Measuring social communication behaviors as a treatment endpoint in individuals with autism spectrum disorder. *Autism, 19*(5), 622–636.

Anderson, D. K., Lord, C., Risi, S., DiLavore, P. S., Shulman, C., Thurm, A., . . . Pickles, A. (2007). Patterns of growth in verbal abilities among children with autism spectrum disorder. *Journal of Consulting and Clinical Psychology, 75*(4), 594.

Arick, J. R., Krug, D. A., Loos, L., & Falco, R. (2004). *The STAR Program: Strategies for Teaching Based on Autism Research: Level III.* Austin, TX: PRO-ED.

Arick, J. R., Young, H. E., Falco, R. A., Loos, L. M., Krug, D. A., Gense, M. H., & Johnson, S. B. (2003). Designing an outcome study to monitor the progress of students with autism spectrum disorders. *Focus on Autism and Other Developmental Disabilities, 18*(2), 75–87.

Baker-Ericzén, M. J., Brookman-Frazee, L., & Stahmer, A. (2005). Stress levels and adaptability in parents of toddlers with and without autism spectrum disorders. *Research and Practice for Persons with Severe Disabilities, 30*(4), 194–204.

Bakhai, A., Chhabra, A., & Wang, D. (2006). Endpoints. In D. Wang & A. Bakhai (Eds.), *Clinical trials: A practical guide to design, analysis and reporting* (pp. 37–45). London: Remedica.

Barker, E. T., Hartley, S. L., Seltzer, M. M., Floyd, F. J., Greenberg, J. S., & Orsmond, G. I. (2011). Trajectories of emotional well-being in mothers of adolescents and adults with autism. *Developmental Psychology, 47*(2), 551.

Bearss, K., Johnson, C., Smith, T., Lecavalier, L., Swiezy, N., Aman, M., . . . Sukhodolsky, D. G. (2015). Effect of parent training vs. parent education on behavioral problems in children with autism spectrum disorder: A randomized clinical trial. *JAMA, 313*(15), 1524–1533.

Bodfish J. W., Symons, F. J., & Lewis, M. H. (1998). *The Repetitive Behavior Scale: A test manual*. Morganton, NC: Western Carolina Center.

Bono, M. A., Daley, T., & Sigman, M. (2004). Relations among joint attention, amount of intervention and language gain in autism. *Journal of Autism and Developmental Disorders, 34*(5), 495–505.

Bopp, K. D., Mirenda, P., & Zumbo, B. D. (2009). Behavior predictors of language development over 2 years in children with autism spectrum disorders. *Journal of Speech, Language, and Hearing Research, 52*(5), 1106–1120.

Boyd, B. A., Hume, K., Mcbee, M. T., Alessandri, M., Gutierrez, A., Johnson, L., . . . Odom, S. L. (2014). Comparative efficacy of LEAP, TEACCH and non-model-specific special education programs for preschoolers with autism spectrum disorders. *Journal of Autism and Developmental Disorders, 44*(2), 366–380.

Boyd, B. A., Watson, L. R., Reszka, S. S., Sideris, J., Alessandri, M., Baranek, G. T., . . . Belardi, K. (2018). Efficacy of the ASAP intervention for preschoolers with ASD: A cluster randomized controlled trial. *Journal of Autism and Developmental Disorders, 48*, 3144–3162.

Bremer, E., Balogh, R., & Lloyd, M. (2015). Effectiveness of a fundamental motor skill intervention for 4-year-old children with autism spectrum disorder: A pilot study. *Autism, 19*(8), 980–991.

Bruner, J. (1985). Child's talk: Learning to use language. *Child Language Teaching and Therapy, 1*(1), 111–114.

Carr, T., Shih, W., Lawton, K., Lord, C., King, B., & Kasari, C. (2016). The relationship between treatment attendance, adherence, and outcome in a caregiver-mediated intervention for low-resourced families of young children with autism spectrum disorder. *Autism, 20*(6), 643–652.

Carter, M., Roberts, J., Williams, K., Evans, D., Parmenter, T., Silove, N., . . . Warren, A. (2011). Interventions used with an Australian sample of preschool children with autism spectrum disorders. *Research in Autism Spectrum Disorders, 5*(3), 1033–1041.

Casenhiser, D. M., Binns, A., McGill, F., Morderer, O., & Shanker, S. G. (2015). Measuring and supporting language function for children with autism: Evidence from a randomized control trial of a social-interaction-based therapy. *Journal of Autism and Developmental Disorders, 45*(3), 846–857.

Casenhiser, D. M., Shanker, S. G., & Stieben, J. (2013). Learning through interaction in children with autism: Preliminary data from asocial-communication-based intervention. *Autism, 17*(2), 220–241.

Chang, Y. C., Shire, S. Y., Shih, W., Gelfand, C., & Kasari, C. (2016). Preschool deployment of evidence-based social communication intervention: JASPER in the classroom. *Journal of Autism and Developmental Disorders, 46*(6), 2211–2223.

Charman, T., Baron-Cohen, S., Swettenham, J., Baird, G., Cox, A., & Drew, A. (2000). Testing joint attention, imitation, and play as infancy precursors to language and theory of mind. *Cognitive Development, 15*(4), 481–498.

Chorpita, B. F., & Weisz, J. R. (2009). *MATCH-ADTC: Modular approach to therapy for children with anxiety, depression, trauma, or conduct problems*. Satellite Beach, FL: PracticeWise.

Cohen, H., Amerine-Dickens, M., & Smith, T. (2006). Early intensive behavioral treatment: Replication of the UCLA model in a community setting. *Journal of Developmental and Behavioral Pediatrics, 27*(2), S145–S155.

Cohrs, A. C., & Leslie, D. L. (2017). Depression in parents of children diagnosed with autism spectrum disorder: A claims-based analysis. *Journal of Autism and Developmental Disorders, 47*(5), 1416–1422.

Dawson, G., Jones, E. J. H., Merkle, K., Venema, K., Lowy, R., Faja, S., . . . Webb, S. J. (2012). Early behavioral intervention is associated with normalized brain activity in young children with autism. *Journal of the American Academy of Child and Adolescent Psychiatry, 51*(11), 1150–1159.

Dawson, G., Rogers, S., Munson, J., Smith, M., Winter, J., Greenson, J., . . . Varley, J. (2010). Randomized, controlled trial of an intervention for toddlers with autism: The Early Start Denver Model. *Pediatrics, 125*(1), e17–e23.

Dawson, R., Lavori, P. W., Luby, J. L., Ryan, N. D., & Geller, B. (2007). Adaptive strategies for treating childhood mania. *Biological Psychiatry, 61*(6), 758–764.

Drew, A., Baird, G., Baron-Cohen, S., Cox, A., Slonims, V., Wheelwright, S., . . . Charman, T. (2002). A pilot randomised control trial of a parent training intervention for pre-school children with autism. *European Child and Adolescent Psychiatry, 11*(6), 266–272.

Eldevik, S., Eikeseth, S., Jahr, E., & Smith, T. (2006). Effects of low-intensity behavioral treatment for children with autism and mental retardation. *Journal of Autism and Developmental Disorders, 36*(2), 211–224.

Estes, A., Munson, J., Rogers, S. J., Greenson, J., Winter, J., & Dawson, G. (2015). Long-term outcomes of early intervention in 6-year-old children with autism spectrum disorder. *Journal of the American Academy of Child and Adolescent Psychiatry, 54*(7), 580–587.

Fenson, L., Dale, P. S., Reznick, J. S., Thal, D., Bates, E., Hartung, J. P., . . . Reilly, J. S. (1991). *Technical manual for the MacArthur Communicative Development Inventories*. San Diego, CA: San Diego State University.

Fernell, E., & Gillberg, C. (2010). Autism spectrum disorder diagnoses in Stockholm preschoolers. *Research in Developmental Disabilities, 31*(3), 680–685.

Fletcher-Watson, S., Petrou, A., Scott-Barrett, J., Dicks, P., Graham, C., O'Hare, A., . . . McConachie, H. (2016). A trial of an iPad™ intervention targeting social communication skills in children with autism. *Autism, 20*(7), 771–782.

Georgiades, S., & Kasari, C. (2018). Reframing optimal outcomes in autism. *JAMA Pediatrics, 172*(8), 716–717.

Georgiades, S., Szatmari, P., Boyle, M., Hanna, S., Duku, E., Zwaigenbaum, L., . . . Smith, I. (2013). Investigating phenotypic heterogeneity in children with autism spectrum disorder: A factor mixture modeling approach. *Journal of Child Psychology and Psychiatry, 54*(2), 206–215.

Ginn, N. C., Clionsky, L. N., Eyberg, S. M., Warner-Metzger, C., & Abner, J. (2017).

Child-directed interaction training for young children with autism spectrum disorders: Parent and child outcomes. *Journal of Clinical Child and Adolescent Psychology, 46*(1), 101–109.

Goods, K. S., Ishijima, E., Chang, Y., & Kasari, C. (2013). Preschool based JASPER intervention in minimally verbal children with autism: Pilot RCT. *Journal of Autism and Developmental Disorders, 43*(5), 1050–1056.

Grahame, V., Brett, D., Dixon, L., McConachie, H., Lowry, J., Rodgers, J., . . . Couteur, A. (2015). Managing repetitive behaviours in young children with autism spectrum disorder (ASD): Pilot randomised controlled trial of a new parent group intervention. *Journal of Autism and Developmental Disorders, 45*(10), 3168–3182.

Green, J., Charman, T., McConachie, H., Aldred, C., Slonims, V., Howlin, P., . . . Barrett, B. (2010). Parent-mediated communication-focused treatment in children with autism (PACT): A randomised controlled trial. *The Lancet, 375*(9732), 2152–2160.

Gulsrud, A. C., Hellemann, G. S., Freeman, S. F. N., & Kasari, C. (2014). Two to ten years: Developmental trajectories of joint attention in children with ASD who received targeted social communication interventions. *Autism Research, 7*(2), 207–215.

Gulsrud, A. C., Hellemann, G., Shire, S., & Kasari, C. (2016). Isolating active ingredients in a parent-mediated social communication intervention for toddlers with autism spectrum disorder. *Journal of Child Psychology and Psychiatry, 57*(5), 606–613.

Gulsrud, A. C., Jahromi, L. B., & Kasari, C. (2010). The co-regulation of emotions between mothers and their children with autism. *Journal of Autism and Developmental Disorders, 40*(2), 227–237.

Gulsrud, A. C., Kasari, C., Freeman, S., & Paparella, T. (2007). Children with autism's response to novel stimuli while participating in interventions targeting joint attention or symbolic play skills. *Autism, 11*(6), 535–546.

Hampton, L. H., Kaiser, A. P., & Roberts, M. Y. (2017). One-year language outcomes in toddlers with language delays: An RCT follow-up. *Pediatrics, 140*(5), e20163646.

Hancock, T. B., & Kaiser, A. P. (2002). The effects of trainer-implemented enhanced milieu teaching on the social communication of children with autism. *Topics in Early Childhood Special Education, 22*(1), 39–54.

Hardan, A. Y., Gengoux, G. W., Berquist, K. L., Libove, R. A., Ardel, C. M., Phillips, J., . . . Minjarez, M. B. (2015). A randomized controlled trial of pivotal response treatment group for parents of children with autism. *Journal of Child Psychology and Psychiatry, 56*(8), 884–892.

Harrop, C., Gulsrud, A., Shih, W., Hovsepyan, L., & Kasari, C. (2017). The impact of caregiver-mediated JASPER on child restricted and repetitive behaviors and caregiver responses. *Autism Research, 10*(5), 983–992.

Hawes, D. J., Dadds, M. R., Brennan, J., Rhodes, T., & Cauchi, A. (2013). Revisiting the treatment of conduct problems in children with callous-unemotional traits. *Australian and New Zealand Journal of Psychiatry, 47*(7), 646–653.

Horner, R. H., Carr, E. G., Halle, J., McGee, G., Odom, S., & Wolery, M. (2005). The use of single-subject research to identify evidence-based practice in special education. *Exceptional Children, 71*(2), 165–179.

Howard, J. S., Sparkman, C. R., Cohen, H. G., Green, G., & Stanislaw, H. (2005). A comparison of intensive behavior analytic and eclectic treatments for young children with autism. *Research in Developmental Disabilities, 26*(4), 359–383.

Howlin, P., Magiati, I., & Charman, T. (2009). Systematic review of early intensive behavioral interventions for children with autism. *American Journal on Intellectual and Developmental Disabilities, 114*(1), 23–41.

Howlin, P., Mawhood, L., & Rutter, M. (2000). Autism and developmental receptive language disorder—a follow-up comparison in early adult life. *Journal of Child Psychology and Psychiatry, 41*(5), 561–578.

Individuals with Disabilities Education Act, 20 U.S.C. § 1400 (2004).

Ingersoll, B. (2010). Brief report: Pilot randomized controlled trial of reciprocal imitation training for teaching elicited and spontaneous imitation to children with autism. *Journal of Autism and Developmental Disorders, 40*(9), 1154–1160.

Ingersoll, B. (2012). Effect of a focused imitation intervention on social functioning in children with autism. *Journal of Autism and Developmental Disorders, 42*(8), 1768–1773.

Ingersoll, B., & Dvortcsak, A. (2010). *Teaching social communication to children with autism: A practitioner's guide to parent training.* New York: Guilford Press.

Ingersoll, B., & Gergans, S. (2007). The effect of a parent-implemented imitation intervention on spontaneous imitation skills in young children with autism. *Research in Developmental Disabilities, 28*(2), 163–175.

Ingersoll, B., Lewis, E., & Kroman, E. (2007). Teaching the imitation and spontaneous use of descriptive gestures in young children with autism using a naturalistic behavioral intervention. *Journal of Autism and Developmental Disorders, 37*(8), 1446–1456.

Ingersoll, B. R., & Wainer, A. L. (2013a). Pilot study of a school-based parent training program for preschoolers with ASD. *Autism, 17*(4), 434–448.

Ingersoll, B., & Wainer A. (2013b). Initial efficacy of Project ImPACT: A parent-mediated social communication intervention for young children with ASD. *Journal of Autism and Developmental Disorders, 43*(12), 2943–2952.

Ingersoll, B., Wainer, A. L., Berger, N. I., Pickard, K. E., & Bonter, N. (2016). Comparison of a self-directed and therapist-assisted telehealth parent-mediated intervention for children with ASD: A pilot RCT. *Journal of Autism and Developmental Disorders, 46*(7), 2275–2284.

Ingersoll, B. R., Wainer, A. L., Berger, N. I., & Walton, K. M. (2017). Efficacy of low intensity, therapist-implemented Project ImPACT for increasing social communication skills in young children with ASD. *Developmental Neurorehabilitation, 20*(8), 502–510.

Jocelyn, L. J., Casiro, O. G., Beattie, D., Bow, J., & Kneisz, J. (1998). Treatment of children with autism: A randomized controlled trial to evaluate a caregiver-based intervention program in community day-care centers. *Journal of Developmental and Behavioral Pediatrics, 19*(5), 326–334.

Jüni, P., Altman, D. G., & Egger, M. (2001). Assessing the quality of controlled clinical trials. *BMJ, 323*(7303), 42–46.

Kaale, A., Fagerland, M. W., Martinsen, E. W., & Smith, L. (2014). Preschool-based social communication treatment for children with autism: 12-month follow-up of a randomized trial. *Journal of the American Academy of Child and Adolescent Psychiatry, 53*(2), 188–198.

Kaale, A., Smith, L., & Sponheim, E. (2012). A randomized controlled trial of preschool-based joint attention intervention for children with autism. *Journal of Child Psychology and Psychiatry, 53*(1), 97–105.

Kaiser, A. P., Hancock, T. B., & Nietfeld, J. P. (2000). The effects of parent-implemented enhanced milieu teaching on the social communication of children who have autism. *Early Education and Development, 11*(4), 423–446.

Kaiser, A. P., & Roberts, M. Y. (2013). Parent-implemented enhanced milieu teaching with preschool children who have intellectual disabilities. *Journal of Speech, Language, and Hearing Research, 56*(1), 295–309.

Kasari, C. (2002). Assessing change in early intervention programs for children with autism. *Journal of Autism and Developmental Disorders, 32*(5), 447–461.

Kasari, C., Freeman, S., & Paparella, T. (2006). Joint attention and symbolic play in young children with autism: A randomized controlled intervention study. *Journal of Child Psychology and Psychiatry, 47*(6), 611–620.

Kasari, C., Freeman, S., Paparella, T., Wong, C., Kwon, S., & Gulsrud, A. (2005). Early intervention on core deficits in autism. *Clinical Neuropsychiatry: Journal of Treatment Evaluation, 2*(6), 380–388.

Kasari, C., Gulsrud, A., Freeman, S., Paparella, T., & Hellemann, G. (2012). Longitudinal follow-up of children with autism receiving targeted interventions on joint attention and play. *Journal of the American Academy of Child and Adolescent Psychiatry, 51*(5), 487–495.

Kasari, C., Gulsrud, A., Paparella, T., Hellemann, G., & Berry, K. (2015). Randomized comparative efficacy study of parent-mediated interventions for toddlers with autism. *Journal of Consulting and Clinical Psychology, 83*(3), 554–563.

Kasari, C., Gulsrud, A. C., Wong, C., Kwon, S., & Locke, J. (2010). Randomized controlled caregiver mediated joint engagement intervention for toddlers with autism. *Journal of Autism and Developmental Disorders, 40*(9), 1045–1056.

Kasari, C., Kaiser, A., Goods, K., Nietfeld, J., Mathy, P., Landa, R., . . . Almirall, D. (2014a). Communication interventions for minimally verbal children with autism: A sequential multiple assignment randomized trial. *Journal of the American Academy of Child and Adolescent Psychiatry, 53*(6), 635–646.

Kasari, C., Lawton, K., Shih, W., Barker, T. V., Landa, R., Lord, C., . . . Senturk, D. (2014b). Caregiver-mediated intervention for low-resourced preschoolers with autism: An RCT. *Pediatrics, 134*(1), e72–e79.

Kasari, C., Paparella, T., Freeman, S., & Jahromi, L. B. (2008). Language outcome in autism: Randomized comparison of joint attention and play interventions. *Journal of Consulting and Clinical Psychology, 76*(1), 125–137.

Kasari, C., & Sigman, M. (1997). Linking parental perceptions to interactions in young children with autism. *Journal of Autism and Developmental Disorders, 27*(1), 39–57.

Kasari, C., Siller, M., Huynh, L. N., Shih, W., Swanson, M., Hellemann, G. S., & Sugar, C. A. (2014c). Randomized controlled trial of parental responsiveness intervention for toddlers at high risk for autism. *Infant Behavior and Development, 37*(4), 711–721.

Kasari, C., & Smith, T. (2013). Interventions in schools for children with autism spectrum disorder: Methods and recommendations. *Autism, 17*(3), 254–267.

Kasari, C., & Smith, T. (2016). Forest for the trees: Evidence-based practices in ASD. *Clinical Psychology: Science and Practice, 23*(3), 260–264.

Kasari, C., Sturm, A., & Shih, W. (2018). SMARTer approach to personalizing intervention for children with autism spectrum disorder. *Journal of Speech, Language, and Hearing Research, 61*(11), 2629–2640.

Kovshoff, H., Hastings, R. P., & Remington, B. (2011). Two-year outcomes for children with autism after the cessation of early intensive behavioral intervention. *Behavior Modification, 35*(5), 427–450.

Kuhlthau, K., Payakachat, N., Delahaye, J., Hurson, J., Pyne, J. M., Kovacs, E., &

Tilford, J. M. (2014). Quality of life for parents of children with autism spectrum disorders. *Research in Autism Spectrum Disorders, 8*(10), 1339–1350.

Landa, R., Holman, K., & Garrett-Mayer, E. (2007). Social and communication development in toddlers with early and later diagnosis of autism spectrum disorders. *Archives of General Psychiatry, 64*(7), 853–864.

Landa, R. J., Holman, K. C., O'Neill, A. H., & Stuart, E. A. (2011). Intervention targeting development of socially synchronous engagement in toddlers with autism spectrum disorder: A randomized controlled trial. *Journal of Child Psychology and Psychiatry, 52*(1), 13–21.

Lawton, K., & Kasari, C. (2012a). Brief report: Longitudinal improvements in the quality of joint attention in preschool children with autism. *Journal of Autism and Developmental Disorders, 42*(2), 307–312.

Lawton, K., & Kasari, C. (2012b). Teacher-implemented joint attention intervention: Pilot randomized controlled study for preschoolers with autism. *Journal of Consulting and Clinical Psychology, 80*(4), 687–693.

Lim, H. A., & Draper, E. (2011). The effects of music therapy incorporated with applied behavior analysis verbal behavior approach for children with autism spectrum disorders. *Journal of Music Therapy, 48*(4), 532–550.

Lord, C., Rutter, M., DiLavore, P. C., & Risi, S. (2008). *ADOS: Autism diagnostic observation schedule.* Boston: Hogrefe.

Lord, C., Wagner, A., Rogers, S., Szatmari, P., Aman, M., Charman, T., . . . Harris, S. (2005). Challenges in evaluating psychosocial interventions for autistic spectrum disorders. *Journal of Autism and Developmental Disorders, 35*(6), 695–708.

Lovaas, O. I. (1987). Behavioral treatment and normal educational and intellectual functioning in young autistic children. *Journal of Consulting and Clinical Psychology, 55*(1), 3.

Maenner, M. J., Shaw, K. A., Baio, J., Washington, A., Patrick, M., DiRienzo, M., . . . Dietz, P. M. (2020). Prevalence of autism spectrum disorder among children aged 8 years—Autism and Developmental Disabilities Monitoring Network, 11 Sites, United States, 2016. *MMWR Surveillance Summaries, 69*(No. SS-4), 1–12.

Magiati, I., Charman, T., & Howlin, P. (2007). A two-year prospective follow-up study of community-based early intensive behavioural intervention and specialist nursery provision for children with autism spectrum disorders. *Journal of Child Psychology and Psychiatry, 48*(8), 803–812.

Mandell, D. S., Stahmer, A. C., Shin, S., Xie, M., Reisinger, E., & Marcus, S. C. (2013). The role of treatment fidelity on outcomes during a randomized field trial of an autism intervention. *Autism, 17*(3), 281–295.

McEachin, J. J., Smith, T., & Lovaas, O. I. (1993). Long-term outcome for children with autism who received early intensive behavioral treatment. *American Journal on Mental Retardation, 97*(4), 359–372.

Mullen, E. M. (1995). *Mullen scales of early learning.* Circle Pines, MN: American Guidance Service.

Mundy, P., Sigman, M., & Kasari, C. (1990). A longitudinal study of joint attention and language development in autistic children. *Journal of Autism and Developmental Disorders, 20*(1), 115–128.

National Research Council. (2001). *Educating children with autism.* Washington, DC: National Academy Press.

Nefdt, N., Koegel, R., Singer, G., & Gerber, M. (2010). The use of a self-directed learning program to provide introductory training in pivotal response treatment to parents of children with autism. *Journal of Positive Behavior Interventions, 12*(1), 23–32.

Odom, S. L., Brown, W. H., Frey, T., Karasu, N., Lee Smith-Canter, L., & Strain, P. S. (2003). Evidence-based practices for young children with autism: Contributions for single-subject design research. *Focus on Autism and Other Developmental Disabilities, 18*(3), 166–175.

Oono, I. P., Honey, E. J., & McConachie, H. (2013). Parent-mediated early intervention for young children with autism spectrum disorders (ASD). *Evidence-Based Child Health: A Cochrane Review Journal, 8*(6), 2380–2479.

Oosterling, I., Visser, J., Swinkels, S., Rommelse, N., Donders, R., Woudenberg, T., . . . Buitelaar, J. (2010). Randomized controlled trial of the focus parent training for toddlers with autism: 1-year outcome. *Journal of Autism and Developmental Disorders, 40*(12), 1447–1458.

Osborne, L. A., McHugh, L., Saunders, J., & Reed, P. (2008). Parenting stress reduces the effectiveness of early teaching interventions for autistic spectrum disorders. *Journal of Autism and Developmental Disorders, 38*(6), 1092–1103.

Pajareya, K., & Nopmaneejumruslers, K. (2011). A pilot randomized controlled trial of DIR/Floortime™ parent training intervention for pre-school children with autistic spectrum disorders. *Autism, 15*(5), 563–577.

Paparella, T., Goods, K. S., Freeman, S., & Kasari, C. (2011). The emergence of nonverbal joint attention and requesting skills in young children with autism. *Journal of Communication Disorders, 44*(6), 569–583.

Patterson, S. Y., Smith, V., & Mirenda, P. (2012). A systematic review of training programs for parents of children with autism spectrum disorders: Single subject contributions. *Autism, 16*(5), 498–522.

Pellecchia, M., Connell, J. E., Beidas, R. S., Xie, M., Marcus, S. C., & Mandell, D. S. (2015). Dismantling the active ingredients of an intervention for children with autism. *Journal of Autism and Developmental Disorders, 45*(9), 2917–2927.

Pickles, A., Le Couteur, A., Leadbitter, K., Salomone, E., Cole-Fletcher, R., Tobin, H., . . . Green, J. (2016). Parent-mediated social communication therapy for young children with autism (PACT): Long-term follow-up of a randomised controlled trial. *The Lancet, 388*(10059), 2501–2509.

Rahman, A., Divan, G., Hamdani, S. U., Vajaratkar, V., Taylor, C., Leadbitter, K., . . . Patel, V. (2016). Effectiveness of the parent-mediated intervention for children with autism spectrum disorder in south Asia in India and Pakistan (PASS): A randomised controlled trial. *The Lancet Psychiatry, 3*(2), 128–136.

Reed, P., Osborne, L. A., & Corness, M. (2007). The real-world effectiveness of early teaching interventions for children with autism spectrum disorder. *Exceptional Children, 73*(4), 417–433.

Rickards, A. L., Walstab, J. E., Wright-Rossi, R., Simpson, J., & Reddihough, D. S. (2007). A randomized, controlled trial of a home-based intervention program for children with autism and developmental delay. *Journal of Developmental and Behavioral Pediatrics, 28*(4), 308–316.

Roberts, J., Williams, K., Carter, M., Evans, D., Parmenter, T., Silove, N., . . . Warren, A. (2011). A randomised controlled trial of two early intervention programs for young children with autism: Centre-based with parent program and home-based. *Research in Autism Spectrum Disorders, 5*(4), 1553–1566.

Roberts, M. Y., & Kaiser, A. P. (2015). Early intervention for toddlers with language delays: A randomized controlled trial. *Pediatrics, 135*(4), 686–693.

Rogers, S. J., Estes, A., Lord, C., Munson, J., Rocha, M., Winter, J., . . . Talbot, M. (2019). A Multisite Randomized Controlled Two-Phase Trial of the Early Start Denver Model Compared to Treatment as Usual. *Journal of the American Academy of Child and Adolescent Psychiatry, 58*(9), 853–865.

Rogers, S. J., Estes, A., Lord, C., Vismara, L., Winter, J., Fitzpatrick, A., . . . Dawson, G. (2012). Effects of a brief Early Start Denver Model (ESDM)–based parent intervention on toddlers at risk for autism spectrum disorders: A randomized controlled trial. *Journal of the American Academy of Child and Adolescent Psychiatry, 51*(10), 1052–1065.

Ruble, L. A., McGrew, J. H., Toland, M. D., Dalrymple, N. J., & Jung, L. A. (2013). A randomized controlled trial of compass web-based and face-to-face teacher coaching in autism. *Journal of Consulting and Clinical Psychology, 81*(3), 566–572.

Sallows, G. O., & Graupner, T. D. (2005). Intensive behavioral treatment for children with autism: Four-year outcome and predictors. *American Journal on Mental Retardation, 110*(6), 417–438.

Scahill, L., Bearss, K., Lecavalier, L., Smith, T., Swiezy, N., Aman, M. G., . . . Johnson, C. (2016). Effect of parent training on adaptive behavior in children with autism spectrum disorder and disruptive behavior: Results of a randomized trial. *Journal of the American Academy of Child and Adolescent Psychiatry, 55*(7), 602–609.

Schertz, H. H., Odom, S. L., Baggett, K. M., & Sideris, J. H. (2013). Effects of joint attention mediated learning for toddlers with autism spectrum disorders: An initial randomized controlled study. *Early Childhood Research Quarterly, 28*(2), 249–258.

Schreibman, L., Dawson, G., Stahmer, A. C., Landa, R., Rogers, S. J., McGee, G. G., . . . Halladay, A. (2015). Naturalistic developmental behavioral interventions: Empirically validated treatments for autism spectrum disorder. *Journal of Autism and Developmental Disorders, 45*(8), 2411–2428.

Schreibman, L., & Stahmer, A. C. (2014). A randomized trial comparison of the effects of verbal and pictorial naturalistic communication strategies on spoken language for young children with autism. *Journal of Autism and Developmental Disorders, 44*(5), 1244–1251.

Schreibman, L., Stahmer, A. C., Barlett, V. C., & Dufek, S. (2009). Brief report: Toward refinement of a predictive behavioral profile for treatment outcome in children with autism. *Research in Autism Spectrum Disorders, 3*(1), 163–172.

Schwartzman, B. C., Wood, J. J., & Kapp, S. K. (2016). Can the five factor model of personality account for the variability of autism symptom expression?: Multivariate approaches to behavioral phenotyping in adult autism spectrum disorder. *Journal of Autism and Developmental Disorders, 46*(1), 253–272.

Sheinkopf, S. J., & Siegel, B. (1998). Home-based behavioral treatment of young children with autism. *Journal of Autism and Developmental Disorders, 28*(1), 15–23.

Sherer, M. R., & Schreibman, L. (2005). Individual behavioral profiles and predictors of treatment effectiveness for children with autism. *Journal of Consulting and Clinical Psychology, 73*(3), 525.

Shih, W., Patterson, S. Y., & Kasari, C. (2016). Developing an adaptive treatment strategy for peer-related social skills for children with autism spectrum disorders. *Journal of Clinical Child and Adolescent Psychology, 45*(4), 469–479.

Shire, S. Y., Chang, Y., Shih, W., Bracaglia, S., Kodjoe, M., & Kasari, C. (2017). Hybrid implementation model of community-partnered early intervention for toddlers with autism: A randomized trial. *Journal of Child Psychology and Psychiatry, 58*(5), 612–622.

Shire, S. Y., Shih, W., Chang, Y. C., Bracaglia, S., Kodjoe, M., & Kasari, C. (2019). Sustained community implementation of JASPER intervention with toddlers with autism. *Journal of Autism and Developmental Disorders, 49*(5), 1863–1875.

Sibbald, B., & Roland, M. (1998). Understanding controlled trials: Why are randomised controlled trials important? *British Medical Journal, 316*(7126), 201.

Siller, M., Hutman, T., & Sigman, M. (2013). A parent-mediated intervention to increase responsive parental behaviors and child communication in children with ASD: A randomized clinical trial. *Journal of Autism and Developmental Disorders, 43*(3), 540–555.

Smith, T., Groen, A. D., & Wynn, J. W. (2000). Randomized trial of intensive early intervention for children with pervasive developmental disorder. *American Journal on Mental Retardation, 105*(4), 269–285.

Smith, T., & Iadarola, S. (2015). Evidence base update for autism spectrum disorder. *Journal of Clinical Child and Adolescent Psychology, 44*(6), 897–922.

Solomon, R., Van Egeren, L. A., Mahoney, G., Huber, M. S. Q., & Zimmerman, P. (2014). PLAY Project Home Consultation intervention program for young children with autism spectrum disorders: A randomized controlled trial. *Journal of Developmental and Behavioral Pediatrics, 35*(8), 475–485.

Sparrow, S., Cicchetti, D., & Balla, D. (2005). *Vineland-II: Vineland Adaptive Behavior Scales: Survey forms manual* (2nd ed.). Circle Pines, MN: American Guidance Services.

Stahmer, A. C., Collings, N. M., & Palinkas, L. A. (2005). Early intervention practices for children with autism: Descriptions from community providers. *Focus on Autism Other Developmental Disabilities, 20*, 66–79.

Stahmer, A. C., Schreibman, L., & Cunningham, A. B. (2011). Toward a technology of treatment individualization for young children with autism spectrum disorders. *Brain Research, 1380*, 229–239.

Strain, P. S., & Bovey, E. H., II. (2011). Randomized, controlled trial of the LEAP model of early intervention for young children with autism spectrum disorders. *Topics in Early Childhood Special Education, 31*(3), 133–154.

Tager-Flusberg, H., & Joseph, R. M. (2003). Identifying neurocognitive phenotypes in autism. *Philosophical Transactions of the Royal Society of London B: Biological Sciences, 358*(1430), 303–314.

Tager-Flusberg, H., & Kasari, C. (2013). Minimally verbal school-aged children with autism spectrum disorder: The neglected end of the spectrum. *Autism Research, 6*(6), 468–478.

Thompson, G. A., McFerran, K. S., & Gold, C. (2014). Family-centred music therapy to promote social engagement in young children with severe autism spectrum disorder: A randomized controlled study. *Child: Care, Health and Development, 40*(6), 840–852.

Tincani, M., Cucchiarra, M. B., Thurman, S., Snyder, M., & McCarthy, C. (2013). Evaluating NRC's recommendations for educating children with autism a decade later. *Child Youth and Care Forum, 43*(3), 315–337.

Tomasello, M., & Farrar, M. (1986). Joint attention and early language. *Child Development, 57*, 1454–1463.

Tonge, B., Brereton, A., Kiomall, M., Mackinnon, A., & Rinehart, N. J. (2014). A randomised group comparison controlled trial of "preschoolers with autism": A parent education and skills training intervention for young children with autistic disorder. *Autism, 18*(2), 166–177.

Turner-Brown, L., Hume, K., Boyd, B. A., & Kainz, K. (2019). Preliminary efficacy of family implemented TEACCH for toddlers: Effects on parents and their toddlers with autism spectrum disorder. *Journal of Autism and Developmental Disorders, 49*(7), 2685–2698.

Vernon, T. W., Holden, A. N., Barrett, A. C., Bradshaw, J., Ko, J. A., McGarry, E. S., . . . German, T. C. (2019). A pilot randomized clinical trial of an enhanced pivotal response treatment approach for young children with autism: The PRISM model. *Journal of Autism and Developmental Disorders, 49*(6), 2358–2373.

Virués-Ortega, J. (2010). Applied behavior analytic intervention for autism in early childhood: Meta-analysis, meta-regression and dose–response meta-analysis of multiple outcomes. *Clinical Psychology Review, 30*(4), 387–399.

Vivanti, G., Dissanayake, C., Duncan, E., Feary, J., Capes, K., Upson, S., . . . Hudry, K. (2019). Outcomes of children receiving Group-Early Start Denver Model in an inclusive versus autism-specific setting: A pilot randomized controlled trial. *Autism, 23*(5), 1165–1175.

Vivanti, G., Paynter, J., Duncan, E., Fothergill, H., Dissanayake, C., Rogers, S. J., & Victorian ASELCC Team. (2014). Effectiveness and feasibility of the Early Start Denver Model implemented in a group-based community childcare setting. *Journal of Autism and Developmental Disorders, 44*(12), 3140–3153.

Welterlin, A., Turner-Brown, L. M., Harris, S., Mesibov, G., & Delmolino, L. (2012). The home TEACCHing program for toddlers with autism. *Journal of Autism and Developmental Disorders, 42*(9), 1827–1835.

Wetherby, A. M., Guthrie, W., Woods, J., Schatschneider, C., Holland, R. D., Morgan, L., & Lord, C. (2014). Parent-implemented social intervention for toddlers with autism: An RCT. *Pediatrics, 134*(6), 1084–1093.

Whalen, C., Moss, D., Ilan, A. B., Vaupel, M., Fielding, P., Macdonald, K., . . . Symon, J. (2010). Efficacy of TeachTown: Basics computer-assisted intervention for the intensive comprehensive autism program in Los Angeles unified school district. *Autism, 14*(3), 179–197.

White, P. J., O'Reilly, M., Streusand, W., Levine, A., Sigafoos, J., Lancioni, G., . . . Aguilar, J. (2011). Best practices for teaching joint attention: A systematic review of the intervention literature. *Research in Autism Spectrum Disorders, 5*(4), 1283–1295.

Whitehouse, A. J. O., Granich, J., Alvares, G., Busacca, M., Cooper, M. N., Dass, A., . . . Anderson, A. (2017). A randomised controlled trial of an iPad-based application to complement early behavioural intervention in autism spectrum disorder. *Journal of Child Psychology and Psychiatry, 58*(9), 1042–1052.

Williams, B. T., Gray, K. M., & Tonge, B. J. (2012). Teaching emotion recognition skills to young children with autism: A randomised controlled trial of an emotion training programme. *Journal of Child Psychology and Psychiatry, 53*(12), 1268–1276.

Wong, C. S. (2013). A play and joint attention intervention for teachers of young children with autism: A randomized controlled pilot study. *Autism, 17*(3), 340–357.

Wong, C., Odom, S., Hume, K., Cox, A., Fettig, A., Kucharczyk, S., . . . Schultz, T. R. (2015). Evidence-based practices for children, youth, and young adults with autism spectrum disorder: A comprehensive review. *Journal of Autism and Developmental Disorders, 45*, 1951–1966.

Wong, V. C. N., & Kwan, Q. K. (2010). Randomized controlled trial for early intervention for autism: A pilot study of the Autism 1–2–3 project. *Journal of Autism and Developmental Disorders, 40*(6), 677–688.

Yoder, P., & Stone, W. L. (2006). Randomized comparison of two communication interventions for preschoolers with autism spectrum disorders. *Journal of Consulting and Clinical Psychology, 74*(3), 426–435.

Young, H. E., Falco, R. A., & Hanita, M. (2016). Randomized, controlled trial of a comprehensive program for young students with autism spectrum disorder. *Journal of Autism and Developmental Disorders, 46*(2), 544–560.

Zablotsky, B., Anderson, C., & Law, P. (2013). The association between child autism symptomatology, maternal quality of life, and risk for depression. *Journal of Autism and Developmental Disorders, 43*(8), 1946–1955.

Zachor, D. A., Ben-Itzchak, E., Rabinovich, A., & Lahat, E. (2007). Change in autism core symptoms with intervention. *Research in Autism Spectrum Disorders, 1*(4), 304–317.

CHAPTER 5

• • • • • • • •

Development of Infant Siblings of Children with Autism Spectrum Disorder

Katarzyna Chawarska, Suzanne L. Macari, Angelina Vernetti, and Ludivine Brunissen

The past decade has witnessed an explosion of studies reporting on the development of younger siblings of children with autism spectrum disorder (ASD), following evidence for the familial aggregation of autism features among first- and second-degree relatives from genetic studies (Hansen et al., 2019; Schendel, Grønborg, & Parner, 2014; Szatmari et al., 2016). The methodological approach employed by prospective infant sibling studies involves the recruitment of younger siblings of children with ASD during presymptomatic stages of the disorder, usually within the first months of life or during pregnancy. The infants are then followed prospectively until the age of 2–3 years, when a diagnosis can be reliably ascertained. The prospective follow-up often involves repeated examination of an array of behavioral and brain development indices in younger siblings of children with ASD and low-risk controls, who usually consist of younger siblings of children who are developing typically. Prospective studies of infant siblings aim to facilitate the identification of the earliest diagnostic indicators (e.g., ASD vs. non-ASD) and predictors of later levels of functioning in order to enhance our understanding of the mechanisms contributing to symptom development. These studies also seek to facilitate the identification of novel treatment targets (Rogers, 2009; Szatmari et al., 2016; Tager-Flusberg, 2010; Yirmiya & Charman, 2011; Zwaigenbaum et al., 2009). By examining differences between sibling pairs who are concordant (i.e., both siblings have ASD) and discordant for ASD (only one sibling in the pair has ASD), researchers also hope to identify factors that may play a protective role against genetic liability for ASD (Szatmari, 2018). Furthermore, by comparing the development of male and female siblings, studies of infant siblings may elucidate factors contributing to sex differences in syndrome expression and prevalence (Chawarska, Macari, Powell, DiNicola, & Shic, 2016; Kleberg, Nyström, Bölte, & Falck-Ytter, 2019; Werling & Geschwind, 2013; Zwaigenbaum et al., 2012).

Relative Recurrence Risk

Although ASD affects approximately 1–2% of all children in the general population (Centers for Disease Control and Prevention, 2012), the relative recurrence risk, or the sibling recurrence risk relative to the risk of ASD for the later-born siblings of nonaffected first-born children, increases approximately fivefold in half-siblings and tenfold in full siblings of children with ASD (Hansen et al., 2019). Although there is robust evidence that the relative recurrence risk of ASD in younger siblings is elevated, the magnitude of this effect is dependent on several factors, including the number of children already affected in the family as well as the sex of both the affected child and the younger sibling. Indeed, the relative recurrence risk more than doubles in families that have more than one child already diagnosed with ASD (32.2–36.3%), compared to families where only one older child is affected (13.5–16.1%) (McDonald, 2020; Ozonoff et al., 2011). The recurrence risk also appears to be higher when the younger sibling is male rather than female (Ozonoff et al., 2011; Palmer et al., 2017; Werling & Geschwind, 2015); these rates are further influenced by the sex of the older affected sibling (Palmer et al., 2017). Specifically, when the older affected sibling is male, the recurrence risk when a younger sibling is also male is approximately 12.9%, compared to 4.2% when the younger sibling is female. However, when the older affected sibling is female, the recurrence risk for a younger male sibling is approximately 16.7%, compared to 7.6% for a younger female sibling (Palmer et al., 2017). Thus, the recurrence risk in families when the older affected sibling is a female with ASD is higher than the risk associated with a male sibling (Palmer et al., 2017; Risch et al., 2014; Robinson, Lichtenstein, Anckarsäter, Happé, & Ronald, 2013).

In addition, a significant minority of high-risk infants is likely to develop mild deficits in social and communication domains, or atypical repetitive behaviors and rigidities, often referred to as the broader autism phenotype (BAP; Bailey, Palferman, Heavey, & Le Couteur, 1998; Ingersoll & Wainer, 2014; Murphy et al., 2000). Siblings who do not develop ASD are also at risk for language and other cognitive delays, attention-deficit/hyperactivity disorder (ADHD), and emotional challenges (Constantino, Zhang, Frazier, Abbacchi, & Law, 2010; Miller, Iosif, Young, Hill, & Ozonoff, 2016a; Miller et al., 2019; Ozonoff et al., 2014). The characteristics of BAP begin to manifest as early as 12 to 18 months of age (Georgiades et al., 2013; Macari et al., 2012; Ozonoff et al., 2014). Therefore, as a group, younger siblings of children with ASD are at elevated risk for developing a range of social and other neurodevelopmental problems that emerge in early childhood and tend to persist in later development (Miller et al., 2016a, 2016b; Miller, Iosif, Young, Hill, & Ozonoff, 2016).

Social and Communication Development

Some of the core symptoms of autism in toddlers include limited attention to faces of interactive partners, poor eye contact, and low frequency of socially directed smiling and vocalization (Chawarska, Klin, Paul, Macari, & Volkmar, 2009; Chawarska, Klin, Paul, & Volkmar, 2007a; Lord, Luyster, Guthrie, & Pickles, 2012b; Lord et al., 2006). These behaviors are functional in typically developing infants by 6 months of age, and thus may be expected to be affected in infants later diagnosed with ASD. Several studies have examined smiling, attention to faces, and socially directed vocalizations in 6-month-old infants at high and low risk for ASD, yielding discrepant results. Two studies (Rozga et al., 2011; Young, Merin, Rogers, & Ozonoff, 2009) employed the still-face paradigm (Tronick, Als, Adamson, Wise, & Brazelton, 1978) in which the infant is observed while interacting with a parent. In this paradigm, the parent is asked either to interact "as usual" or to cease interaction altogether but remain in a face-to-face position ("still face"). In another observational study (Ozonoff et al., 2010), the infant interacted with an examiner while undergoing a series of object-based developmental tasks from the Mullen Scales of Early Learning (MSEL; Mullen, 1995). A free-play setting with a parent served as another context for observation of infant social and communicative behavior in a few other studies (Gangi et al., 2018; Rozga et al., 2011; Schwichtenberg, Kellerman, Young, Miller, & Ozonoff, 2019). Finally, in a most recent study, infants were observed during a face-to-face interaction with an examiner who delivered a series of standard bids for social engagement consisting of episodes of speaking to the infant, singing, playing peek-a-boo, tickling the infant, or presenting the infant with a toy (Macari et al., 2020).

Studies employing the still-face paradigm with the mother (Rozga et al., 2011; Young et al., 2009), a free-play session with the mother (Gangi et al., 2018; Rozga et al., 2011; Schwichtenberg et al., 2019), or that observed the infant in the context of a developmental assessment (Ozonoff et al., 2010) yielded largely null results. At 6 months of age, infants later diagnosed with ASD did not differ from non-ASD siblings or low-risk controls with regard to social smiling, attention to faces, or social vocalizations (Ozonoff et al., 2010; Rozga et al., 2011; Schwichtenberg et al., 2019). However, a number of factors, including the social partner and evaluation context, are likely to influence infant behavior and thus the likelihood of observing ASD-specific deficits. Utilizing a parent as the partner, though ecologically valid, has the disadvantage of inviting variability in the partner's behavior. In addition, infants and their mothers develop a unique interactional style over the first months of life. Thus, there may be methodological benefits to using an unfamiliar, trained examiner as the social partner. The context of engagement is also critically important. During structured developmental testing, the focus is often on objects, and thus the situation may not tap into infants' potential social vulnerabilities. A free-play session leaves room for significant differences in the content of the interaction. Therefore, a structured interaction that presses for social behavior may be more effective at eliciting subtle vulnerabilities in social attention and interaction patterns in infants later diagnosed with ASD.

To investigate this possibility, Macari and colleagues (Macari et al., 2020) conducted a study in which 6-, 9-, and 12-month-old infants' attention to faces of interactive partners was observed in response to standardized and graduated bids for social engagement by an examiner. All involved eye contact and positive affect, but the bids also included child-directed speech ("motherese"), singing, a peek-a-boo game, a tickling game, or a toy demonstration. Infants who were later diagnosed with ASD showed diminished attention to the faces of the interactive partners compared to non-ASD siblings or low-risk controls, but the effect was highly dependent on context. The context that separated infants later diagnosed with ASD from the comparison groups consisted of standard bids for social engagement involving child-directed speech, with or without physical contact. Interestingly, no group differences were observed during the social interaction probes when the examiner sang a song to the infant, engaged in a peek-a-boo game with the infant, or presented the infant with an attractive toy. The study suggests that behavioral differences associated with a later diagnosis of autism are present as early as 6 months, but they are highly context specific, which may explain why less stringent manipulation of the types of social bids or inclusion of objects in previous studies might have obscured the existing differences. The findings of diminished attention to faces of real-world interactive partners in the presence of direct gaze and speech (Macari et al., 2020) are consistent with other studies of high-risk infants with ASD (Chawarska, Macari, & Shic, 2013; Shic, Macari, & Chawarska, 2014), as well as toddlers with ASD (Chawarska, Macari, & Shic, 2012; Shic, Wang, Macari, & Chawarska, 2019) in response to videotaped interactive partners.

In addition to these observational studies involving microanalytic coding of social communication behavior offline, some studies have utilized a structured assessment of autism symptoms scored by a clinician. The Autism Observation Scale for Infants (AOSI; Bryson, Zwaigenbaum, McDermott, Rombough, & Brian, 2008) measures ASD-related symptoms during infancy. In one study (Zwaigenbaum et al., 2005), AOSI total scores did not differentiate infants with ASD from non-ASD peers at 6 months, whereas in another study (Gammer et al., 2015), 7-month-old high-risk siblings later diagnosed with ASD scored significantly worse than low-risk controls but not worse than nonaffected high-risk siblings.

By 12 months, high-risk infants later diagnosed with ASD present with overt vulnerabilities, spanning the core features of autism. Deficits in language, including speech-like vocalizations (Paul, Fuerst, Ramsay,

Chawarska, & Klin, 2011) and canonical babbling (Patten et al., 2014) were observed in affected infants at this age and often are among parents' earliest concerns (Chawarska et al., 2007b; Ozonoff et al., 2009; Sacrey et al., 2015; Talbott, Nelson, & Tager-Flusberg, 2015). When assessed formally using the MSEL, 12-month-old infants with ASD displayed lower levels of expressive and receptive language than controls (Lazenby et al., 2016; Ozonoff et al., 2014). Social communication and social responsivity are also clearly impacted by 12 months, including diminished positive affect (Filliter et al., 2015), responding to name (Miller et al., 2017; Nadig et al., 2007), inventory of gestures (Mitchell et al., 2006; Talbott et al., 2015), requesting, eye contact, social smiling, imitating, showing, and initiating joint attention (Macari et al., 2012; Ozonoff et al., 2010; Rowberry et al., 2015; Rozga et al., 2011; Zwaigenbaum et al., 2005). During a play-based communication assessment, 12-month-old infants later diagnosed with ASD exhibited lower rates of initiation of joint attention (pointing and showing) and lower response to joint attention bids (distal pointing), as well as fewer requests and protests as compared to nonaffected high-risk infants and low-risk controls (Rozga et al., 2011). Differences between siblings later diagnosed with ASD and siblings without ASD can also be detected at 12 months, based on parental report. A study utilizing the First Year Inventory (Reznick, Baranek, Reavis, Watson, & Crais, 2007) suggests that siblings later diagnosed with ASD had higher scores in the Social Communication domain, particularly with regard to imitation, compared to siblings without ASD but with other developmental challenges and typically developing siblings (Rowberry et al., 2015). Parents did not note any differences at this age regarding restrictive and repetitive behavior symptoms (Rowberry et al., 2015).

These findings suggest that, already at 12 months, as a group, infant siblings later diagnosed with ASD begin to show atypical features related to core and co-occurring symptoms of ASD. Importantly, however, delays and atypical features at this age can also be observed in infant siblings who are not eventually diagnosed with ASD. For instance, Macari and colleagues (2012) examined the severity of autism symptoms using the Autism Diagnostic Observation Schedule—Toddler Module (ADOS-T) (Lord, Luyster, Gotham, & Guthrie, 2012a) in a sample of high- and low-risk infants followed through 24 months of age. While those diagnosed later with ASD exhibited elevated scores on the ADOS-T compared to those with other atypical outcomes and typically developing infants, those with atypical outcomes also had elevated ADOS-T scores compared to typically developing infants, and this pattern persisted at 18 and 24 months (Macari et al., 2012). These results are consistent with other reports utilizing direct observation (AOSI) and parent report (FYI; Georgiades et al., 2013; Rowberry et al., 2015). However, a significant minority of infants who did not ultimately receive a diagnosis of ASD also exhibited delays and atypical features in key diagnostic areas at 12 months as measured by the ADOS-T (Macari et al., 2012) or AOSI (Georgiades et al., 2013). This suggests that the genetic vulnerability to ASD is expressed in a variable manner, with many high-risk infants showing a range of autism-related symptoms early in life and the deficits becoming less pronounced as the children grow older.

Repetitive Behaviors and Restricted Interests

Certain types of restrictive and repetitive behaviors in young children are common and developmentally appropriate. However, while most repetitive behaviors diminish by 12 months of age in typically developing toddlers (Thelen, 1979), they persist past childhood in individuals with autism. Restrictive and repetitive behaviors (RRBs) constitute a core feature of autism and include a broad range of behaviors, from circumscribed interests and rituals to motor stereotypies and adherence to routines. However, RRBs remain perhaps one of the most understudied and least understood domains of the ASD phenotype. Given the familial liability associated with ASD, prospective studies of infants at high familial risk for ASD can help shed light on the developmental progression of RRBs and their relevance as an early-risk marker for a later autism diagnosis.

To date, several prospective sibling studies have examined object-focused repetitive behaviors and motor mannerisms in high-risk infants. Findings from four observational studies, during which different types of RRBs were coded from videotaped play-based assessments, suggest that some features of RRBs manifest as early as 12 or 18 months of age in high-risk siblings (Christensen et al., 2011; Damiano, Nahmias, Hogan-Brown, & Stone, 2013; Elison et al., 2014; Loh et al., 2007). However, whether atypical RRBs in early development are predictive of later diagnostic outcomes appears to be highly dependent on RRB type. In a study of high- and low-risk 18-month-olds engaged in free play with a standard set of toys, Christensen et al. (2011) observed that high-risk siblings exhibited greater levels of nonfunctional repetitive play with objects than low-risk toddlers. Yet, within the high-risk group, levels of repetitive play did not differ based on diagnostic outcomes (i.e., ASD, other delays, no other delays) at 36 months. In contrast, 12-month-old infants later diagnosed with ASD could be differentiated from their high-risk and low-risk peers based on some kinds of repetitive behavior with objects: rotating, spinning, and unusual visual exploration of objects occurred significantly more frequently in infants with ASD than in infants with other delays or in those without concerns at 24 or 36 months of age, but developmentally appropriate actions such as banging, shaking, and mouthing of objects were observed equally at 12 months across all outcome groups (Ozonoff et al., 2008).

In another observational study, repetitive object manipulation and stereotyped motor behaviors were coded from recordings of the Communication and Symbolic Behavior Scales (CSBS-DP) using the Repetitive and Stereotyped Movement Scales (RSMS) in high- and low-risk 12-month olds (Elison et al., 2014). The CSBS-DP is a widely used assessment of social and communicative behaviors in infants, composed of six standardized interactions between the examiner and the infant (Wetherby & Prizant, 2002). At 12 months of age, high-risk siblings, including those who met the criteria for ASD at 24 months and those who did not, demonstrated more motor mannerisms and repetitive object manipulation than the low-risk group. There was no difference in repetitive object manipulation between high-risk siblings based on diagnostic outcome, but the high-risk siblings who went on to develop ASD displayed more motor mannerisms than the non-affected high-risk siblings. In a similar study, Damiano et al. (2013) measured the rate and number of different types (i.e., inventory) of repetitive and stereotyped movements (RSMs) using the RSMS based on coded videotapes of a play-based assessment structured around requesting, directing attention, and motor imitation (Stone, Coonrod, & Ousley, 2000; Stone, Coonrod, Turner, & Pozdol (2004). Similar to Christensen et al.'s (2011) and Elison et al.'s (2014) findings, high-risk siblings at 15 months displayed higher rates of RSMs, including body movements and object actions, than low-risk controls, irrespective of diagnostic outcome 18 months later. Furthermore, preliminary evidence suggests that a greater inventory of RSMs may be evident only for those high-risk siblings who are later diagnosed with ASD, but not unaffected high-risk siblings.

Finally, Loh et al. (2007) examined four postures and nine repetitive movements during standardized observational assessments at 12 and 18 months and found that only one behavior—"arm waving" at 18 months—differentiated high-risk siblings who developed ASD from both nonaffected high-risk siblings and low-risk controls. Two other behaviors—"arm waving" at 12 months and "hands to ears" at 18 months—were observed more frequently in the high-risk group as a whole compared to the low-risk group. Therefore, while the frequency of RRBs does appear to reliably differentiate high-risk siblings from low-risk controls in early life, only some specific RRBs seem to predict a future ASD diagnosis in high-risk siblings.

However, in a multisite longitudinal study of parent-reported patterns of RRBs at 12 and 24 months, Wolff and colleagues (2014) observed that RRBs in high-risk siblings later diagnosed with ASD were elevated compared to both high- and low-risk toddlers without the disorder at the 12-month time point on all six subtypes of the Repetitive Behavior Scales—Revised (RBS-R). Furthermore, high-risk siblings without ASD were intermediate to low-risk toddlers and high-risk siblings with ASD in the rates of RRBs displayed. It would therefore appear that, unlike observational measures, parent-report measures can distinguish high-risk siblings with

ASD from nonaffected high-risk siblings based on a wide range of RRBs. In addition, RRBs in high-risk siblings were present across a broad range of measures of general cognitive ability, which suggests that RRBs are largely unrelated to cognitive ability at early stages of development. However, total RBS-R scores were negatively correlated with measures of adaptive behavior and socialization scores in high-risk siblings later diagnosed with ASD. The authors point to a possible trade-off between RRBs and the acquisition of social skills, whereby the persistence of RRBs may limit opportunities for engaging in flexible and adaptive social interactions, while difficulties in socialization may also restrict toddlers' ability to develop functional play skills, leading to the emergence of nonfunctional play and RRBs. It may therefore be that higher rates of RRBs early in development play a contributing role in the emergence of ASD in high-risk siblings by hampering developmental plasticity (Chawarska et al., 2013; Elison et al., 2013a, 2013b), but further research into the association between repetitive behaviors and socialization among high-risk toddlers is needed.

Lastly, Chawarska et al.'s (2014) large-scale study aimed at identifying specific behavioral features predictive of diagnostic outcomes (ASD, atypical development, and typical development) in high-risk siblings paints a more nuanced picture. By applying Classification and Regression Trees (CART) analysis to individual items of the Autism Diagnostic Observation Schedule (ADOS) in 18-month-old high-risk siblings, the authors identified three distinct combinations of features predictive of ASD outcome. Notably, children who exhibited a lack of giving objects to others, repetitive interests and stereotyped behaviors, and intact eye contact were over three times more likely to have ASD than other high-risk siblings. These findings suggest that diagnostic outcomes are related not just to rates or types of RRBs, but to complex associations between RRBs and other specific behavioral features.

Taken together, these findings suggest that RRBs tend to aggregate in families and emerge as early as 12 or 18 months of age in high-risk siblings. However, the association between RRBs and diagnostic outcomes in high-risk siblings remains unresolved. RRBs include a very broad category of motor and cognitive behaviors subject to different developmental pathways, which are, almost certainly, of vastly different predictive value for a later autism diagnosis in high-risk siblings. It could be that our classification and coding of RRBs in infancy, a time in development when RRBs are especially common in the general population, is not sensitive and specific enough to pick up on subtle differences between high-risk siblings who go on to develop ASD and nonaffected high-risk siblings. Findings from Chawarska et al. (2014) suggest that various developmental pathways may result in an ASD diagnosis in high-risk siblings, each of which has its own distinct combinations of early markers, which sometimes include elevated rates of RRBs. Future studies should focus on testing the familial aggregation of different RRB subtypes and identifying combinations of behavioral features, including RRBs, at various age levels. This can help differentiate high-risk siblings based on future diagnostic outcomes and develop sensitive ASD screening tools for high-risk siblings at different stages of development.

Emotional Development

Research in high-risk infants has focused almost exclusively on identifying early brain and behavioral markers of core symptoms and their underlying mechanisms (Chawarska et al., 2013; Elsabbagh et al., 2012; Emerson et al., 2017; Hazlett et al., 2012, 2017; Shic et al., 2014; Wagner, Luyster, Moustapha, Tager-Flusberg, & Nelson, 2018; Wolff et al., 2014). Similarly, preventive (Green et al., 2015; Pickles et al., 2016) or early intervention treatments (Kasari, Gulsrud, Paparella, Hellemann, & Berry, 2015; Kasari et al., 2014; Schreibman et al., 2015) have focused on addressing core social impairments. However, in addition to social and communicative challenges, a large proportion of children with ASD develop a range of internalizing (e.g., depressive mood, anxiety) or externalizing (e.g., aggression, impulsivity) symptoms (Gadow, DeVincent, & Schneider, 2008; Leyfer et al., 2006; Salazar et al., 2015; Simonoff et al., 2008; Wood & Gadow, 2010). These conditions are also common among unaffected siblings of children with ASD, compounding their already elevated risk for social vulnerabilities (Charman et al., 2016; Georgiades et al., 2013; Howlin, Moss, Savage, Bolton, & Rutter, 2015; Jokiranta-Olkoniemi et al., 2016; Messinger et al., 2013; Miller et al., 2016, 2019; Ozonoff et al., 2011). The presence of comorbid conditions among children with ASD and their siblings impacts their social and adaptive functioning (Chiang & Gau, 2016; Rosen, Mazefsky, Vasa, & Lerner, 2018), increases family stress (Hayes & Watson, 2013), and is associated with less optimal outcomes (McGuire et al., 2016). Research in the general population demonstrates that precursors of internalizing and externalizing disorders can be identified in the first 2 years of life, are indexed by attenuated positive and accentuated negative emotional reactivity (Abulizi et al., 2017; Chronis-Tuscano et al., 2009; Finsaas, Bufferd, Dougherty, Carlson, & Klein, 2018; Kagan, Reznick, & Snidman, 1987; Lonigan, Vasey, Phillips, & Hazen, 2004; Mäntymaa et al., 2012; Moffitt, 1990; Nelson, Martin, Hodge, Havill, & Kamphaus, 1999; Nigg, 2006; Prior, Smart, Sanson, & Oberklaid, 2000; Rubin, Burgess, Dwyer, & Hastings, 2003; Volbrecht & Goldsmith, 2010), and can be targeted for intervention using parent training and dyadic psychotherapeutic interventions (Barlow, Bennett, Midgley, Larkin, & Wei, 2015; Blizzard, Barroso, Ramos, Graziano, & Bagner, 2018; Girard, Wallace, Kohlho, Morgan, & McNeil, 2018; Lowell, Carter, Godoy, Paulicin, & Briggs-Gowan, 2011;

Webster-Stratton & Reid, 2003; Zisser & Eyberg, 2010). Identification of infants and toddlers at risk for developing emotional vulnerabilities among siblings of children with ASD may hasten access to empirically validated early interventions targeting the prevention and amelioration of emotional vulnerabilities.

Data regarding the emotional development of infant siblings are scarce, and available studies focus only on parent-report measures of temperament such as the Infant Behavior Questionnaire (IBQ; Gartstein & Rothbart, 2003) or the Early Childhood Behavior Questionnaire (ECBQ; Putnam, Gartstein, & Rothbart, 2006; Putnam, Rothbart, & Gartstein, 2008). Parents reported that 6- and 12-month-old high-risk siblings later diagnosed with ASD show lower intensity of positive affectivity (surgency) compared to siblings without ASD and low-risk controls (Paterson et al., 2019) as well as lower emotional and behavioral regulation capacities compared to unaffected siblings and low-risk controls (Clifford, Hudry, Elsabbagh, Charman, & Johnson, 2013 [at 14 months]; Paterson et al., 2019). In another study, however, surgency was higher in 7-month-old infants with ASD and low-risk controls compared to non-ASD siblings (Clifford et al., 2013). Negative affect was observed to be elevated in infants with ASD at 6, 12, and 24 months (Paterson et al., 2019) in one study, but only at 24 months in another (Clifford et al., 2013), and in both cases, levels were not different from those reported for high-risk infants without ASD. At 24 months, high-risk infants diagnosed with ASD exhibited poor regulation compared to low-risk infants and high-risk infants without ASD (Paterson et al., 2019) in one study, but in another study, parental ratings of regulation as well as surgency and negative affect were not different from those of high-risk infants who were not diagnosed with ASD (Clifford et al., 2013). Thus, the findings to date suggest that temperamental vulnerabilities among siblings of children with ASD are in some cohorts and domains specific to those who are diagnosed with ASD but in other domains, vulnerabilities are expressed in unaffected siblings as well.

Although helpful in gauging temperamental characteristics of at-risk infants, parent-report measures have a number of limitations (Briggs-Gowan, Carter, & Schwab-Stone, 1996; Gartstein & Marmion, 2008) and have been known to capture unique but incomplete representations of the child's emotionality and temperament (Gagne & Goldsmith, 2011; Gagne, Van Hulle, Aksan, Essex, & Goldsmith, 2011). To date, there have been no direct observational or experimental studies of emotional reactivity in high-risk infants, though studies of emotional development in clinic-referred toddlers with ASD are just beginning to emerge. Such studies typically utilize standardized in vivo probes aimed at eliciting discrete emotions of fear, anger, or joy derived from the Laboratory Temperament Assessment Battery (LabTAB; Gagne et al., 2011), a tool developed to study development of temperament. Although parent-report studies in general reveal elevated levels of negative affectivity in high-risk infants compared to low-risk/typically developing controls, direct studies of emotional expression in toddlers with ASD paint a more complex picture. Specifically, they demonstrate that toddlers with ASD may have a diametrically different response to probes aimed to elicit fear and anger and that their response may be modulated by the social load of the emotion-eliciting events (Macari et al., 2018; Scherr, Hogan, Hatton, & Roberts, 2017). In a large sample of toddlers, the ASD group exhibited *decreased* intensity of fear in response to nonsocial threatening stimuli such as a mechanical spider compared to developmentally delayed (DD) and typically developing (TD) controls (Macari et al., 2018). In contrast, in response to social fear-eliciting probes (i.e., a stranger), young children with ASD exhibited more intense fear reactivity compared to TD and fragile X groups (Scherr et al., 2017). However, the ASD group demonstrated *increased* intensity of anger and frustration in response to goal blockage compared to the developmentally delayed group, but not typically developing controls (Macari et al., 2018). Several studies have examined positive emotional reactivity in toddlers with ASD. In response to nonsocial induction probes derived from the LabTAB (e.g., bubbles), toddlers with ASD exhibited similar levels of joy intensity compared to the DD and TD controls (Macari et al., 2018). However, in social contexts, the intensity of joy appeared to be diminished in preschoolers with ASD (Kasari, Sigman, Mundy, & Yirmiya, 1990; Joseph & Tager-Flusberg, 1997).

Understanding the emotional development of infants at risk for ASD is essential from clinical and theoretical standpoints. In the general population, early atypical negative and positive emotional reactivity is associated with later psychopathology. For instance, low levels of fear in infancy have been linked to later internalizing *and* externalizing symptoms, whereas elevated levels of fear were linked to internalizing symptoms (Colder, Mott, & Berman, 2002; Putnam & Stifter, 2005). With regard to trigger specificity, extreme fear of strangers in infancy is a precursor to the development of social anxiety (De Rosnay, Cooper, Tsigaras, & Murray, 2006; Kagan et al., 1987). Augmented anger in response to goal blockage has been associated with later externalizing problems and in some studies has predicted internalizing problems as well (Gartstein, Putnam, & Rothbart, 2012). Low levels of joy are associated with depression in middle childhood (Dougherty, Klein, Durbin, Hayden, & Olino, 2010; Ghassabian et al., 2014), while excessive levels of joy (i.e., exuberance) predict later externalizing problems (Ghassabian et al., 2014). Despite its high relevance to long-term outcomes and overall quality of life, there is extremely limited evidence regarding the early emotional development of infant siblings and predictors of internalizing and externalizing problems in this highly vulnerable population.

At present, the relationship between atypical emotional reactivity and social disability in affected children is not clear. Correlation analyses revealed no associations between the severity of autism symptoms and temperamental negative affectivity characteristics (Macari, Koller, Campbell, & Chawarska, 2017) or the intensity of emotional responses to negatively valenced events (Macari et al., 2018). This suggests that social and negative emotionality challenges in the early stages of ASD may arise from distinct etiological factors (Hawks, Marrus, Glowinski, & Constantino, 2019; Macari et al., 2018; Micalizzi, Ronald, & Saudino, 2016) and that emotional vulnerabilities contribute independently to shaping the complex phenotype of children at familial risk for ASD. Future studies will need to examine the extent to which infant siblings exhibit atypical emotional profiles in the first year of life, in addition to the links between their early temperamental and emotional reactivity and later core and comorbid psychopathology.

For more information on studies of emotional development in toddlers with ASD, see Macari et al. (Chapter 3, this volume).

Development of Attention: Evidence from Eye-Tracking Studies

Atypical attention patterns are highly prevalent from the earliest point at which ASD can currently be reliably diagnosed. When describing the syndrome for the first time, Leo Kanner (Kanner, 1943) noted that children with autism exhibit deficits in social orienting: "Comings and goings, even of the mother, did not seem to register. Conversation going on in the room elicited no interest" (pp. 245–247). Subsequent observational and experimental work has indicated that social attention deficits (i.e., the ability to select and encode information about others) represent one of the earliest symptoms of ASD (Chawarska et al., 2012; Jones, Carr, & Klin, 2008; Pierce et al., 2016). It has also been found that individual differences in social attention may contribute to some of the observed heterogeneity in levels of functioning and outcomes observed in ASD (Campbell, Shic, Macari, & Chawarska, 2014b; Elsabbagh et al., 2014; Norbury, 2014). Despite the prominence of impaired social attention in ASD, neither the mechanisms that give rise to such deficits nor their role in autistic psychopathology are well understood.

Given the strong links between gaze and attention (Deubel & Schneider, 1996), measurement of gaze allocation in response to social and nonsocial stimuli represents one of the most promising paradigms for studying development of attention in ASD. Gaze behavior studies typically involve eye-tracking technology. Eye tracking, which consists of tracking the reflection of a light source (commonly near infrared) directly toward the eyes, along with other ocular features such as the pupil, is used to extrapolate and map the direction of someone's gaze onto visual stimuli. The eye-tracking approach is highly versatile and can be used to study multiple facets of attention, including visual orienting, attentional shifting, and selective attention, as well as perception, learning, and memory in young, disabled, and largely nonverbal participants for whom instructions are difficult to follow.

In the past decade, studies utilizing eye movements have shown great promise for elucidating the processes associated with atypical social attention in ASD (see Falck-Ytter, Bölte, & Gredebäck, 2013; Guillon, Hadjikhani, Baduel, & Rogé, 2014; and Senju & Johnson, 2009, for reviews) and revealing profiles of normative and atypical performance in young children. Although toddlers with ASD detect faces among distractors as rapidly as controls (Elsabbagh et al., 2013), unlike typically developing and developmentally delayed controls, they disengage their attention from faces more quickly (Chawarska, Klin, & Volkmar, 2003; Chawarska, Volkmar, & Klin, 2010). These findings suggest that faces trigger reflexive orienting in toddlers with ASD as they do in unaffected children. However, faces do not appear to hold their attention (Cohen, 1972), presumably due to limited depth of processing or engagement with these stimuli (Bloom & Mudd, 1991; Coin & Tiberghien, 1997). When examining an image of a novel face, toddlers with ASD employ atypical face-scanning strategies and require more time to extract the invariant features necessary for identity recognition (Bradshaw, Shic, & Chawarska, 2011; Chawarska & Shic, 2009). Notably, in experiments targeting elementary face-processing skills such as capture or recognition, the stimuli are typically presented in rapid succession. Attention paid to these stimuli is externally supported by the sudden onset of the target stimuli on the screen or presentation of "attention getters" (e.g., audiovisual central fixation stimuli prior to the target onset). Such design features serve to increase the number of valid trials from individual participants and rely heavily on exogenous (i.e., reflexive, bottom-up) orienting (Petersen & Posner, 2012). However, they do not provide information about endogenous (i.e., spontaneous, top-down) orienting (Petersen & Posner, 2012) to social stimuli. Thus, they may underestimate attentional deficits in ASD and may not be helpful in explaining atypical spontaneous gaze behaviors in natural environments (Henderson, 2007; Kingstone, Smilek, & Eastwood, 2008; Tatler, 2014).

Studies of the gaze behaviors of toddlers with ASD in response to dynamic multimodal social stimuli typically employ the free-viewing paradigm, during which a child is presented with video recordings of a variety of social scenes in the absence of explicit instructions. That is, the toddlers are free to select the elements of the scene for processing as they wish, while their spatial and temporal attentional patterns are recorded and later analyzed. When toddlers with ASD view people trying to engage their attention through eye contact and child-directed speech (Chawarska et al., 2012; Shic et al., 2019), social games, and overtures (Jones et al.,

2008), or when they observe interacting adults (Nakano et al., 2010; von Hofsten, Uhlig, Adell, & Kochukhova, 2009), they tend to look less at faces than children with other developmental outcomes. They also are less likely to look at objects attended to by others (Bedford et al., 2012), and they show limited attention to the goal-oriented activities of others (Shic, Bradshaw, Klin, Scassellati, & Chawarska, 2011). Limited attention to faces in toddlers with ASD does not appear to stem from active avoidance of faces, direct gaze, or child-directed speech (Moriuchi, Klin, & Jones, 2016; Shic et al., 2019). Instead, the evidence points to the limited salience of faces or to a failure to recognize or appreciate their informational and emotional value for guiding attentional selection (Tatler, Hayhoe, Land, & Ballard, 2011). Moreover, limited attention to faces in toddlers with ASD appears highly context specific; that is, the deficits are most pronounced when either child-directed speech (i.e., children view people who speak but do not make eye contact) or both direct gaze and child-directed speech (i.e., children view people who both speak and make eye contact with them) are present (Shic et al., 2019). In the same study, no differences between toddlers with ASD and developmentally delayed and typically developing controls have been found when children were exposed to silent faces without eye contact or silent faces with eye contact. These results suggest that poor attention to faces and limited sensitivity to speech are linked during the early syndromal stages of the disorder. Shic and colleagues (2019) also reported that lesser sensitivity to gaze and verbal cues was associated with greater impairment in terms of autism symptoms, as well as verbal and nonverbal ability, concurrently and 1–2 years later. Although the mechanisms related to poor attention to faces in ASD remain to be elucidated, these results suggest that enhancing sensitivity to audiovisual speech may be a particularly efficacious target for early intervention in ASD for improving social and language outcomes.

Given the marked attentional abnormalities observed in the second year of life, that is, at the time when symptoms of ASD become apparent, a question arises: Can attentional deficits in infant siblings of children with ASD be identified in the first year of life, prior to the onset of the behavioral symptoms of ASD? Several studies have examined elementary (e.g., attention capture) and more complex (e.g., selective attention) aspects of attention using eye-tracking methods. The studies revealed several normative facets of attention in infants later diagnosed with ASD (Elsabbagh et al., 2013; Bedford et al., 2012; Jones & Klin, 2013). Typical level of attention directed at the eyes was reported in 2-month-old (Jones & Klin, 2013) as well as in 6-month-old infants later diagnosed with ASD (Chawarska et al., 2013; Shic et al., 2014). Similarly, 6- to 10-month-olds with a later diagnosis of ASD show typical attention capture by faces presented in an array of objects (Elsabbagh et al., 2012), as well as reflexive orienting to gaze cues, another relatively low-level and early-emerging aspect of social cognition

(Bedford et al., 2012). These findings are consistent with reports of attention capture by faces (O'Loughlin, Macari, Shic, & Chawarska, 2012) and reports of orienting to gaze cues (Chawarska et al., 2003) in toddlers with ASD and add to the growing evidence that the very elementary attentional processing of social stimuli may be intact in young children with ASD.

However, a number of studies reported atypical attentional functioning on multiple levels. While gaze following appeared intact, 13-month-old infants at risk for ASD looked less at congruent objects previously gazed at by a person (Bedford et al., 2012). In line with this apparent impairment in exogenous social orienting, several eye-tracking studies reported on deficits in attention to complex dynamic social stimuli (Chawarska et al., 2013; Shic et al., 2014). The paradigms captured the infant's endogenous strategies for selecting and attending to targets in the environment they find most relevant in the context of a free-viewing paradigm. Two studies examined selective social attention in 6-month-old infants later diagnosed with ASD. Chawarska and colleagues (2013) studied attention to a person engaged in several activities, and Shic and colleagues (2014) compared gaze behaviors in response to static, smiling, and speaking faces. As in other studies (Rozga et al., 2011; Young et al., 2009), 6-month-old siblings later diagnosed with ASD modulated their scanning strategies in a context-dependent manner. That is, just like their typically and atypically developing high-risk siblings and low-risk peers, they attended to the person's face when she spoke and to her hands when she made a sandwich (Chawarska et al., 2013), or they monitored the mouth region of a speaker more than the mouth region on a static image (Shic et al., 2014). In both studies, however, the siblings later diagnosed with ASD spent more time looking away from the screen altogether, suggesting that one of the prodromal features of autism likely consists of a general deficit in the regulation of visual attention to complex social scenes. In addition, infants later diagnosed with ASD spent less time fixating on the person's face (Chawarska et al., 2013; Shic et al., 2014). Recent studies examining social attention in more complex live settings or emotionally valenced social stimuli found further atypicalities and fewer gaze-alternating behaviors in siblings at risk for ASD at 10 months of age (Thorup, Nyström, Gredebäck, Bölte, & Falck-Ytter, 2016; Thorup et al., 2018). Similarly, when examining visual responses to social stimuli involving emotional content such as fearful and happy faces, 12-month-old infants later diagnosed with ASD showed reduced disengagement of attention compared to their TD peers, which further demonstrates the possibility of impairments related to the modulation of gaze and attentional shifting. These are two essential factors for the regulation of visual exchanges with social partners (Wagner, Keehn, Tager-Flusberg, & Nelson, 2019).

In addition to poor modulation of attention in infants at risk for ASD, the developmental age at which social attention is examined in siblings at risk for autism appears to explain some of the discrepancies observed among eye-tracking studies. Indeed, although looking at the eye region appeared to be present at 2 months of age, Jones and Klin (2013) revealed a decline in eye looking from 2 to 18 months of age. Similarly, Bradshaw and colleagues (2019) recently revealed poorer overall attention to animated (faces and voices) and inanimate stimuli (rattle and ball) from 2 to 3 months of age in siblings at risk for ASD compared to their typically developing peers. However, these differences were no longer present at 4 and 5 months of age (Bradshaw et al., 2019), potentially revealing vulnerabilities at important phases of neurodevelopment in infants at risk for autism. Even though all these atypical attentional features were found months before ASD can be reliably diagnosed, they were consistent with attentional difficulties noted in toddlers newly diagnosed with ASD before or around their second birthday (Chawarska et al., 2012; Pierce et al., 2016; Shic et al., 2019).

The extant evidence points to pervasive deficits in selective attention during prodromal and early syndromal stages of ASD. Given that attention gates learning can improve selective attention, it can prove beneficial to the development of social and nonsocial cognition in ASD (Wang et al., 2020b). However, poor understanding of the mechanisms underlying selective attention deficits in ASD hinders treatment efficacy. To address this limitation, several studies have begun investigating the role of value learning in selective attention in ASD (Wang, DiNicola, Heymann, Hampson, & Chawarska, 2018b, Wang, Chang, & Chawarska, 2020a). Value learning system constitutes one of the components of the reward neural circuitry and supports leaning about relevance of objects in the real-world environment, thus enabling an individual to direct attentional resources toward objects that are informative while ignoring those that carry little adaptive value (Gottlieb, Hayhoe, Hikosaka, & Rangel, 2014). A recent study utilizing a novel eye-tracking gaze-contingent task identified deficits in value-driven attentional selection in the social domain and enhanced value-driven attentional selection in the nonsocial domain in ASD (Wang et al., 2020a). The study demonstrated links between atypical value learning in social and nonsocial domains and selective attention in ASD. If present early, atypical value learning in social and nonsocial domains may have a profound impact on the development of neural systems supporting development of social attention and cognition in ASD. This hypothesis would be best addressed through prospective studies of infant siblings where development of value learning systems and their links with emerging atypical attention and autistic psychopathology can be evaluated directly.

Thus, real-world and eye-tracking studies suggest that attention to social patterns, particularly to faces, is impaired not only during the early syndromal stages of the disorder, but also during the prodromal stage, with deficits becoming apparent as early as 6 months of age. Extant, albeit still limited, evidence suggests that impaired attention to faces is present particularly when the infants interact face to face with a person making eye contact and speaking. Importantly, the deficits observed in infants later diagnosed with ASD are consistent with those observed in clinic-referred toddlers with ASD. This provides evidence not only for the continuity of these impairments from the prodromal to the syndromal stage of the disorder, but also for the generalizability of findings from prospective sibling samples to clinic-referred samples. Free-viewing eye-tracking protocols have yielded highly promising discriminative and predictive biomarkers. Given the high heterogeneity in social attention present in ASD (Campbell et al., 2014b; Wang, Campbell, Macari, Chawarska, & Shic, 2018a), future investigation into functional subtypes within the autism spectrum based on attention to gaze and speech cues will facilitate the development of stratification biomarkers in the early stages of ASD. There is also a pressing need to complement this work with an investigation into markers of ASD based on a process-oriented approach that may provide more direct insights into mechanisms underlying atypical social attention in ASD (Fitzpatrick, 2018; Wang et al., 2018b; Wang et al., 2020a).

For more information on neuroanatomical and neurophysiological development, see Sifre, Piven, and Elison (Chapter 6, this volume).

Cognitive, Language, and Motor Development

Delays in the development of language and cognition are very common among toddlers with ASD, though there is a marked heterogeneity among toddlers with regard to the degree and type of delays. While some children experience delays across verbal and nonverbal domains, it is also rather common to observe a large split between verbal and nonverbal skills (Barbaro & Dissanayake, 2012; Chawarska et al., 2007b; for more information, see Macari et al., Chapter 3, this volume). Most commonly, the split reflects the nonverbal skill advantage and, much less commonly, the verbal skill advantage. These uniformly delayed or atypical split profiles are rarely observed in the first year of life. At 6 months, infants later diagnosed with ASD tend to have scores in the verbal and nonverbal domains largely in the normative range, as captured by the MSEL (Chawarska et al., 2013; Landa & Garrett-Mayer, 2006; Ozonoff et al., 2010). When differences from low-risk controls begin to emerge, they are typically not specific to siblings who are later diagnosed with ASD, but are shared with siblings showing BAP features (Estes et al., 2015).

Delays in nonverbal skills are typically not very pronounced at the group level among 12-month-old infants later diagnosed with ASD (Estes et al., 2015; Macari et al., 2012; Ozonoff et al., 2010). However, verbal and fine motor skills tend to be lower in high-risk infants, but their specificity to ASD is not very strong. Indeed, although 12-month-old infants with ASD exhibit lower scores on the receptive and expressive language scales of the

MSEL (Mullen, 1995) compared to typical controls (Mitchell et al., 2006; Zwaigenbaum et al., 2005), similar deficits are observed among high-risk infants without ASD (Estes et al., 2015; Landa & Garrett-Mayer, 2006; Macari et al., 2012). Language delays persist at 24 months in siblings with and without ASD alike (Estes et al., 2015; Marrus et al., 2018). The prevalence of language delays is 3–4 times greater in siblings without ASD than in low-risk controls (e.g., 15.6 vs. 5.7%, respectively; Marrus et al., 2018). Similar to toddlers with ASD (Paul, Chawarska, Klin, & Volkmar, 2017), high-risk siblings without ASD show particular vulnerabilities in the understanding of language (receptive language), despite intact language production (expressive language; Marrus et al., 2018).

With regard to motor development, performance on standardized tests of fine and motor skills of infants later diagnosed with ASD also appears to be largely in the normative range at 6 months of age (Iverson et al., 2019), suggesting that the motor deficits reported in older children with ASD (e.g., Ament et al., 2015) are likely to emerge later, in the second and third years of life (West, Leezenbaum, Northrup, & Iverson, 2019). Interestingly, although minor vulnerabilities in fine motor skills have been reported in the first year of life, these do not appear to be specific to infants who later develop ASD. In a large multisite study, at 6 months, high-risk infants were more likely to fail some items on the fine motor scale than low-risk infants, and their performance on the scale was predictive of the severity of autism symptoms at 36 months but not of diagnostic outcome (Iverson et al., 2019).

Thus, frank delays among infant siblings later diagnosed with ASD or their unaffected siblings are not readily observable in the first year of life. Delays in language development, nonverbal cognition, and motor skills begin to emerge around, and intensify, after the first birthday. However, even at 2 years of age, the observed delays are not specific to ASD; indeed, they are also frequently observed in siblings without an ASD diagnosis.

For more information on the developmental profiles of toddlers with ASD, see Macari et al. (Chapter 3, this volume).

Clinical Care of Siblings at Familial Risk for ASD

As reviewed in previous sections, social, language, cognitive, and motor delays as indexed by standardized tests are not readily apparent in the first year of life in infants at familial risk for ASD. When these features begin to emerge in the second year, they are present in both ASD and non-ASD siblings. For these reasons, differentiating siblings with ASD from those exhibiting BAP features in the second year of life can be complex and requires consideration of infants' profiles of strengths and challenges across multiple domains to achieve a reliable diagnostic classification (Ozonoff et al., 2015; see also Campi, Lord, and Grzadzinski, Chapter 2, this volume). Studies that follow high-risk siblings into preschool age suggest that an early diagnosis of ASD among siblings of children with ASD is typically stable (Ozonoff et al., 2015; Zwaigenbaum et al., 2016), even at 18 months of age. In a multisite study, ASD diagnosis ascertained at 18 months and at 24 months was confirmed at 36 months in 93% and 82% of subjects, respectively. However, many siblings are initially missed and not diagnosed until the age of 3 years or later (Ozonoff et al., 2015; Zwaigenbaum et al., 2016). For instance, expert clinicians missed as many as 63% of ASD cases at 18 months and 41% of cases at 24 months (Ozonoff et al., 2015). Those who are missed are less likely to have marked language or cognitive delays and have less severe autism symptoms (Ozonoff et al., 2015; Zwaigenbaum et al., 2016). One explanation for the missed cases in the second year of life is that symptoms of ASD emerge and intensify at different ages in different children (e.g., early- versus later-onset groups; Landa, Holman, & Garrett-Mayer, 2007), which would suggest that the appropriate approach to early detection is repeated screening and surveillance. However, delays and atypical features are typically present early on in high-risk siblings who do not receive a diagnosis until 2–3 years of age, as well as in toddlers ascertained from general pediatric practices and universal screenings (Bacon et al., 2018; Øien et al., 2018; Ozonoff et al., 2015). This could point to an alternative explanation, whereby the current diagnostic practices for young children are based on how social disability presents in less cognitively able toddlers (Chawarska et al., 2014). Future studies will need to determine whether and how early screening and diagnostic instruments for ASD need to be further calibrated to improve detection of ASD in toddlers who do not experience marked developmental delays and to help differentiate ASD from BAP (Chawarska et al., 2014).

Although experimental studies suggest that the prognostic features of ASD may be detectable in the first year of life on the behavioral, neurobehavioral, neurophysiological, and neuroanatomical levels, the sensitivity and specificity of the features are either weak or unknown, or the feasibility of their use in the general population still remains to be determined. Thus, these features are not currently recommended as diagnostic or prognostic indicators, either to rule in or rule out an ASD diagnosis or to determine the future level of impairment. However, these studies suggest that processes related to ASD are already unfolding within the first postnatal months, perhaps even earlier, and it is a matter of time until more reliable brain and behavioral markers of ASD are identified.

Although determining the ultimate ASD status of siblings of children with ASD in the first 2 to 3 years of life may be challenging, there is overwhelming evidence suggesting that siblings, as a group, experience enduring vulnerabilities in social, emotional, language, behavioral, attentional, and cognitive domains. As such, their clinical needs should be addressed in a timely manner, regardless of their current diagnostic classification. This pertains not only to social difficulties but also to language and cognitive delays, to emotional and regulatory challenges that may foreshadow the emergence of other neurodevelopmental problems such as ADHD, anxiety, or behavioral challenges. Close clinical follow-up achieved through prospective studies of infant siblings may indeed facilitate early detection of vulnerabilities and initiation of treatment. Consistent with this notion, a recent review of 11 prospective infant sibling studies suggests that toddlers with ASD ascertained through these studies have higher developmental levels and lower severity of autism symptoms compared to clinic-referred toddlers with ASD and toddlers identified through universal screening (Micheletti et al., 2020). Although other factors such as ascertainment biases and genetic factors (e.g., multiplex versus simplex status) cannot be fully ruled out, it is also plausible that prospective follow-up results in a "surveillance effect" that contributed to more optimal developmental outcomes in infant siblings. That is, by being exposed to expert clinical teams and observations of clinical assessment procedures, parents may learn new ways of interacting with and scaffolding their infants' development. Moreover, infants and toddlers who are lagging behind may benefit from early referrals to intervention services. It is also likely that participation in prospective studies of infant siblings provides parents with much-needed educational and emotional support, contributing to the developmental gains of their infants (Brian, Bryson, Zwaigenbaum, Cosgrove, & Roberts, 2018).

For more information on screening, see Campi, Lord, and Grzadzinski (Chapter 2, this volume). For more information about intervention during prodromal and early syndromal stages, see Pizzano and Kasari (Chapter 4, this volume) and Green (Chapter 8, this volume). For information regarding long-term outcomes of infants at risk, see Miller and Ozonoff (Chapter 7, this volume).

Conclusions and Future Directions

The emerging evidence from prospective studies of infants at risk for ASD suggests that features of autism begin to emerge early in the first year of life and that genetic liability for ASD confers risk for not only social but also affective, behavioral, and emotional difficulties later in life. Genetic risk factors also result in a range of clinically consequential developmental challenges among siblings who do not eventually meet the diagnostic criteria for ASD. In addition to generating important insights into the timing and processes contributing to the development of autism symptoms, the prospective studies of infant siblings also generate readily translatable clinical findings useful for addressing therapeutic needs of the vulnerable sibling population and their families.

However, much work remains to be done. Although behavioral, neurobehavioral, and neurophysiological studies suggest that differences between infants who are later diagnosed with ASD and their unaffected counterparts are present by 6 months of age, further refinement of research paradigms and measurement methods is necessary to increase the predictive accuracy of identified biomarkers. Moreover, most of the markers described in the literature were detected at 6 months or thereafter largely because studies focused on the first postnatal months are still very rare. Lowering the age at which siblings are recruited into prospective studies will help to elucidate primary impairments and their underlying mechanisms on neurobehavioral, physiological, electrophysiological, and neuroimaging levels. Furthermore, many ASD cases among high-risk siblings go undetected despite undergoing comprehensive evaluations at 18 or 24 months. The factors leading to delayed diagnosis in a large number of siblings are not well understood, and their elucidation may lead to the development of more precise screening, diagnostic instruments, and assessment practices. Although there is compelling evidence linking the sex of siblings and recurrence risk, less is known about behavioral and brain markers of risk and resilience as well as differences in developmental trajectories and outcomes in male and female at-risk siblings. The evidence in this area is only beginning to emerge (Bedford et al., 2016; Campbell, Chang, & Chawarska, 2014a; Chawarska et al., 2016; Halladay et al., 2015; Kleberg et al., 2019; Messinger et al., 2015; Zwaigenbaum et al., 2012), and future work needs to focus not only on siblings affected by ASD but also on those who experience other developmental challenges but do not develop ASD and those who are developing typically. The latter groups are particularly important for determining factors that may protect otherwise genetically vulnerable siblings from developing the social disability syndrome (Szatmari, 2018). Finally, the infant sibling paradigm provides a unique opportunity for examining the interaction of genetic and familial risk factors shaping their complex developmental trajectories. Multiple studies have documented an increased liability for anxiety, depression, and elevated stress levels, as well as remarkable resiliency and coping strategies among parents of children with ASD. However, our understanding of how these factors influence the developmental outcomes of younger siblings of children of autism remains very limited.

Although extremely valuable, prospective infant sibling studies have a number of limitations (Szatmari et al., 2016). Repeated evaluations over the course of the first 2–3 years may generate practice or habituation effects, altering patterns of brain and behavioral findings in unpredictable ways. Close clinical monitoring, parent education, and early referral for services may alter the overall developmental outcomes of siblings, limiting the generalizability of findings from prospective studies to a broader population of clinic-referred toddlers (Micheletti et al., 2020). Finally, it is not clear whether behavioral and biological findings from families with more than one child with ASD (multiplex cases) generalize to children in families with only one affected child (simplex cases), in whom the disorder might arise through partially different genetic mechanisms and result in distinct phenotypes (Dissanayake, Searles, Barbaro, Sadka, & Lawson, 2019; Leppa et al., 2016; Ruzzo et al., 2018; Sanders et al., 2012). Thus, future studies are needed to verify whether the phenotypic characteristics of infants in multiplex families are consistent with those observed in simplex cases as well. These challenges will need to be tackled as the research on infant siblings of children with ASD enters its second decade.

REFERENCES

Abulizi, X., Pryor, L., Michel, G., Melchior, M., Van Der Waerden, J., & on behalf of the EDEN Mother–Child Cohort Group. (2017). Temperament in infancy and behavioral and emotional problems at age 5.5: The EDEN mother–child cohort. *PLOS ONE, 12*(2), e0171971.

Ament, K., Mejia, A., Buhlman, R., Erklin, S., Caffo, B., Mostofsky, S., & Wodka, E. (2015). Evidence for specificity of motor impairments in catching and balance in children with autism. *Journal of Autism and Developmental Disorders, 45*(3), 742–751.

Bacon, E. C., Courchesne, E., Barnes, C. C., Cha, D., Pence, S., Schreibman, L., . . . Pierce, K. (2018). Rethinking the idea of late autism spectrum disorder onset. *Development and Psychopathology, 30*(2), 553–569.

Bailey, A., Palferman, S., Heavey, L., & Le Couteur, A. (1998). Autism: The phenotype in relatives. *Journal of Autism and Developmental Disorders, 28*(5), 369–392.

Barbaro, J., & Dissanayake, C. (2012). Developmental profiles of infants and toddlers with autism spectrum disorders identified prospectively in a community-based setting. *Journal of Autism and Developmental Disorders, 42*(9), 1939–1948.

Barlow, J., Bennett, C., Midgley, N., Larkin, S. K., & Wei, Y. (2015). Parent–infant psychotherapy for improving parental and infant mental health. *Cochrane Database of Systematic Reviews, 2015*(1), CD010534.

Bedford, R., Elsabbagh, M., Gliga, T., Pickles, A., Senju, A., Charman, T., . . . BASIS Team. (2012). Precursors to social and communication difficulties in infants at-risk for autism: Gaze following and attentional engagement. *Journal of Autism and Developmental Disorders, 42*(10), 2208–2218.

Bedford, R., Jones, E. J., Johnson, M. H., Pickles, A., Charman, T., & Gliga, T. (2016). Sex differences in the association between infant markers and later autistic traits. *Molecular Autism, 7*(1), 21.

Blizzard, A. M., Barroso, N. E., Ramos, F. G., Graziano, P. A., & Bagner, D. M. (2018). Behavioral parent training in infancy: What about the parent–infant relationship? *Journal of Clinical Child and Adolescent Psychology, 47*(Supp. 1), S341–S353.

Bloom, L. C., & Mudd, S. A. (1991). Depth of processing approach to face recognition: A test of two theories. *Journal of Experimental Psychology: Learning, Memory, and Cognition, 17*(3), 556–565.

Bradshaw, J., Klin, A., Evans, L., Klaiman, C., Saulnier, C., & McCracken, C. (2019). Development of attention from birth to 5 months in infants at risk for autism spectrum disorder. *Development and Psychopathology, 23*, 1–11.

Bradshaw, J., Shic, F., & Chawarska, K. (2011). Brief report: Face-specific recognition deficits in young children with autism spectrum disorders. *Journal of Autism and Developmental Disorders, 41*(10), 1429–1435.

Brian, J., Bryson, S. E., Zwaigenbaum, L., Cosgrove, S., & Roberts, W. (2018). Supporting the families of high-risk infants who have an older sibling with ASD: Collaboration, consultation, and care. In M. Siller & L. Morgan (Eds.), *Handbook of parent-implemented interventions for very young children with autism* (pp. 45–57). New York: Springer.

Briggs-Gowan, M. J., Carter, A. S., & Schwab-Stone, M. (1996). Discrepancies among mother, child, and teacher reports: Examining the contributions of maternal depression and anxiety. *Journal of Abnormal Child Psychology, 24*(6), 749–765.

Bryson, S. E., Zwaigenbaum, L., McDermott, C., Rombough, V., & Brian, J. (2008). The Autism Observation Scale for Infants: Scale development and reliability data. *Journal of Autism and Developmental Disorders, 38*(4), 731–738.

Campbell, D. J., Chang, J., & Chawarska, K. (2014a). Early generalized overgrowth in autism spectrum disorder: Prevalence rates, gender effects, and clinical outcomes. *Journal of the American Academy of Child and Adolescent Psychiatry, 53*(10), 1063–1073.

Campbell, D. J., Shic, F., Macari, S., & Chawarska, K. (2014b). Gaze response to dyadic bids at 2 years related to outcomes at 3 years in autism spectrum disorders: A subtyping analysis. *Journal of Autism and Developmental Disorders, 44*(2), 431–442.

Centers for Disease Control and Prevention. (2012). Prevalence of autism spectrum disorders—Autism and Developmental Disabilities Monitoring Network, 14 sites, United States, 2008. *MMWR Surveillance Summaries, 61*(SS03), 1–19

Charman, T., Young, G. S., Brian, J., Carter, A., Carver, L. J., Chawarska, K., . . . Zwaigenbaum, L. (2016). Non-ASD outcomes at 36 months in siblings at familial risk for autism spectrum disorder (ASD): A Baby Siblings Research Consortium (BSRC) study. *Autism Research, 10*(1), 169–178.

Chawarska, K., Klin, A., Paul, R., Macari, S., & Volkmar, F. (2009). A prospective study of toddlers with ASD: Short-term diagnostic and cognitive outcomes. *Journal of Child Psychology and Psychiatry, 50*(10), 1235–1245.

Chawarska, K., Klin, A., Paul, R., & Volkmar, F. (2007a). Autism spectrum disorder in the second year: Stability and change in syndrome expression. *Journal of Child Psychology and Psychiatry, 48*(2), 128–138.

Chawarska, K., Klin, A., & Volkmar, F. (2003). Automatic attention cueing through eye movement in 2-year-old children with autism. *Child Development, 74*(4), 1108–1122.

Chawarska, K., Macari, S., Powell, K., DiNicola, L., & Shic, F. (2016). Enhanced social attention in female infant siblings at risk for autism. *Journal of the American Academy of Child and Adolescent Psychiatry, 55*(3), 188–195.

Chawarska, K., Macari, S., & Shic, F. (2012). Context modulates attention to social scenes in toddlers with autism. *Journal of Child Psychology and Psychiatry, 53*(8), 903–913.

Chawarska, K., Macari, S., & Shic, F. (2013). Decreased spontaneous attention to social scenes in 6-month-old infants later diagnosed with autism spectrum disorders. *Biological Psychiatry, 74*(3), 195–203.

Chawarska, K., Paul, R., Klin, A., Hannigen, S., Dichtel, L., & Volkmar, F. (2007b). Parental recognition of developmental problems in toddlers with autism spectrum disorders. *Journal of Autism and Developmental Disorders, 37*(1), 62–72.

Chawarska, K., & Shic, F. (2009). Looking but not seeing: Atypical visual scanning and recognition of faces in 2- and 4-year-old children with autism spectrum disorder. *Journal of Autism and Developmental Disorders, 39*(12), 1663–1672.

Chawarska, K., Shic, F., Macari, S., Campbell, D. J., Brian, J., Landa, R., . . . Bryson, S. (2014). 18-month predictors of later outcomes in younger siblings of children with autism spectrum disorder: A Baby Siblings Research Consortium study. *Journal of the American Academy of Child and Adolescent Psychiatry, 53*(12), 1317–1327.

Chawarska, K., Volkmar, F., & Klin, A. (2010). Limited attentional bias for faces in toddlers with autism spectrum disorders. *Archives of General Psychiatry, 67*(2), 178–185.

Chiang, H. L., & Gau, S. S. F. (2016). Comorbid psychiatric conditions as mediators to predict later social adjustment in youths with autism spectrum disorder. *Journal of Child Psychology and Psychiatry, 57*(1), 103–111.

Christensen, L., Hutman, T., Rozga, A., Young, G. S., Ozonoff, S., Rogers, S. J., . . . Sigman, M. (2011). Play and developmental outcomes in infant siblings of children with autism. *Journal of Autism and Developmental Disorders, 40*(8), 946–957.

Chronis-Tuscano, A., Degnan, K. A., Pine, D. S., Perez-Edgar, K., Henderson, H. A., Diaz, Y., . . . Fox, N. A. (2009). Stable early maternal report of behavioral inhibition predicts lifetime social anxiety disorder in adolescence. *Journal of the American Academy of Child and Adolescent Psychiatry, 48*(9), 928–935.

Clifford, S. M., Hudry, K., Elsabbagh, M., Charman, T., & Johnson, M. H. (2013). Temperament in the first 2 years of life in infants at high-risk for autism spectrum disorders. *Journal of Autism and Developmental Disorders, 43*(3), 673–686.

Cohen, L. B. (1972). Attention-getting and attention-holding processes of infant visual preferences. *Child Development, 43*(3), 869–879.

Coin, C., & Tiberghien, G. (1997). Encoding activity and face recognition. *Memory, 5*(5), 545–568.

Colder, C. R., Mott, J. A., & Berman, A. S. (2002). The interactive effects of infant activity level and fear on growth trajectories of early childhood behavior problems. *Development and Psychopathology, 14*(1), 1–23.

Constantino, J. N., Zhang, Y., Frazier, T., Abbacchi, A. M., & Law, P. (2010). Sibling recurrence and the genetic epidemiology of autism. *American Journal of Psychiatry, 167*(11), 1349.

Damiano, C. R., Nahmias, A., Hogan-Brown, A. L., & Stone, W. L. (2013). What do repetitive and stereotyped movements mean for infant siblings of children with autism spectrum disorders? *Journal of Autism and Developmental Disorders, 43*(6), 1326–1335.

De Rosnay, M., Cooper, P. J., Tsigaras, N., & Murray, L. (2006). Transmission of social anxiety from mother to infant: An experimental study using a social referencing paradigm. *Behaviour Research and Therapy, 44*(8), 1165–1175.

Deubel, H., & Schneider, W. X. (1996). Saccade target selection and object recognition: Evidence for a common attentional mechanism. *Vision Research, 36*(12), 1827–1837.

Dissanayake, C., Searles, J., Barbaro, J., Sadka, N., & Lawson, L. P. (2019). Cognitive and behavioral differences in toddlers with autism spectrum disorder from multiplex and simplex families. *Autism Research, 12*(4), 682–693.

Dougherty, L. R., Klein, D. N., Durbin, C. E., Hayden, E. P., & Olino, T. M. (2010). Temperamental positive and negative emotionality and children's depressive symptoms: A longitudinal prospective study from age three to age ten. *Journal of Social and Clinical Psychology, 29*(4), 462–488.

Elison, J. T., Paterson, S. J., Wolff, J. J., Reznick, J. S., Sasson, N. J., Gu, H., . . . Infant Brain Imaging Study (IBIS) Network. (2013a). White matter microstructure and atypical visual orienting in 7-month-olds at risk for autism. *American Journal of Psychiatry, 170*, 899–908.

Elison, J. T., Wolff, J. J., Heimer, D. C., Paterson, S. J., Gu, H., Hazlett, H. C., . . . Infant Brain Imaging Study (IBIS) Network. (2013b). Frontolimbic neural circuitry at 6 months predicts individual differences in joint attention at 9 months. *Developmental Science, 16*(2), 186–197.

Elison, J. T., Wolff, J. J., Reznick, J. S., Botteron, K. N., Estes, A. M., Gu, H., . . . Zwaigenbaum, L. (2014). Repetitive behavior in 12-month-olds later classified with autism spectrum disorder. *Journal of the American Academy of Child and Adolescent Psychiatry, 53*(11), 1216–1224.

Elsabbagh, M., Bedford, R., Senju, A., Charman, T., Pickles, A., & Johnson, M. H. (2014). What you see is what you get: Contextual modulation of face scanning in typical and atypical development. *Social Cognitive and Affective Neuroscience, 9*(4), 538–543.

Elsabbagh, M., Gliga, T., Pickles, A., Hudry, K., Charman, T., Johnson, M. H., & BASIS Team. (2013). The development of face orienting mechanisms in infants at-risk for autism. *Behavioural Brain Research, 251*, 147–154.

Elsabbagh, M., Mercure, E., Hudry, K., Chandler, S., Pasco, G., Charman, T., . . . BASIS Team. (2012). Infant neural sensitivity to dynamic eye gaze is associated with later emerging autism. *Current Biology, 22*(4), 338–342.

Emerson, R. W., Adams, C., Nishino, T., Hazlett, H. C., Wolff, J. J., Zwaigenbaum, L., . . . Piven, J. (2017). Functional neuroimaging of high-risk 6-month-old infants predicts a diagnosis of autism at 24 months of age. *Science Translational Medicine, 9*(393), pii.

Estes, A., Zwaigenbaum, L., Gu, H., John, T. S., Paterson, S., Elison, J. T., . . . Infant Brain Imaging Study (IBIS) Network. (2015). Behavioral, cognitive, and adaptive development in infants with autism spectrum disorder in the first 2 years of life. *Journal of Neurodevelopmental Disorders, 7*(1), 24.

Falck-Ytter, T., Bölte, S., & Gredebäck, G. (2013). Eye tracking in early autism research. *Journal of Neurodevelopmental Disorders, 5*(1), 28.

Filliter, J. H., Longard, J., Lawrence, M. A., Zwaigenbaum, L., Brian, J., Garon, N., . . . Bryson, S. E. (2015). Positive affect in infant siblings of children diagnosed with autism spectrum disorder. *Journal of Abnormal Child Psychology, 43*(3), 567–575.

Finsaas, M. C., Bufferd, S. J., Dougherty, L. R., Carlson, G. A., & Klein, D. N. (2018). Preschool psychiatric disorders: Homotypic and heterotypic continuity through middle childhood and early adolescence. *Psychological Medicine, 48*(13), 1–10.

Fitzpatrick, P. (2018). The future of autism research: Dynamic and process-oriented approaches. *Journal of the American Academy of Child and Adolescent Psychiatry, 57*(1), 16–17.

Gadow, K. D., DeVincent, C., & Schneider, J. (2008). Predictors of psychiatric symptoms in children with an autism spectrum disorder. *Journal of Autism and Developmental Disorders, 38*(9), 1710–1720.

Gagne, J. R., & Goldsmith, H. H. (2011). A longitudinal analysis of anger and inhibitory control in twins from 12 to 36 months of age. *Developmental Science, 14*(1), 112–124.

Gagne, J. R., Van Hulle, C. A., Aksan, N., Essex, M. J., & Goldsmith, H. (2011). Deriving childhood temperament measures from emotion-eliciting behavioral episodes: Scale construction and initial validation. *Psychological Assessment, 23*(2), 337–353.

Gammer, I., Bedford, R., Elsabbagh, M., Garwood, H., Pasco, G., Tucker, L., . . . BASIS Team. (2015). Behavioural markers for autism in infancy: Scores on the Autism Observational Scale for Infants in a prospective study of at-risk siblings. *Infant Behavior and Development, 38,* 107–115.

Gangi, D. N., Schwichtenberg, A., Iosif, A.-M., Young, G. S., Baguio, F., & Ozonoff, S. (2018). Gaze to faces across interactive contexts in infants at heightened risk for autism. *Autism, 22*(6), 763–768.

Gartstein, M. A., & Marmion, J. (2008). Fear and positive affectivity in infancy: Convergence/discrepancy between parent-report and laboratory-based indicators. *Infant Behavior and Development, 31*(2), 227–238.

Gartstein, M. A., Putnam, S. P., & Rothbart, M. K. (2012). Etiology of preschool behavior problems: Contributions of temperament attributes in early childhood. *Infant Mental Health Journal, 33*(2), 197–211.

Gartstein, M. A., & Rothbart, M. K. (2003). Studying infant temperament via the revised infant behavior questionnaire. *Infant Behavior and Development, 26*(1), 64–86.

Georgiades, S., Szatmari, P., Zwaigenbaum, L., Bryson, S., Brian, J., Roberts, W., . . . Garon, N. (2013). A prospective study of autistic-like traits in unaffected siblings of probands with autism spectrum disorder. *JAMA Psychiatry, 70*(1), 42–48.

Ghassabian, A., Szekely, E., Herba, C. M., Jaddoe, V. W., Hofman, A., Oldehinkel, A. J., . . . Tiemeier, H. (2014). From positive emotionality to internalizing problems: The role of executive functioning in preschoolers. *European Child and Adolescent Psychiatry, 23*(9), 729–741.

Girard, E. I., Wallace, N. M., Kohlho, J. R., Morgan, S. S., & McNeil, C. B. (2018). *Parent–child interaction therapy with toddlers.* New York: Springer.

Gottlieb, J., Hayhoe, M., Hikosaka, O., & Rangel, A. (2014). Attention, reward, and information seeking. *Journal of Neuroscience, 34*(46), 15497–15504.

Green, J., Charman, T., Pickles, A., Wan, M. W., Elsabbagh, M., Slonims, V., . . . BASIS Team. (2015). Parent-mediated intervention versus no intervention for infants at high risk of autism: A parallel, single-blind, randomised trial. *The Lancet Psychiatry, 2*(2), 133–140.

Guillon, Q., Hadjikhani, N., Baduel, S., & Rogé, B. (2014). Visual social attention in autism spectrum disorder: Insights from eye tracking studies. *Neuroscience and Biobehavioral Reviews, 42,* 279–297.

Halladay, A. K., Bishop, S., Constantino, J. N., Daniels, A. M., Koenig, K., Palmer, K., . . . Szatmari, P. (2015). Sex and gender differences in autism spectrum disorder: Summarizing evidence gaps and identifying emerging areas of priority. *Molecular Autism, 6*(1), 36.

Hansen, S. N., Schendel, D. E., Francis, R. W., Windham, G. C., Bresnahan, M., Levine, S. Z., . . . Parner, E. T. (2019). Recurrence risk of autism in siblings and cousins: A multinational, population-based study. *Journal of the American Academy of Child and Adolescent Psychiatry, 58*(9), 866–875.

Hawks, Z. W., Marrus, N., Glowinski, A. L., & Constantino, J. N. (2019). Early origins of autism comorbidity: Neuropsychiatric traits correlated in childhood are independent in infancy. *Journal of Abnormal Child Psychology, 47*(2), 369–379.

Hayes, S. A., & Watson, S. L. (2013). The impact of parenting stress: A meta-analysis of studies comparing the experience of parenting stress in parents of children with and without autism spectrum disorder. *Journal of Autism and Developmental Disorders, 43*(3), 629–642.

Hazlett, H. C., Gu, H., Munsell, B. C., Kim, S. H., Styner, M., Wolff, J. J., . . . Statistical Analysis. (2017). Early brain development in infants at high risk for autism spectrum disorder. *Nature, 542*(7641), 348.

Hazlett, H. C., Poe, M. D., Lightbody, A. A., Styner, M., MacFall, J. R., Reiss, A. L., & Piven, J. (2012). Trajectories of early brain volume development in fragile X syndrome and autism. *Journal of the American Academy of Child and Adolescent Psychiatry, 51*(9), 921–933.

Henderson, J. M. (2007). Regarding scenes. *Current Directions in Psychological Science, 16*(4), 219–222.

Howlin, P., Moss, P., Savage, S., Bolton, P., & Rutter, M. (2015). Outcomes in adult life among siblings of individuals with autism. *Journal of Autism and Developmental Disorders, 45*(3), 707–718.

Ingersoll, B., & Wainer, A. (2014). The broader autism phenotype. In F. R. Volkmar, R. Paul, S. J. Rgers, & K. A. Pelphrey, *Handbook of autism and pervasive developmental disorders, fourth edition.* Hoboken, NJ: Wiley.

Iverson, J. M., Shic, F., Wall, C. A., Chawarska, K., Curtin, S., Estes, A., . . . Young, G. S. (2019). Early motor abilities in infants at heightened versus low risk for ASD: A Baby Siblings Research Consortium (BSRC) study. *Journal of Abnormal Psychology, 128*(1), 69.

Jokiranta-Olkoniemi, E., Cheslack-Postava, K., Sucksdorff, D., Suominen, A., Gyllenberg, D., Chudal, R., . . . Sourander, A. (2016). Risk of psychiatric and neurodevelopmental disorders among siblings of probands with autism spectrum disorders. *JAMA Psychiatry, 73*(6), 622–629.

Jones, W., Carr, K., & Klin, A. (2008). Absence of preferential looking to the eyes of approaching adults predicts level of social disability in 2-year-old toddlers with autism spectrum disorder. *Archives of General Psychiatry, 65*(8), 946–954.

Jones, W., & Klin, A. (2013). Attention to eyes is present but in decline in 2–6-month-old infants later diagnosed with autism. *Nature, 504*(7480), 427–431.

Joseph, R. M., & Tager-Flusberg, H. (1997). An investigation of attention and affect in children with autism and Down syndrome. *Journal of Autism and Developmental Disorders, 27*(4), 385–396.

Kagan, J., Reznick, J., & Snidman, N. (1987). The physiology and psychology of behavioral inhibition in children. *Child Development, 58*(6), 1459–1473.

Kanner, L. (1943). Autistic disturbances of affective contact. *Nervous Child, 2*(3), 217–250.

Kasari, C., Gulsrud, A., Paparella, T., Hellemann, G., & Berry, K. (2015). Randomized comparative efficacy study of parent-mediated interventions for toddlers with autism. *Journal of Consulting and Clinical Psychology, 83*(3), 554.

Kasari, C., Kaiser, A., Goods, K., Nietfeld, J., Mathy, P., Landa, R., . . . Almirall, D. (2014). Communication interventions for minimally verbal children with autism: A sequential multiple assignment randomized trial. *Journal of the American Academy of Child and Adolescent Psychiatry, 53*(6), 635–646.

Kasari, C., Sigman, M., Mundy, P., & Yirmiya, N. (1990). Affective sharing in the context of joint attention interactions of normal, autistic, and mentally retarded children. *Journal of Autism and Developmental Disorders, 20*(1), 87–100.

Kingstone, A., Smilek, D., & Eastwood, J. D. (2008). Cognitive ethology: A new approach for studying human cognition. *British Journal of Psychology, 99*(3), 317–340.

Kleberg, J. L., Nyström, P., Bölte, S., & Falck-Ytter, T. (2019). Sex differences in social attention in infants at risk for autism. *Journal of Autism and Developmental Disorders, 49*(4), 1342–1351.

Landa, R., & Garrett-Mayer, E. (2006). Development in infants with autism spectrum disorders: A prospective study. *Journal of Child Psychology and Psychiatry, 47*(6), 629–638.

Landa, R. J., Holman, K. C., & Garrett-Mayer, E. (2007). Social and communication development in toddlers with early and later diagnosis of autism spectrum disorders. *Archives of General Psychiatry, 64*(7), 853–864.

Lazenby, D. C., Sideridis, G. D., Huntington, N., Prante, M., Dale, P. S., Curtin, S., . . . Tager-Flusberg, H. (2016). Language differences at 12 months in infants who develop autism spectrum disorder. *Journal of Autism and Developmental Disorders, 46*(3), 899–909.

Leppa, V. M., Kravitz, S. N., Martin, C. L., Andrieux, J., Le Caignec, C., Martin-Coignard, D., . . . Geschwind, D. H. (2016). Rare inherited and de novo CNVs reveal complex contributions to ASD risk in multiplex families. *American Journal of Human Genetics, 99*(3), 540–554.

Leyfer, O. T., Folstein, S. E., Bacalman, S., Davis, N. O., Dinh, E., Morgan, J., . . . Lainhart, J. E. (2006). Comorbid psychiatric disorders in children with autism: Interview development and rates of disorders. *Journal of Autism and Developmental Disorders, 36*(7), 849–861.

Loh, A., Soman, T., Brian, J., Bryson, S. E., Roberts, W., Szatmari, P., . . . Zwaigenbaum, L. (2007). Stereotyped motor behaviors associated with autism in high-risk infants: A pilot videotape analysis of a sibling sample. *Journal of Autism and Developmental Disorders, 37*(1), 25–36.

Lonigan, C. J., Vasey, M. W., Phillips, B. M., & Hazen, R. A. (2004). Temperament, anxiety, and the processing of threat-relevant stimuli. *Journal of Clinical Child and Adolescent Psychology, 33*(1), 8–20.

Lord, C., Luyster, R., Gotham, K., & Guthrie, W. (2012a). *Autism Diagnostic Observation Schedule (ADOS-2) manual (Part II): Toddler module.* Los Angeles: Western Psychological Services.

Lord, C., Luyster, R., Guthrie, W., & Pickles, A. (2012b). Patterns of developmental trajectories in toddlers with autism spectrum disorder. *Journal of Consulting and Clinical Psychology, 80*(3), 477–489.

Lord, C., Risi, S., DiLavore, P. S., Shulman, C., Thurm, A., & Pickles, A. (2006). Autism from 2 to 9 years of age. *Archives of General Psychiatry, 63*(6), 694–701.

Lowell, D. I., Carter, A. S., Godoy, L., Paulicin, B., & Briggs-Gowan, M. J. (2011). A randomized controlled trial of Child FIRST: A comprehensive home-based intervention translating research into early childhood practice. *Child Development, 82*(1), 193–208.

Macari, S., Campbell, D., Gengoux, G., Saulnier, C., Klin, A., & Chawarska, K. (2012). Predicting developmental status from 12 to 24 months in infants at risk for autism spectrum disorder: A preliminary report. *Journal of Autism and Developmental Disorders, 42*(12), 2636–2647.

Macari, S., DiNicola, L., Kane-Grade, F., Prince, E., Vernetti, A., Powell, K., . . . Chawarska, K. (2018). Emotional expressiveness in toddlers with autism spectrum disorder. *Journal of the American Academy of Child and Adolescent Psychiatry, 57*(11), 828–836.

Macari, S. L., Koller, J., Campbell, D. J., & Chawarska, K. (2017). Temperamental markers in toddlers with autism spectrum disorder. *Journal of Child Psychology and Psychiatry, 58*(7), 819–828.

Macari, S., Milgramm, A., Reed, J., Shic, F., Powell, K., Macris, D. M., & Chawarska, K. (2020). Context-specific dyadic attention vulnerabilities during the first year in infants later developing autism spectrum disorder. *Journal of the American Academy of Child and Adolescent Psychiatry.* [Epub ahead of print]

Mäntymaa, M., Puura, K., Luoma, I., Latva, R., Salmelin, R. K., & Tamminen, T. (2012). Predicting internalizing and externalizing problems at five years by child and parental factors in infancy and toddlerhood. *Child Psychiatry and Human Development, 43*(2), 153–170.

Marrus, N., Hall, L., Paterson, S., Elison, J., Wolff, J., Swanson, M., . . . Hazlett, H. (2018). Language delay aggregates in toddler siblings of children with autism spectrum disorder. *Journal of Neurodevelopmental Disorders, 10*(1), 29.

McDonald, N. M., Senturk, D., Scheffler, A., Brian, J. A., Carver, L. J., Charman, T., . . . Jeste, S. S. (2020). Developmental trajectories of infants with multiplex family risk for autism: A Baby Siblings Research Consortium study. *JAMA Neurology, 77*(1), 73–81.

McGuire, K., Fung, L. K., Hagopian, L., Vasa, R. A., Mahajan, R., Bernal, P., . . . Hardan, A. Y. (2016). Irritability and problem behavior in autism spectrum disorder: A practice pathway for pediatric primary care. *Pediatrics, 137*(Suppl. 2), S136–S148.

Messinger, D., Young, G. S., Ozonoff, S., Dobkins, K., Carter, A., Zwaigenbaum, L., . . . Sigman, M. (2013). Beyond autism: A Baby Siblings Research Consortium study of high-risk children at three years of age. *Journal of the American Academy of Child and Adolescent Psychiatry, 52*(3), 300–308.

Messinger, D. S., Young, G. S., Webb, S. J., Ozonoff, S., Bryson, S. E., Carter, A., . . . Curtin, S. (2015). Early sex differences are not autism-specific: A Baby Siblings Research Consortium (BSRC) study. *Molecular Autism, 6*(1), 1–12.

Micalizzi, L., Ronald, A., & Saudino, K. J. (2016). A genetically informed cross-lagged analysis of autistic-like traits and affective problems in early childhood. *Journal of Abnormal Child Psychology, 44*(5), 937–947.

Micheletti, M., McCracken, C., Constantino, J. N., Mandell, D., Jones, W., & Klin, A. (2020). Research review: Outcomes of 24- to 36-month-old children with autism spectrum disorder vary by ascertainment strategy: A systematic review and meta-analysis. *Journal of Child Psychology and Psychiatry, 61*(1), 4–17.

Miller, M., Iosif, A.-M., Hill, M., Young, G. S., Schwichtenberg, A., & Ozonoff, S. (2017). Response to name in infants developing autism spectrum disorder: A prospective study. *Journal of Pediatrics, 183,* 141–146.

Miller, M., Iosif, A.-M., Young, G. S., Bell, L. J., Schwichtenberg, A., Hutman, T., & Ozonoff, S. (2019). The dysregulation profile in preschoolers with and without a family history of autism spectrum disorder. *Journal of Child Psychology and Psychiatry, 60*(5), 516–523.

Miller, M., Iosif, A.-M., Young, G. S., Hill, M. M., & Ozonoff, S. (2016a). Early detection of ADHD: Insights from infant siblings of children with autism. *Journal of Clinical Child and Adolescent Psychology, 47*(5), 737–744.

Miller, M., Iosif, A.-M., Young, G. S., Hill, M., Phelps Hanzel, E., Hutman, T., . . .

Ozonoff, S. (2016b). School-age outcomes of infants at risk for autism spectrum disorder. *Autism Research, 9*(6), 632–642.

Mitchell, S., Brian, J., Zwaigenbaum, L., Roberts, W., Szatmari, P., Smith, I., & Bryson, S. (2006). Early language and communication development of infants later diagnosed with autism spectrum disorder. *Journal of Developmental and Behavioral Pediatrics, 27*(Suppl. 2), S69–S78.

Moffitt, T. (1990). Juvenile delinquency and attention deficit disorder: Boys' developmental trajectories from age 3 to age 15. *Child Development, 61*(3), 893–910.

Moriuchi, J. M., Klin, A., & Jones, W. (2016). Mechanisms of diminished attention to eyes in autism. *American Journal of Psychiatry, 174*(1), 26–35.

Mullen, E. (1995). *Mullen Scales of Early Learning AGS edition.* Circle Pines, MN: American Guidance Serivce.

Murphy, M., Bolton, P., Pickles, A., Fombonne, E., Piven, J., & Rutter, M. (2000). Personality traits of the relatives of autistic probands. *Psychological Medicine, 30*(6), 1411–1424.

Nadig, A. S., Ozonoff, S., Young, G. S., Rozga, A., Sigman, M., & Rogers, S. J. (2007). A prospective study of response to name in infants at risk for autism. *Archives of Pediatrics and Adolescent Medicine, 161*(4), 378–383.

Nakano, T., Tanaka, K., Endo, Y., Yamane, Y., Yamamoto, T., Nakano, Y., . . . Kitazawa, S. (2010). Atypical gaze patterns in children and adults with autism spectrum disorders dissociated from developmental changes in gaze behaviour. *Proceedings of the Royal Society B: Biological Sciences, 277*(1696), 2935–2943.

Nelson, B., Martin, R., Hodge, S., Havill, V., & Kamphaus, R. (1999). Modeling the prediction of elementary school adjustment from preschool temperament. *Personality and Individual Differences, 26*(4), 687–700.

Nigg, J. T. (2006). Temperament and developmental psychopathology. *Journal of Child Psychology and Psychiatry, 47*(3–4), 395–422.

Norbury, C. F. (2014). Sources of variation in developmental language disorders: Evidence from eye-tracking studies of sentence production. *Philosophical Transactions of the Royal Society B: Biological Sciences, 369*(1634), 20120393.

Øien, R. A., Schjølberg, S., Volkmar, F. R., Shic, F., Cicchetti, D. V., Nordahl-Hansen, A., . . . Chawarska, K. (2018). Clinical features of children with autism who passed 18-month screening. *Pediatrics, 141*(6), e20173596.

O'Loughlin, K., Macari, S., Shic, F., & Chawarska, K. (2012). *Attention capture by and preference for faces with direct gaze in toddlers with ASD, DD, and TD.* Paper presented at the International Meeting for Autism Research (IMFAR 2012), Toronto, Ontario, Canada.

Ozonoff, S., Iosif, A., Baguio, F., Cook, I. D., Hill, M. M., Hutman, T., . . . Young, G. S. (2010). A prospective study of the emergence of early behavioral signs of autism. *Journal of the American Academy of Child and Adolescent Psychiatry, 49*(3), 258–268.

Ozonoff, S., Macari, S., Young, G. S., Goldring, S., Thompson, M., & Rogers, S. J. (2008). Atypical object exploration at 12 months of age is associated with autism in a prospective sample. *Autism, 12*(5), 457–472.

Ozonoff, S., Young, G. S., Belding, A., Hill, M., Hill, A., Hutman, T., . . . Iosif, A. M. (2014). The broader autism phenotype in infancy: When does it emerge? *Journal of the American Academy of Child and Adolescent Psychiatry, 53*(4), 398–407.

Ozonoff, S., Young, G. S., Carter, A., Messinger, D., Yirmiya, N., Zwaigenbaum, L.,

. . . Stone, W. L. (2011). Recurrence risk for autism spectrum disorders: A Baby Siblings Research Consortium study. *Pediatrics, 128*(3), e488–e495.

Ozonoff, S., Young, G. S., Landa, R. J., Brian, J., Bryson, S., Charman, T., . . . Iosif, A. M. (2015). Diagnostic stability in young children at risk for autism spectrum disorder: A Baby Siblings Research Consortium study. *Journal of Child Psychology and Psychiatry, 56*(9), 988–998.

Ozonoff, S., Young, G. S., Steinfeld, M. B., Hill, M., Cook, I., Hutman, T., . . . Sigman, M. (2009). How early do parent concerns predict later autism diagnosis? *Journal of Developmental and Behavioral Pediatrics, 30*(5), 365–375.

Palmer, N., Beam, A., Agniel, D., Eran, A., Manrai, A., Spettell, C., . . . Cohane, I. (2017). Association of sex with recurrence of autism spectrum disorder among siblings. *JAMA Pediatrics, 171*(11), 1107–1112.

Paterson, S. J., Wolff, J. J., Elison, J. T., Winder-Patel, B., Zwaigenbaum, L., Estes, A., . . . Infant Brain Imaging Study (IBIS) Network. (2019). The importance of temperament for understanding early manifestations of autism spectrum disorder in high-risk infants. *Journal of Autism and Developmental Disorders, 49*(7), 2849–2863.

Patten, E., Belardi, K., Baranek, G. T., Watson, L. R., Labban, J. D., & Oller, D. K. (2014). Vocal patterns in infants with autism spectrum disorder: Canonical babbling status and vocalization frequency. *Journal of Autism and Developmental Disorders, 44*(10), 2413–2428.

Paul, R., Chawarska, K., Klin, A., & Volkmar, F. (2017). Dissociations in the development of early communication in autism spectrum disorders. In R. Paul (Ed.), *Language disorders from a developmental perspective: Essays in honor of Robin S. Chapman* (pp. 163–194). Hove, UK: Psychology Press.

Paul, R., Fuerst, Y., Ramsay, G., Chawarska, K., & Klin, A. (2011). Out of the mouths of babes: Vocal production in infant siblings of children with ASD. *Journal of Child Psychology and Psychiatry, 52*(5), 588–598.

Petersen, S. E., & Posner, M. I. (2012). The attention system of the human brain: 20 years after. *Annual Review of Neuroscience, 35,* 73.

Pickles, A., Le Couteur, A., Leadbitter, K., Salomone, E., Cole-Fletcher, R., Tobin, H., . . . Green, J. (2016). Parent-mediated social communication therapy for young children with autism (PACT): Long-term follow-up of a randomised controlled trial. *The Lancet, 388*(10059), 2501–2509.

Pierce, K., Marinero, S., Hazin, R., McKenna, B., Barnes, C. C., & Malige, A. (2016). Eye tracking reveals abnormal visual preference for geometric images as an early biomarker of an autism spectrum disorder subtype associated with increased symptom severity. *Biological Psychiatry, 79*(8), 657–666.

Prior, M., Smart, D., Sanson, A., & Oberklaid, F. (2000). Does shy-inhibited temperament in childhood lead to anxiety problems in adolescence? *Journal of the American Academy of Child and Adolescent Psychiatry, 39*(4), 461–468.

Putnam, S. P., Gartstein, M. A., & Rothbart, M. K. (2006). Measurement of fine-grained aspects of toddler temperament: The Early Childhood Behavior Questionnaire. *Infant Behavior and Development, 29*(3), 386–401.

Putnam, S. P., Rothbart, M. K., & Gartstein, M. A. (2008). Homotypic and heterotypic continuity of fine-grained temperament during infancy, toddlerhood, and early childhood. *Infant and Child Development, 17*(4), 387–405.

Putnam, S. P., & Stifter, C. A. (2005). Behavioral approach–inhibition in toddlers: Prediction from infancy, positive and negative affective components, and relations with behavior problems. *Child Development, 76*(1), 212–226.

Reznick, J., Baranek, G. T., Reavis, S., Watson, L. R., & Crais, E. R. (2007). A parent-report instrument for identifying one-year-olds at risk for an eventual diagnosis of autism: The First Year Inventory. *Journal of Autism and Developmental Disorders, 37*(9), 1691–1710.

Risch, N., Hoffmann, T. J., Anderson, M., Croen, L. A., Grether, J. K., & Windham, G. C. (2014). Familial recurrence of autism spectrum disorder: Evaluating genetic and environmental contributions. *American Journal of Psychiatry, 171*(11), 1206–1213.

Robinson, E. B., Lichtenstein, P., Anckarsäter, H., Happé, F., & Ronald, A. (2013). Examining and interpreting the female protective effect against autistic behavior. *Proceedings of the National Academy of Sciences of the USA, 110*(13), 5258–5262.

Rogers, S. J. (2009). What are infant siblings teaching us about autism in infancy? *Autism Research, 2*, 125–137.

Rosen, T. E., Mazefsky, C. A., Vasa, R. A., & Lerner, M. D. (2018). Co-occurring psychiatric conditions in autism spectrum disorder. *International Review of Psychiatry, 30*(1), 40–61.

Rowberry, J., Macari, S., Chen, G., Campbell, D., Leventhal, J. M., Weitzman, C., & Chawarska, K. (2015). Screening for autism spectrum disorders in 12-month-old high-risk siblings by parental report. *Journal of Autism and Developmental Disorders, 45*(1), 221–229.

Rozga, A., Hutman, T., Young, G. S., Rogers, S. J., Ozonoff, S., Dapretto, M., & Sigman, M. (2011). Behavioral profiles of affected and unaffected siblings of children with autism: Contribution of measures of mother–infant interaction and nonverbal communication. *Journal of Autism and Developmental Disorders, 41*(3), 287–301.

Rubin, K. H., Burgess, K. B., Dwyer, K. M., & Hastings, P. D. (2003). Predicting preschoolers' externalizing behaviors from toddler temperament, conflict, and maternal negativity. *Developmental Psychology, 39*(1), 164–176.

Ruzzo, E. K., Perez-Cano, L., Jung, J.-Y., Wang, L.-k., Kashef-Haghighi, D., Hartl, C., . . . Wall, D. P. (2018). Whole genome sequencing in multiplex families reveals novel inherited and *de novo* genetic risk in autism. *bioRxiv*. [Epub ahead of print]

Sacrey, L.-A. R., Zwaigenbaum, L., Bryson, S., Brian, J., Smith, I. M., Roberts, W., . . . Armstrong, V. (2015). Can parents' concerns predict autism spectrum disorder?: A prospective study of high-risk siblings from 6 to 36 months of age. *Journal of the American Academy of Child and Adolescent Psychiatry, 54*(6), 470–478.

Salazar, F., Baird, G., Chandler, S., Tseng, E., O'Sullivan, T., Howlin, P., . . . Simonoff, E. (2015). Co-occurring psychiatric disorders in preschool and elementary school-aged children with autism spectrum disorder. *Journal of Autism and Developmental Disorders, 45*(8), 2283–2294.

Sanders, S. J., Murtha, M. T., Gupta, A. R., Murdoch, J. D., Raubeson, M. J., Willsey, A. J., . . . State, M. W. (2012). *De novo* mutations revealed by whole-exome sequencing are strongly associated with autism. *Nature, 485*(7397), 237–241.

Schendel, D. E., Grønborg, T. K., & Parner, E. T. (2014). The genetic and environmental contributions to autism: Looking beyond twins. *JAMA, 311*(17), 1738–1739.

Scherr, J. F., Hogan, A. L., Hatton, D., & Roberts, J. E. (2017). Stranger fear and early risk for social anxiety in preschoolers with fragile X syndrome contrasted to autism spectrum disorder. *Journal of Autism and Developmental Disorders, 47*(12), 3741–3755.

Schreibman, L., Dawson, G., Stahmer, A. C., Landa, R., Rogers, S. J., McGee, G. G.,

. . . Halladay, A. (2015). Naturalistic developmental behavioral interventions: Empirically validated treatments for autism spectrum disorder. *Journal of Autism and Developmental Disorders, 45*(8), 2411–2428.

Schwichtenberg, A., Kellerman, A. M., Young, G. S., Miller, M., & Ozonoff, S. (2019). Mothers of children with autism spectrum disorders: Play behaviors with infant siblings and social responsiveness. *Autism, 23*(4), 821–833.

Senju, A., & Johnson, M. H. (2009). Atypical eye contact in autism: Models, mechanisms and development. *Neuroscience and Biobehavioral Reviews, 33*(8), 1204–1215.

Shic, F., Bradshaw, J., Klin, A., Scassellati, B., & Chawarska, K. (2011). Limited activity monitoring in toddlers with autism spectrum disorder. *Brain Research, 1380,* 246–254.

Shic, F., Macari, S., & Chawarska, K. (2014). Speech disturbs face scanning in 6-month-old infants who develop autism spectrum disorder. *Biological Psychiatry, 75*(3), 231–237.

Shic, F., Wang, Q., Macari, S. L., & Chawarska, K. (2019). The role of limited salience of speech in selective attention to faces in toddlers with autism spectrum disorders. *Journal of Child Psychology and Psychiatry.* [Epub ahead of print]

Simonoff, E., Pickles, A., Charman, T., Chandler, S., Loucas, T., & Baird, G. (2008). Psychiatric disorders in children with autism spectrum disorders: Prevalence, comorbidity, and associated factors in a population-derived sample. *Journal of the American Academy of Child and Adolescent Psychiatry, 47*(8), 921–929.

Stone, W. L., Coonrod, E. E., & Ousley, O. Y. (2000). Brief report: Screening tool for autism in two-year-olds (STAT): Development and preliminary data. *Journal of Autism and Developmental Disorders, 30*(6), 607.

Stone, W. L., Coonrod, E. E., Turner, L. M., & Pozdol, S. L. (2004). Psychometric properties of the STAT for early autism screening. *Journal of Autism and Developmental Disorders, 34*(6), 691–701.

Szatmari, P. (2018). Risk and resilience in autism spectrum disorder: A missed translational opportunity? *Developmental Medicine and Child Neurology, 60*(3), 225–229.

Szatmari, P., Chawarska, K., Dawson, G., Georgiades, S., Landa, R., Lord, C., . . . Halladay, A. (2016). Prospective longitudinal studies of infant siblings of children with autism: Lessons learned and future directions. *Journal of the American Academy of Child and Adolescent Psychiatry, 55*(3), 179–187.

Tager-Flusberg, H. (2010). The origins of social impairments in autism spectrum disorder: Studies of infants at risk. *Neural Networks, 23*(8–9), 1072–1076.

Talbott, M. R., Nelson, C. A., & Tager-Flusberg, H. (2015). Maternal gesture use and language development in infant siblings of children with autism spectrum disorder. *Journal of Autism and Developmental Disorders, 45*(1), 4–14.

Tatler, B. W. (2014). Eye movements from laboratory to life. In M. Horsley, N. Toom, B. A. Knight, & R. Reilly (Eds.), *Current trends in eye tracking research* (pp. 17–35). Cham, Switzerland: Springer.

Tatler, B. W., Hayhoe, M. M., Land, M. F., & Ballard, D. H. (2011). Eye guidance in natural vision: Reinterpreting salience. *Journal of Vision, 11*(5), 5.

Thelen, E. (1979). Rhythmical stereotypies in normal human infants. *Animal Behaviour, 27,* 699–715.

Thorup, E., Nyström, P., Gredebäck, G., Bölte, S., & Falck-Ytter, T. (2016). Altered gaze following during live interaction in infants at risk for autism: An eye tracking study. *Molecular Autism, 7*(1), 12.

Thorup, E., Nyström, P., Gredebäck, G., Bölte, S., Falck-Ytter, T., & EASE Team. (2018). Reduced alternating gaze during social interaction in infancy is associated with elevated symptoms of autism in toddlerhood. *Journal of Abnormal Child Psychology, 46*(7), 1547–1561.

Tronick, E., Als, H., Adamson, L., Wise, S., & Brazelton, T. B. (1978). The infant's response to entrapment between contradictory messages in face-to-face interaction. *Journal of the American Academy of Child psychiatry, 17*(1), 1–13.

Volbrecht, M. M., & Goldsmith, H. H. (2010). Early temperamental and family predictors of shyness and anxiety. *Developmental Psychology, 46*(5), 1192–1205.

von Hofsten, C., Uhlig, H., Adell, M., & Kochukhova, O. (2009). How children with autism look at events. *Research in Autism Spectrum Disorders, 3*(2), 556–569.

Wagner, J., Keehn, B., Tager-Flusberg, H., & Nelson, C. (2019). Attentional bias to fearful faces in infants at high risk for autism spectrum disorder. *Emotion.* [Epub ahead of print]

Wagner, J., Luyster, R. J., Moustapha, H., Tager-Flusberg, H., & Nelson, C. A. (2018). Differential attention to faces in infant siblings of children with autism spectrum disorder and associations with later social and language ability. *International Journal of Behavioral Development, 42*(1), 83–92.

Wang, Q., Campbell, D. J., Macari, S. L., Chawarska, K., & Shic, F. (2018a). Operationalizing atypical gaze in toddlers with autism spectrum disorders: A cohesion-based approach. *Molecular Autism, 9*(1), 25.

Wang, Q., Chang, J., & Chawarska, K. (2020a). Atypical value-driven selective attention in young children with autism spectrum disorder. *JAMA Network Open, 3*(5), e204928.

Wang, Q., DiNicola, L., Heymann, P., Hampson, M., & Chawarska, K. (2018b). Impaired value learning for faces in preschoolers with autism spectrum disorder. *Journal of the American Academy of Child and Adolescent Psychiatry, 57*(1), 33–40.

Wang, Q., Wall, C. A., Barney, E. C., Bradshaw, J. L., Macari, S. L., Chawarska, K., & Shic, F. (2020b). Promoting social attention in 3-year-olds with ASD through gaze-contingent eye tracking. *Autism Research, 13*(1), 61–73.

Webster-Stratton, C., & Reid, M. J. (2003). The incredible years parents, teachers and children training series: A multifaceted treatment approach for young children with conduct problems. In A. E. Kazdin & J. R. Weisz (Eds.), *Evidence-based psychotherapies for children and adolescents* (pp. 224–240). New York: Guilford Press.

Werling, D. M., & Geschwind, D. H. (2013). Understanding sex bias in autism spectrum disorder. *Proceedings of the National Academy of Sciences of the USA, 110*(13), 4868–4869.

Werling, D. M., & Geschwind, D. H. (2015). Recurrence rates provide evidence for sex-differential, familial genetic liability for autism spectrum disorders in multiplex families and twins. *Molecular Autism, 6*(1), 27.

West, K. L., Leezenbaum, N. B., Northrup, J. B., & Iverson, J. M. (2019). The relation between walking and language in infant siblings of children with autism spectrum disorder. *Child Development, 90*(3), e356–e372.

Wetherby, A. M., & Prizant, B. M. (2002). *Communication and symbolic behavior scales: Developmental profile.* Baltimore: Brookes.

Wolff, J. J., Botteron, K. N., Dager, S. R., Elison, J. T., Estes, A. M., Gu, H., . . . IBIS Network. (2014). Longitudinal patterns of repetitive behavior in toddlers with autism. *Journal of Child Psychology and Psychiatry, 55*(8), 945–953.

Wood, J. J., & Gadow, K. D. (2010). Exploring the nature and function of anxiety in youth with autism spectrum disorders. *Clinical Psychology: Science and Practice, 17*(4), 281–292.

Yirmiya, N., & Charman, T. (2011). The prodrome of autism: Early behavioral and biological signs, regression, peri- and post-natal development and genetics. *Journal of Child Psychology and Psychiatry, 51*(4), 432–458.

Young, G. S., Merin, N., Rogers, S. J., & Ozonoff, S. (2009). Gaze behavior and affect at 6 months: Predicting clinical outcomes and language development in typically developing infants and infants at risk for autism. *Developmental Science, 12*(5), 798–814.

Zisser, A., & Eyberg, S. M. (2010). Treating oppositional behavior in children using parent–child interaction therapy. In J. R. Weisz & A. E. Kazdin (Eds.), *Evidence-based psychotherapies for children and adolescents* (2nd ed., pp. 179–193). New York: Guilford Press.

Zwaigenbaum, L., Bryson, S. E., Brian, J., Smith, I. M., Roberts, W., Szatmari, P., . . . Vaillancourt, T. (2016). Stability of diagnostic assessment for autism spectrum disorder between 18 and 36 months in a high-risk cohort. *Autism Research, 9*(7), 790–800.

Zwaigenbaum, L., Bryson, S., Lord, C., Rogers, S., Carter, A., Carver, L., . . . Yirmiya, N. (2009). Clinical assessment and management of toddlers with suspected autism spectrum disorder: Insights from studies of high-risk infants. *Pediatrics, 123*(5), 1383–1391.

Zwaigenbaum, L., Bryson, S., Rogers, T., Roberts, W., Brian, J., & Szatmari, P. (2005). Behavioral manifestations of autism in the first year of life. *International Journal of Developmental Neuroscience, 23*(2–3), 143–152.

Zwaigenbaum, L., Bryson, S. E., Szatmari, P., Brian, J., Smith, I. M., Roberts, W., . . . Roncadin, C. (2012). Sex differences in children with autism spectrum disorder identified within a high-risk infant cohort. *Journal of Autism and Developmental Disorders, 42*(12), 2585–2596.

CHAPTER 6

• • • • • • • •

Brain and Behavioral Development in High-Risk Infants

CONSIDERING THE ROLE OF SENSORIMOTOR, ATTENTIONAL, AND REWARD NETWORKS

Robin Sifre, Joseph Piven, and Jed T. Elison

O ver the past decade, a growing body of work on high-risk (HR) infant siblings has informed a greater understanding of the early manifestations of autism. The recurrence risk of autism spectrum disorder (ASD) has been estimated to be between 8 and 20% (Messinger et al., 2015; Ozonoff et al., 2011; Sandin et al., 2014), enabling researchers to track and study the early development of HR infant siblings of children with autism. These studies shed light on the early developmental time course of autism through prospectively measuring the unfolding of brain development, visual attention, motor development, language development, and social orienting behaviors in HR infants. Accumulating evidence from this body of research paints a picture of early atypicalities in brain development and sensorimotor/attentional experiences, cascading into increasingly atypical social engagement over the first 2 years of life.

One hypothesis advanced in this field is that this pattern of increasing divergence from typically developing (TD) peers may reflect a disruption in brain development during a critical transition period. Models of typical early social engagement have proposed that, in the first months of life, infants reflexively direct their attention toward social stimuli and conspecifics, entreating further interaction and creating rich opportunities for learning via reciprocal social engagement (Lavelli & Fogel, 2005). Because of these rich social learning opportunities, orienting mechanisms are thought to transition from reflexive and largely subcortically mediated mechanisms to experience-dependent and largely cortically mediated mechanisms (Morton & Johnson, 1991; Simion, Di Giorgio, Leo, & Bardi, 2011). While infants' reflexive attentional systems are initially biased toward broadly tuned conspecific social stimuli, as these stimuli are continuously sampled and reinforced, social information processing becomes more specialized and finely tuned. Infants who later develop autism, however, may fail to properly make this transition. Some have suggested that this may be due to early disruptions in brain development that lead to poor sampling of information, particularly when information is highly complex and dynamic, as is the case when infants are faced with social stimuli (Johnson, Jones, & Gliga, 2015). Others have focused on a failure to transition from perceptual biases to social stimuli and to interactive visual social *engagement* dependent on rewarding social experiences with a caregiver (Klin, Shultz, & Jones, 2015). Thus, while infants later diagnosed with autism may perform similarly to their peers on tasks that require reflexive social orienting early in life, as social engagement becomes increasingly complex and reliant on experience-dependent and top-down endogenous attentional mechanisms, differences in engagement become amplified (Jones & Klin, 2013; Miller et al., 2017; Nadig et al., 2007). Recent evidence demonstrating that social information seeking is a highly heritable trait—with the most highly heritable characteristics (attention to the eyes and mouth) being those that are affected in autism—suggests that these differences in early environmental sampling may be driven by genetic mechanisms (Constantino et al., 2017). It should be noted that, while conceptually compelling, direct neural evidence from human infants to support this subcortical-to-cortical control transition is sparse.

In this chapter, we expand and build on this theoretical model of how atypical social engagement unfolds in the first years of life in infants with ASD, with a focus on how atypical neural development in early life may give rise to atypical sensory-processing and attentional development in infancy. We will present neural and behavioral evidence in support of this model, which includes a body of work on brain and behavioral development in HR infants, documenting early atypical neural development in domain-general sensorimotor processing areas at a time that coincides with deficits in the flexible allocation of attention (Piven, Elison, & Zylka, 2018). We then consider the development of visual selective attention in infancy, and its role in typical and atypical development of experience-dependent visual social engagement.

After presenting evidence from infant sibling paradigms in favor of this model, we argue in support of expanding these models. Specifically, we present evidence suggesting that these models should be expanded to include a focus on the intersection between sensorimotor and reward circuitry. This may be especially important for 6- to 12-month-old infants, as these infants begin to learn about the world and become better equipped to inhibit their attention from perceptually salient stimuli in order to orient to information they find rewarding and semantically salient. *Semantic salience* refers to stimuli that infants must *learn* are salient, important, or rewarding, but may lack inherent perceptual salience (e.g., bright colors, moving objects). We will consider how *reward-enhanced attention*—or, attention orienting in the context of semantically salient stimuli—increasingly biases these infants' attention. Finally, we speculate on how delays or disruptions in transitioning toward reward-enhanced attention in infants at high risk for ASD (HR-ASD) might influence emerging symptoms. While semantically salient stimuli may be socially salient (e.g., biological motion, fearful faces, or other evolutionarily driven signals), we hope to advance a more nuanced approach to social information processing that accounts for how specific types of social information—such as one's own name—may become prioritized and acquire semantic salience or special meaning over time.

Evidence of Atypical Brain Development in At-Risk Infants

We open with a selective review of magnetic resonance imaging (MRI)-based brain development studies. While a sizable literature utilizing electroencephalography/event-related potentials and other neuroscience methodologies (e.g., near-infrared spectroscopy) in HR siblings exists, the vast majority of these studies do not report findings stratified by diagnostic outcome (for exceptions, see Elsabbagh et al., 2012; Finch, Seery, Talbott, Nelson, & Tager-Flusberg, 2017; Levin, Varcin, O'Leary, Tager-Flusberg, & Nelson, 2017; Orekhova et al., 2014). Results of HR versus low-risk (LR) non-ASD differences are challenging to interpret as group differences could be due to inherited familial risk in the HR group as a whole, or could be driven by a subgroup of HR individuals who will later meet diagnostic criteria. Therefore, we focus on prospective longitudinal studies that include stratification of HR infants by diagnostic outcome. Further, we focus on MRI-based methods as we attempt to offer a conceptualization of early brain and behavior development based on regionally specific patterns of connectivity.

Structural Imaging Studies

Increased head size (Kanner, 1943; Lainhart et al., 1997; Stevenson, Schroer, Skinner, Fender, & Simensen, 1997) and total brain volume (Piven et al., 1992, 1995) have long been noted in a subset of children and adults with ASD. In TD humans, total brain volume increases rapidly in the first years of life, with 75% of adult volume reached by 2 years of age (Markant & Thomas, 2013). There is evidence that this rapid growth may be further accelerated in HR-ASD infants compared to their TD peers. While cross-sectional studies that define enlargement as greater than 1.5 standard deviations above the mean of LR controls estimate that 15% of children with ASD have brain enlargement (Piven et al., 2018), longitudinal studies suggest that accelerated brain growth may be a common characteristic of the early emergence of autism.

The first MRI evidence of brain enlargement in ASD before 18–24 months was published on a sample of 55 infants (n = 10 HR-ASD), imaged at three time points (6–9, 12–15, and 18–24 months; Shen et al., 2013). Compared to the LR non-ASD and HR-negative groups, HR-ASD infants had significantly larger total cerebral volume at 12–15 months, an effect that persisted at 18–24 months. The same study reported increased extra-axial cerebrospinal fluid (CSF) in HR-ASD infants relative to the HR-negative and LR infants at all time points, with extra-axial fluid at 6 months predicting autism severity at 24 months. This finding of increased extra-axial fluid in HR-ASD infants was then reproduced in a separate study with improved image-processing techniques and a much larger sample size (n = 122 LR, and 221 HR infants, 47 of whom were HR-ASD). Again, differences emerged at 6 months and were driven primarily by those who were more severely affected (Shen et al., 2017). These studies demonstrate that increased extra-axial CSF may represent a novel biomarker of ASD observable as early as 6 months of age. Interestingly, infants with "benign extra-axial fluid of infancy" and HR-ASD infants bear some clinical similarities: namely, rapid head growth in the first year of life, co-occurrence with seizures, and higher rate in boys than girls (Shen et al., 2013). Determining the nature of the association between mechanisms accounting for increased extra-axial CSF and other volumetric measurements, be they causal or correlational, is an important avenue for future research.

Cortical gray matter volume can be decomposed into measures of cortical thickness and surface area, tissue features that are controlled by separable genetic mechanisms (Panizzon et al., 2009). In a study leveraging a piecewise longitudinal mixed model on 106 HR (15 HR-ASD) infants who contributed data at 6, 12, and 24 months, it was found that HR-ASD infants demonstrated increased rate of change in surface area (SA) from 6 to 12 months (SA expansion), followed by increased rate of change in total brain volume from 12 to 24 months (Hazlett et al., 2017). Individual differences in the rate of total brain volume change from 12 to 24 months predicted Autism Diagnostic Observation Schedule (ADOS) severity scores on the social-affective subscale. Hazlett et al. (2017) then implemented a deep learning algorithm, relying primarily on SA metrics taken at 6 and 12 months of age, and were able to classify subsequent diagnoses of ASD in HR infants with 88% sensitivity and 95% specificity. From a clinical perspective, these findings are noteworthy in that they demonstrate that a deep learning algorithm trained on MRI data had the sensitivity to detect 30 out of 34 HR-ASD infants, as well as the specificity to correctly identify 138 out of the 145 HR-negative infants correctly. Substantively, these results further support the idea that very early postnatal hyperexpansion of cortical surface area likely plays a significant role in the early development of ASD.

Taken together, these studies show that HR-ASD infants demonstrate total brain volume overgrowth in the second year of life and that this effect is preceded by elevated levels of extra-axial CSF (Shen et al., 2013, 2017) and increased SA expansion (Hazlett et al., 2017). These early disruptions in brain development, including increased levels of extra-axial fluid and SA growth, correspond with the developmental time window in which early attentional differences begin to manifest in HR-ASD infants. Furthermore, the observed SA hyperexpansion in HR-ASD infants was observed in cortical areas associated with sensorimotor processing (Hazlett et al., 2017), which has been implicated in the early pathogenesis of ASD (Piven et al., 2018). Thus, it is possible that these early differences may disrupt early sensorimotor/attentional processes, which may have cascading effects on social and cognitive development.

Diffusion-Weighted MRI

In addition to rapid increases in gray matter, postnatal brain development is also characterized by a rapid increase in white matter in the first year of life, after which the rate of change decreases (Hermoye et al., 2006). White matter fiber bundles provide structural connections between brain regions, and understanding their development in HR-ASD infants is of interest because the integrity of these connections may index neural efficiency (Lewis et al., 2017). Furthermore, there is ample evidence relating abnormalities in brain connectivity to atypical behavior in adults with ASD (for a review, see Lewis et al., 2017). Understanding whether these patterns are present in infancy—similar to the surface area hyperexpansion detailed in the last section—or whether they emerge later in life is critical for understanding the contribution of white matter atypicalities to the early ASD phenotype.

Diffusion tensor imaging (DTI) studies measure the diffusivity patterns of water in the brain and enable researchers to index the development of white matter (Sadeghi et al., 2013). Studies using DTI have revealed atypical white matter structure in HR-ASD infants as early as 6 months (Wolff et al., 2012, 2015, 2017). One study examining white matter development in HR-ASD and HR-negative infants from 6 to 24 months found group differences in fractional anisotropy (FA) trajectories in 12 out of the 15 tracts of interest (Wolff et al., 2012). While both HR-ASD and HR-negative infants demonstrated a positive increase in FA from 6 to 24 months, the linear change was greater for HR-negative infants such that HR-ASD infants had higher FA at 6 months but lower FA at 24 months. Another study examining fiber tract organization in a larger sample (217 HR infants, 44 HR-ASD—largely encompassing the sample from Wolff et al., 2012) at 6, 12, and 24 months focused on white matter development in cerebellar, striatal, and cortical tracts, and their association with restricted and repetitive behaviors (RRBs) as measured by Repetitive Behavior Scale—Revised (RBS-R) scores, and responses to sensory stimuli as measured by the Sensory Experiences Questionnaire (SEQ; Wolff et al., 2017). While both HR-ASD and HR-negative infants demonstrated a significant correlation between RBS-R and SEQ scores, scores in the HR-ASD group were positively associated with FA development in the genu and in the mid-cerebellar and superior cerebellar peduncles. The association between these behaviors and FA in the midcerebellar and superior cerebellar peduncles aligns with past work implicating the cerebellum in repetitive behaviors and sensory processing, while the association with FA in the genu may be attributable to its indirect involvement in cerebellar circuits via frontal cortical regions. Critically, these effects were specific to SEQ and RBS-R scores, as there was no relationship between FA development in these tracts and ADOS social affect scores. For HR-negative infants, the relationship between FA development and RBS-R and SEQ scores was not statistically robust. However, the estimated relationship between FA and RRBs suggested that genu and splenium FA were *negatively* correlated with RRBs. Thus, diagnostic status may moderate the relationship between white matter development and emerging RRBs.

Whole-brain analyses have also elucidated disorder-specific atypical white matter connectivity by highlighting network inefficiencies in HR-ASD infants, as measured by efficiency metrics of white matter connections between brain regions (Lewis et al., 2014, 2017). These network analyses measure a set of connections in the brain, rather than examining each connection individually, and use "efficiency" as a metric. Efficiency is the capacity to exchange information across the network, and it can be measured for the entire network (e.g., global efficiency) or for subnetworks (e.g., local efficiency). At 24 months, HR-ASD infants show reduced local and global efficiency relative to LR- and HR-negative infants, primarily in posterior regions (Lewis et al., 2014), with local efficiency in the left temporal and occipital lobes predicting ADOS severity scores. A follow-up study including 116 infants with longitudinal data was then able to track the emergence of these network inefficiencies (Lewis et al., 2017). It was found that inefficiencies emerge by 6 months, at which point they were most pronounced in the right auditory cortex and superior and middle temporal gyri. Inefficiencies were also noted in the left primary auditory cortex and by 12 months in the left insula. There were also reductions in global efficiency observable by 12 months in Broca's area. Notably, while inefficiency in primary and secondary auditory networks at 6 months predicted autism severity at 24 months, over the next 6 months of life networks involved in visual, somatosensory, motor, and higher-level processing (Broca's and Wernicke's areas) also predicted symptom severity. This pattern of findings suggests that early sensory processing inefficiencies may have cascading effects on more complex networks and, ultimately, on social and cognitive outcomes. An alternative explanation, however, might be that that these later-emerging network inefficiencies in frontal areas arise independently from the earlier inefficiencies observed in the sensory processing regions.

In addition to whole-brain analyses (Lewis et al., 2014, 2017) and studies examining multiple fiber tracts (Wolff et al., 2012, 2017), important work has been published using DTI to elucidate differences in the corpus callosum (Elison et al., 2013; Wolff et al., 2015), a bundle of axonal fibers that connect the left and right cerebral hemispheres. The corpus callosum is topographically organized, such that anterior corpus callosum fibers (the genu) connect to prefrontal cortices; the body of the corpus callosum is composed of fibers from the premotor, motor, parietal, and superior temporal cortices; and the posterior region (the splenium) connects to the inferior temporal and occipital cortices (Frazier & Hardan, 2010). Thus, the corpus callosum represents many long-range white matter connections across the brain and therefore may play an important role in the atypical connectivity patterns in ASD. Imaging studies on children and adults with autism have repeatedly found decreased corpus callosum sizes (Frazier & Hardan, 2010; Piven, Bailey, Ranson, & Arndt, 1997), with corpus callosum size being negatively associated with symptom severity (Hardan et al., 2009; Prigge et al., 2013). In addition to the corpus callosum being atypical in adults and children with ASD, it is known to undergo robust axonal pruning early in life (LaMantia & Rakic, 1990), suggesting that it might be especially relevant to the early development of ASD.

Longitudinal trajectories of corpus callosum development were examined in 270 HR (57 HR-ASD) and 108 LR infants (Wolff et al., 2015). It was found that thickness of the anterior corpus callosum was significantly greater for HR-ASD compared to LR infants, with group differences being greatest at 6 months and diminishing by 24 months. Differences in thickness were driven by increased radial diffusivity in the corpus callosum, a measure sensitive to axon composition, density, and myelination, suggesting that developmental difference in corpus callosum thickness varied as a function of white matter microstructure. Follow-up analysis of the corpus callosum segmented into 25 regions was carried out to investigate group differences with more spatial specificity. Intriguingly, with increased spatial specificity, the differences between HR-ASD and LR infants were most robust at 6 and 12 months. At 6 months, they were most robust in areas implicated in the prefrontal, supplementary motor, and posterior–parietal connectivity, and at 12 months increased effects were seen in regions implicated with primary motor connectivity, while the posterior differences became less robust. In conjunction with the extant literature on adults, which indicated smaller corpora callosa, these findings suggest that axonal overgrowth followed by atypical experience-dependent axonal elimination may contribute to ASD symptomologies. Although these differences in corpus callosum thickness and white matter morphology are intriguing, they are difficult to interpret, as HR-ASD infants only trended toward increased thickness compared to HR-negative ($p = .07$), while HR-negative and LR infants were indistinguishable.

There may also be early functional differences in the corpus callosum for HR-ASD infants. One study investigated the relationship between visual orienting at 7 months and white matter development in the splenium of the corpus callosum (Elison et al., 2013). Given its connections to the striate and extrastriate visual areas, the splenium plays a critical role in efficient and flexible visual orienting in adults (Niogi, Mukherjee, Ghajar, & McCandliss, 2010). It was found that this relationship between white matter development in the splenium and visual orienting was moderated by group status. In other words, while there were significant associations between radial diffusivity in the splenium of the corpus callosum and visual orienting in LR infants, the relationship was not significant for HR-ASD infants. Thus, there appears to be a lack of functional coupling between white matter development and visual orienting behavior in HR-ASD infants, which may account for the observed deficits in visual orienting already observable at this age. A more recent study revealed that, contrary to findings from children and adults, language production at 24 months varied as a function of splenium development (Swanson et al., 2017). Taken together, these findings on white matter in the corpus callosum suggest that the association between white matter structure and function of the corpus callosum is a dynamic process (Johnson, 2000) and that functional differences in white matter tracts in HR-ASD infants warrant further study.

In sum, studies using DTI have demonstrated clear and early differences in white matter development in HR-ASD infants. These findings suggest early axonal overgrowth followed by atypical experience-dependent pruning (Wolff et al., 2012, 2015), which may lead to observed whole-brain network structural inefficiencies (Lewis et al., 2014, 2017) as well as atypical functioning of specific white matter tracts (e.g., Elison et al., 2013; Wolff et al., 2015). Notably, these differences emerge as early as 6 months, with some of the most robust differences observed in the structure or function of sensorimotor areas. This suggests that atypical white matter development may play a critical role in the early etiology of ASD, leading to cascading effects on later social development.

Functional Connectivity

Functional connectivity MRI (fcMRI) is another imaging tool that has been used to predict diagnostic outcomes in HR infants. Functional connectivity measures the temporal correlation in activity between at least two sources in the brain (Deco, Jirsa, & McIntosh, 2011). While structural connectivity as measured through diffusion-weighted imaging is a good predictor of functional connectivity, the opposite is not necessarily true; functional connectivity can be observed between two regions that are not anatomically connected. Intriguingly, these functional networks persist even while individuals are asleep (Mitra et al., 2017), and primitive rest-ing state networks can be observed as early as 2 weeks (Gao et al., 2009). Furthermore, by applying machine learning techniques to fcMRI data, researchers have been able to predict individual diagnostic outcomes for a variety of syndromes (see Emerson et al., 2017, for a review). Given that functional connectivity can be measured in sleeping infants and has utility in capturing diagnostic status for a variety of syndromes, researchers have been interested in examining early measures of functional connectivity in HR-ASD infants.

In a cohort of 58 6-month-old HR infants, Emerson et al. (2017) selected 230 regions to create functional connectivity matrices based on their rele-vance to ASD-related behaviors as determined through a meta-analysis and extensive work on functional areal parcellations in adults. A correlation matrix was generated for these regions, producing 26,335 pairs of regions. These coefficients were then correlated with behavioral performance at 24 months. Of those functional regions of interest (ROIs) pairs that were associated with later behavior and that also yielded statistically significant group differences, approximately 4% were identified for the machine learn-ing classification. The machine learning algorithm, using cross-validation techniques, correctly predicted 9 of the 11 infants who received an ASD diagnosis at 24 months. These results suggest that altered functional con-nectivity is present from 6 months in HR-ASD infants and that these early differences in functional connectivity may play a role in the emergence of future symptomology. In addition to these differences in functionally and spatially disparate networks across the brain, as alluded to above, a small proportion of functional connections were shown to be associated with behavioral outcomes at 24 months (based on scores on the Communica-tion and Symbolic Behavior Scales, Mullen Scales of Early Learning, and Repetitive Behavior Scale—Revised). Thus, further interrogation of these networks may provide more insight into how early connectivity differences in specific networks may lead to downstream behavioral effects. One of the implicated networks that was most strongly correlated with Communica-tion and Symbolic Behavior Scales Developmental Profile scores connected the dorsal striatum to the parietal lobe and postcentral gyrus. This suggests that connectivity between a reward-processing area and an area implicated in visual attention orienting may be implicated in ASD early in develop-ment, and that further study of the intersection between reward processing and attention warrants further study in HR infants.

Summary of Studies on Brain Development in HR Infants

In sum, specific neural markers of early-emerging ASD such as increased extra-axial cerebrospinal fluid (Shen et al., 2017), elevated FA (Wolff et al., 2012), and local white matter network inefficiencies (Lewis et al., 2017) are observable as early as 6 months, while other differences such as surface area hyperexpansion and total brain volume change (Hazlett et al., 2017; Shen et al., 2017) emerge over the first 2 years of life. Markers of atypical brain development present early in life tend to compound over time, such that HR-ASD infants increasingly diverge from their HR-negative or LR peers over time.

Many of the neural regions and networks implicated in these studies can be linked to sensory and sensorimotor processing areas (Hazlett et al., 2017; Lewis et al., 2017; Wolff et al., 2017). While the earliest signs of abnormal brain development precede the later-emerging symptoms that define ASD (Lewis et al., 2017; Shen et al., 2017; Wolff et al., 2012), as symptoms emerge in the second year of life, brain development becomes increasingly atypical. One intriguing possibility is that early disruptions in these sensorimotor processing areas lead to disruption in sensorimotor/ attentional experiences early in life, and these disruptions may have cascading developmental effects on experience-dependent cortical specialization. Specifically, atypical development in sensorimotor networks may cause the early attentional deficits observed in HR-ASD infants, which in turn may lead the individual to sample information from the environment in an atypical manner and, through iterative processes, drive the autistic behaviors that consolidate around 24 months (Piven et al., 2018).

In summary, these findings on early brain development have both important clinical implications as well as implications for our mechanistic understanding of the early development of ASD. However, there are still limitations in this field that should be addressed with further research. First, there are no studies reporting brain development in HR-ASD infants younger than 6 months. While there is indeed rapid brain development from 6 to 24 months, imaging evidence suggests that massive amounts of structural and functional change are happening before 6 months. Substantial structural change has been reported in the first 3 months of life (Holland et al., 2014), and there is evidence that functional networks become more integrated during this period as well, notably in fronto-parietal control networks and the default mode network (Gao et al., 2015). Given the rapid changes in brain development occurring before 6 months, fetal and neonatal imaging studies are needed to elucidate potential differences in development during this period of rapid change.

Second, while many longitudinal imaging studies have found predictive associations between brain development and autism severity (e.g., Emerson et al., 2017; Hazlett et al., 2017; Lewis et al., 2014; Shen et al., 2017), for other studies the association between brain and behavior is moderated by diagnostic group (Elison et al., 2013, Wolff et al., 2017). It should be noted that studies predicting subsequent symptom severity have largely focused on whole-brain or network analyses, whereas those suggesting different functional couplings have examined brain–behavior relationships among specific ROIs, selected based on their hypothesized functions, and have also looked at more specific behavioral outcomes (e.g., visual selective attention, RRBs). Further work clarifying the association between atypical brain development—examining both global measures of brain development and hypothesis-driven ROIs—and symptomology is needed.

Finally, although there are many brain differences found at or beginning at 6 months (Emerson et al., 2017; Hazlett et al., 2017; Lewis et al., 2014; Wolff et al., 2015) that predict future symptom severity, it is challenging to find autism-specific behavioral differences this early. Indeed, this may help explain why there may be such clinical utility in elucidating neural differences at this age. However, while distal associations with symptom severity are critical for construct validity, future studies investigating what these brain differences index earlier in development are needed.

The next section reviews behavioral markers of autism in the first year of life, many of which involve atypical attentional and sensorimotor processes that may be driven by the early neural differences reviewed above.

Attentional and Behavioral Markers of Autism in the First Years of Life

Prospective longitudinal studies have demonstrated differences in brain development as early as 6 months. In addition to these neural differences, behavioral (Miller et al., 2017; Nadig et al., 2007; Ozonoff et al., 2010) and attentional (Bedford et al., 2012; Chawarska, Macari, & Shic, 2013; Elison et al., 2013; Jones & Klin, 2013; Shic, Macari, & Chawarska, 2014; Wass et al., 2015) differences in the first 2 years of life have also been documented. The following sections review this body of literature, documenting attentional and behavioral differences in HR-ASD infants in the first 2 years of life.

Basic Attentional Differences in HR-ASD Infants

There is emerging evidence that basic attentional processes may differ in HR-ASD infants as early as 6 to 7 months (Elison et al., 2013; Wass et al., 2015). For example, 6- to 9-month-old HR-ASD infants show decreased median fixation durations compared to LR infants, with fixation duration at 6 to 9 months predicting ADOS scores at 36 months (Wass et al., 2015). Although these results are intriguing, HR-negative infants did not differ from either LR or HR-ASD infants in median fixation durations, suggesting that the findings are not disorder-specific. The only disorder-specific effect observed in visual orientation before 12 months has been found using the gap-overlap task, in which HR-ASD infants demonstrated longer latencies in the overlap condition (thought to index attentional orienting) than both HR-negative and LR infants (Elison et al., 2013). These findings suggest that domain-general attentional processes enabling infants to flexibly allocate attention and orient to salient information may be disrupted at an early age, at a developmental stage co-occurring with atypical brain development in regions implicated in sensory processing such as the precuneus and middle occipital area (Lewis et al., 2017; Wolff et al., 2017; Hazlett et al., 2017). These brain and behavioral differences may impact how HR-ASD infants sample information from the environment, which likely has adverse influences on the development of top-down attentional processes, as well as how infants deploy attention during complex situations such as social interactions.

An increasing body of evidence, reviewed in the next section, suggests deficits in early visual social engagement in HR-ASD infants. Visual social engagement requires the flexible allocation of attention and is thought to transition from more reflexive and subcortically mediated mechanisms in the first months of life to more experience-dependent and cortically mediated mechanisms (Morton & Johnson, 1991; Simion et al., 2011). This transition to experience-dependent mechanisms, in which infants begin to volitionally attend to information, requires that that information be continously sampled and reinforced. Because of its complexity, social information may be particularly vulnerable to interruptions in the fidelity of sampling and reinforcement over time. It might therefore be speculated that the domain-general attentional deficits outlined above may interrupt the fidelity of this sampling and may have cascading effects leading to the deficits in visual social engagement observed in infants and toddlers with ASD.

Visual Social Engagement

In addition to the differences in attentional skills outlined above, eye-tracking studies have demonstrated that HR-ASD infants show socially specific visual engagement deficits. At 6 months, HR-ASD infants spend less time attending to dynamic visual social stimuli than HR-negative and LR infants; during the time that they *do,* they spend a smaller proportion of time engaged with people and faces (Chawarska et al., 2013). These deficits in sustained engagement may be exacerbated with increasing stimulus complexity. For example, 6-month-old HR-ASD infants spend less time looking at the inner features of faces than LR and HR-negative infants, but only when faces are speaking (Shic et al., 2014). One study examined gaze following, an attentional skill conceptually linked to joint attention, by measuring how frequently infants looked at an object to which a caregiver directed her gaze (Bedford et al., 2012). Although there were no group differences at 7 months, by 13 months HR-ASD and HR-atypical infants spent less time looking at the referred-to object than HR-negative and LR infants.

While atypical visual social engagement has been observed by 6 months, these deficits may start even earlier. Longitudinal eye-tracking data densely sampled at 2, 3, 4, 5, 6, 9, 12, 15, 18, and 24 months demonstrated that, while HR-ASD and LR infants spent comparable amounts of time looking at the eyes of a caregiver onscreen at 2 months, their looking behavior diverged from 2 to 6 months (Jones & Klin, 2013). Specifically, the groups showed different trajectories in the amount of time spent looking at eyes: While the LR group *increased* the amount of time spent looking at the eyes from 2 to 6 months, the HR-ASD group *decreased* the amount of time spent looking at the eyes from 2 to 24 months. These differences in longitudinal trajectories—most notably from 2 to 6 months—resulted in the HR-ASD group spending approximately half as much time engaged with the eyes than the LR group by 24 months. These trajectories were disorder-specific; while the HR-negative group's trajectories overlapped with those of the LR group, the HR-ASD group clearly differed from the LR infants.

Behavioral Differences in HR-ASD Infants

In addition to differences ascertained through eye-tracking studies, behavioral differences in the first years of life have also been reported. By 6 months, the most severely affected group of HR-ASD infants (as determined by ADOS scores at 24 months) show less advanced Gross Motor and Visual Reception skills, as ascertained through the Mullen Scales of Early Learning, than LR infants (Estes et al., 2015). One prospective study (Nadig et al., 2007) examined infants' responses to their own names; this orienting response to a semantically salient auditory stimulus is thought to include a preattentive "detection" stage during which a response occurs only if the subject deems the stimulus to be contextually salient (Tateuchi, Itoh, & Nakada, 2012). While infants had similar responses to name calls at 6 months, by 12 months only 86% of HR infants responded to their name, while all LR infants did (Nadig et al., 2007). A follow-up study then examined this behavior across diagnostic outcome groups at 6, 9, 12, 15, and 24 months (Miller et al., 2017). While all groups had similar and relatively low rates of responding to name at 6 months, the HR-negative and LR groups improved in this behavior over time while the HR-ASD did not improve. These differences in developmental trajectories led to observable group differences at 9 months. Critically, while social behaviors have been found to become increasingly divergent from 6 to 12 months (Ozonoff et al., 2010), and the most severely affected infants show differences in their Gross Motor and Visual Receptive Mullen scores at 6 months (Estes et al., 2015), diminished response to name is the only disorder-specific overt behavioral marker of ASD found before 12 months of age to date.

Summary of Eye-Tracking and Behavioral Findings

Longitudinal measures of infants' time spent looking at the eyes (Jones & Klin, 2013) and responding to name (Miller et al., 2017) reveal that, while early trajectories of HR-ASD and LR infants may initially overlap, they become increasingly divergent over time. These increasingly divergent trajectories during the first year of life complement the literature on brain development in ASD, which implicates robust differences in sensory processing areas, as well as emerging network inefficiencies (Hazlett et al., 2017; Lewis et al., 2017; Wolff et al., 2017).

Differences in visual engagement among HR-ASD infants can be observed as early as 6 to 7 months (Chawarska et al., 2013; Elison et al., 2013; Shic et al., 2014), while the earliest nonvisual behavioral marker (responding to name) is observable at 9 months (Miller et al., 2017). Intriguingly, these behavioral differences tend to be implicated in flexibly and efficiently allocating attention (Elison et al., 2013) or in attending to self-relevant (Miller et al., 2017; Nadig et al., 2007) or socially salient information (Bedford et al., 2012; Chawarska et al., 2013; Jones & Klin, 2013; Shic et al., 2014). In other words, all these processes influence how HR-ASD infants filter information and select what to attend to, thus impacting their early experiences of the world and subsequent experience-dependent development. As previously discussed, many of the neural regions and networks found to be atypical in HR-ASD infants can be linked to sensory and sensorimotor processes (Hazlett et al., 2017; Lewis et al., 2017; Wolff et al., 2017). While drawing connections between disparate studies should be done cautiously, it is possible that these early neural disruptions may underlie the attentional and sensory-processing atypicalities documented in behavioral studies on HR-ASD infants. Indeed, further longitudinal studies examining the link between atypical brain development in sensory-processing areas and subsequent atypical attentional and sensory-processing outcomes in the same sample of infants are needed.

The next section outlines literature highlighting the bidirectional influences between these flexible attentional systems, and learning and memory in typically developing infants. We then present a conceptual model in which reward learning and salience tagging represent the interface of these two systems, and we consider how these mechanisms may impact the transition from predominantly stimulus-driven/automatic orienting to volitional attendance to self-relevant information. These models of how attention develops in LR, TD samples promise to inform a more comprehensive conceptualization of implications for the early development of ASD.

The Development of Visual Selective Attention in the First Years of Life

Infants live in a visually noisy world, and prioritizing attention to meaningful information is arguably the most important task they face in efficiently learning about their surroundings (Markant & Amso, 2013). In the first few months of life, infants are driven primarily by low-level visually salient information (e.g., bright lights, colors, motion), but at around 4 to 6 months selective visual attention mechanisms emerge, allowing for the suppression of competing information (Amso & Scerif, 2015). This ability to selectively attend to relevant, salient information, while inhibiting attention from potentially equally salient distractors, is critical for the development of learning and memory. One such example is inhibition of return (IOR; Posner & Cohen, 1984), or the ability to suppress attention to locations that were previously attended to. IOR has been interpreted as an attentional biasing effect that encourages the visual exploration of novel locations, and its emergence in infancy plays a critical role in attention and learning. One example of this phenomenon is that 9-month-old infants show deeper encoding of objects seen in the context of IOR-based attention (e.g., when their attention was initially biased *away* from the object, with enough time to then shift covert attention back to the object) compared to when their attention was simply biased toward the object (Markant & Amso, 2013). This suggests that when infants engage in an attentional mechanism that requires attention suppression, they encode information more deeply. Furthermore, individual differences in object encoding at 4 months can be predicted by whether infants have developed more mature IOR-based orienting (Markant & Amso, 2016). These findings suggest that the developmental onset of IOR (an attentional mechanism) acts as a catalyst for the development of more sophisticated memory-encoding abilities.

While early attentional systems influence the development of memory systems, this relationship becomes increasingly bidirectional over developmental time. Amso and Scerif (2015) propose a hierarchical organization of infants' visual development, in which visual input is first gained through exogenous orienting to perceptually salient or biologically salient information. Visual areas then feed forward into higher-level regions, acting as developmental catalysts for further top-down modulation of these same visual pathways. Johnson et al. (2015) posit similar mechanisms to explain the development of ASD. Sensory input entrains the cortex in a posterior-to-anterior fashion, such that early in development, cortical organization is dependent on thalamic sensory input. Thus, in the first months of life, there is a period of cortical specialization during which the cortex is sensitive to reorganization via sensory thalamic input. However, if the environment is sampled with poor fidelity, as may be the case with ASD (with complex stimuli such as social stimuli suffering the most from poor sampling), then this may lead to delays in brain development and ultimately to atypical and/ or disorganized brain structure and function. Furthermore, atypical cortical development may be observed initially in posterior regions (Elison et al., 2013; Hazlett et al., 2017), with disorganization becoming more diffuse over time (Lewis et al., 2017).

In both of these hypotheses, early atypical brain development influences sensory experiences and initiates cascading developmental effects, influencing memory and top-down attentional systems. These sensory experiences are mediated by attentional mechanisms—specifically, by exogenous orienting to stimuli, by developmental competencies in selective attention, and finally by self-relevant information biasing individuals' saliency maps. In the case of HR-ASD infants, early atypical attentional mechanisms may lead infants to sample environmental information in a species-atypical manner, which in turn may lead to atypical cortically mediated top-down attentional control. This in turn can influence how individuals seek out information later in development. In other words, differences in what is considered self-relevant or semantically salient are not only the result of early atypical attentional and neural development, but also serve to maintain atypicalities in the low-level visual processing of stimuli and therefore maintain atypical attentional orienting, memory encoding, and cortical specialization.

In the next section, we outline empirical evidence in infants, children, and adults, demonstrating that semantically salient and rewarding information can bias not only *what* individuals selectively attend to but *how* those semantic stimuli become perceptually enhanced. We will then discuss how enhanced or degraded perception of a stimulus dependent on semantic salience can maintain and exacerbate attentional deficits.

How Semantic Salience Biases Attention

Stimuli that are imbued with semantic salience can bias visual attention in a fashion similar to perceptually salient information. For example, when adults search for an object in a familiar scene and therefore know its location, two things occur: First, their response time decreases as a function of their prior experience, and second, these decreased response times are paired with event-related potentials reflecting top-down cortical enhancement of object perception (Summerfield, Rao, Garside, & Nobre, 2011). In other words, changing the contextual salience of the scene due to prior experience enhances the visual perception of that item and its remembered spatial location, an effect that is both cortically and subcortically driven (Green et al., 2017).

Reward seems to be a particularly strong modulator of semantic salience. It has long been known that task-relevant goals to seek out rewarding stimuli exert endogenous control on attention (Awh, Belopolsky, & Theeuwes, 2012; Hickey, Chelazzi, & Theeuwes, 2010; Theeuwes & Belopolsky, 2012). More recently, however, there has been a shift in focus to how reward enhances bottom-up stimulus saliency (Bourgeois, Chelazzi, & Vuilleumier, 2016; Failing & Theeuwes, 2014). When participants learn to associate a stimulus property (i.e., the color red) with a monetary reward and complete a target-selection task in which the rewarded feature is present as a distractor, previously rewarded stimulus features bias attention despite being task-irrelevant (Awh et al., 2012; Della Libera & Chelazzi, 2009). These attentional biases toward rewarding stimuli are accompanied by an increased P1 amplitude contralateral to the rewarding stimulus, even when an individual's task goals are *diametrically opposed* to attending to the stimulus (Hickey et al., 2010). Learned reward associations modulate activity in the intraparietal sulcus (Awh et al., 2012; Bisley & Goldberg, 2010), a region that is integral to the dorsal/frontoparietal-visual selective attention network, and is implicated in calculating salience maps for attention to act upon (Bisley & Goldberg, 2010; Corbetta & Shulman, 2002). Thus, by engaging visual selective attention mechanisms, learned reward history can actually modulate a stimulus's saliency as an attentional cue and *change how a stimulus is perceived.*

fNIRS (functional near-infrared spectroscopy) data has demonstrated that expectation of a visual stimulus—even in its absence—modulates activity in the occipital cortex in 6-month-old infants (Emberson, Richards, & Aslin, 2015). This suggests that cortically driven perceptual enhancement of semantically salient stimuli occurs in the first year of life. Unsurprisingly, reward appears to be a strong modulator of semantic salience in infants as well as adults. One example of reward-enhanced salience comes from a study by Tummeltshammer, Mareschal, and Kirkham (2014), in which 6- and 8-month-old infants were taught to associate a neutral stimulus with a rewarding video. Both 6- and 8-month-olds were able to attend to the reward stimulus in the presence of a nonsalient distractor. However, when a salient distractor was present (a face), only 8-month-olds could inhibit attention to the face. These findings suggest that reward-enhanced attention is present early in infancy and interacts with the development of other top-down attentional control mechanisms. Furthermore, this developmental pattern suggests that reward-enhanced attention may act similarly to exogenous and stimulus-driven attentional mechanisms, and "compete" with top-down attentional control mechanisms that mature later in development.

Research on infants' *response to name* demonstrates that reward-enhanced and semantic-enhanced perception occurs across stimulus modalities. The ability to attend to and perceive one's name in the presence of distracting noise develops from 5 to 13 months, with infants becoming increasingly sensitive to the sound of their own name even in the presence of distracting noise (Newman, 2005). Thus, while an infant's name holds semantic salience as early as 5 months of age, the ability to attend to it in the presence of loud distractors develops over the first year of life. This developmental change is likely due to a combination of enhanced distractor suppression competencies, as well one's own name acquiring increasing semantic meaning and self-relevance over time as infants continuously hear it in a rewarding and contingent social context.

Semantic Salience, Reward, and Autism

This chapter has reviewed evidence from infant sibling studies demonstrating that HR-ASD infants begin to diverge from their LR, TD peers in the first year of life, in terms of both brain development and behavior. Brain-imaging studies have implicated neural regions and networks linked to sensory and sensorimotor processing areas (Hazlett et al., 2017; Lewis et al., 2017; Wolff et al., 2017) and to network inefficiencies in the brain during this early time (Emerson et al., 2017; Lewis et al., 2017; Wolff et al., 2012). Early behavior studies have implicated atypical domain-general attentional mechanisms at 7 months (Elison et al., 2013), with socially specific visual engagement deficits emerging at around the same time (Chawarska et al., 2013; Shic et al., 2014) or unfolding over the first years of life (Bedford et al., 2012; Jones & Klin, 2013).

We have also summarized evidence from the literature on LR non-ASD infants that suggests that the ability to imbue privileged stimuli with semantic salience (either through reward or continuous reinforcement) and to bias attention toward these stimuli is a critical attentional mechanism that helps infants attend to prioritized information while filtering out distractors. By enhancing the perceptual features of semantically salient or rewarding stimuli, reward-enhanced attention helps these stimulus features filter through noise.

Understanding how these processes work may be a critical step toward understanding the early unfolding of ASD. Early deficits in stimulus processing may not necessarily be social-specific but may exist in systems that imbue stimuli with semantic salience, processes that enable infants to have reward-enhanced orienting, or both. One interesting example of this is a study in which preschoolers were taught to learn object-reward associations for social (face) or nonsocial (fractal images) objects (Wang, DiNicola, Heymann, Hampson, & Chawarska, 2018). While TD preschoolers showed enhanced reward learning in the social compared to nonsocial condition, preschoolers with ASD performed comparably across both conditions and showed less reward learning in the social condition compared to TD preschoolers. Critically, the ASD toddlers showed preferential attention to the rewarded object within each category, suggesting that while they are able to learn reward-object associations, their performance is poorer in social contexts.

There is growing consensus that further research on the mechanisms underlying value learning may be critical for understanding the etiology of ASD (Fitzpatrick, 2018). Social information processing may be particularly vulnerable to atypicalities or delays in these attentional and reward processes. This possibility is supported by evidence that the diminished anterior cingulate gyrus and ventral striatal activity that adults with ASD demonstrate during reward tasks is exacerbated in social-reward tasks and is correlated with social ability (for a review, see Dichter, Damiano, & Allen, 2012). There may therefore be a sensitive period for the development of processes that enable infants to imbue stimuli with semantic salience, and orient to semantic salience, that occurs before the transition to experience-dependent social information processing. Critically, atypical reward- or salience-enhanced attention can then serve to maintain the early atypical sensory experiences in toddlers with ASD, with these iterative processes resulting in emerging ASD symptomology. A visual representation of this theoretical model can be found in Figure 6.1.

There are, of course, limitations to this theoretical framework. While there may be a link between the body of work implicating neural regions and networks associated with sensory and sensorimotor processing areas, and the body of work implicating differences in attention and reward processing in ASD infants, further hypothesis-driven studies explicitly testing this link are needed. Furthermore, as studies documenting circumscribed interests in HR-ASD infants and toddlers (Leekam, Prior, & Uljarevic, 2011) make clear, reward processing is intact in certain contexts. While this may be analogous to hypotheses about domain-general attentional deficits in ASD, which are then exacerbated in social contexts when the environment is less predictable (e.g., Johnson et al., 2015), understanding the differences in reward processing and reward-modulated attention in ASD in social versus nonsocial contexts is needed. For more information on development of attention in infant siblings, see Chawarska, Macari, Vernetti, and Brunissen (Chapter 5, this volume).

REFERENCES

Amso, D., & Scerif, G. (2015). The attentive brain: Insights from developmental cognitive neuroscience. *Nature Reviews Neuroscience, 16*(10), 606–619.

Awh, E., Belopolsky, A. V., & Theeuwes, J. (2012). Top-down versus bottom-up attentional control: A failed theoretical dichotomy. *Trends in Cognitive Sciences, 16*(8), 437–443.

Bedford, R., Elsabbagh, M., Gliga, T., Pickles, A., Senju, A., Charman, T., & Johnson, M. H. (2012). Precursors to social and communication difficulties in infants at-risk for autism: Gaze following and attentional engagement. *Journal of Autism and Developmental Disorders, 42*(10), 2208–2218.

Bisley, J. W., & Goldberg, M. E. (2010). Attention, intention, and priority in the parietal lobe. *Annual Review of Neuroscience, 33*(1), 1–21.

Bourgeois, A., Chelazzi, L., & Vuilleumier, P. (2016). How motivation and reward learning modulate selective attention. *Progress in Brain Research, 229*, 325–342.

Chawarska, K., Macari, S., & Shic, F. (2013). Decreased spontaneous attention to social scenes in 6-month-old infants later diagnosed with autism spectrum disorders. *Biological Psychiatry, 74*(3), 195–203.

Constantino, J. N., Kennon-McGill, S., Weichselbaum, C., Marrus, N., Haider, A., Glowinski, A. L., . . . Jones, W. (2017). Infant viewing of social scenes is under genetic control and is atypical in autism. *Nature, 547*(7663), 340–344.

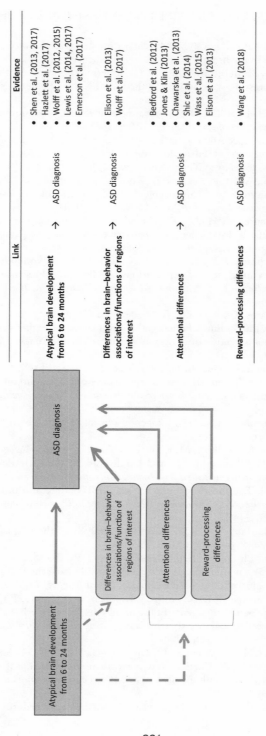

Link		Evidence
Atypical brain development from 6 to 24 months → ASD diagnosis		• Shen et al. (2013, 2017) • Hazlett et al. (2017) • Wolff et al. (2012, 2015) • Lewis et al. (2014, 2017) • Emerson et al. (2017)
Differences in brain–behavior associations/functions of regions of interest → ASD diagnosis		• Elison et al. (2013) • Wolff et al. (2017)
Attentional differences → ASD diagnosis		• Bedford et al. (2012) • Jones & Klin (2013) • Chawarska et al. (2013) • Shic et al. (2014) • Wass et al. (2015) • Elison et al. (2013)
Reward-processing differences → ASD diagnosis		• Wang et al. (2018)

FIGURE 6.1. Diagrammatic representation of theoretical model. Solid lines indicate empirical evidence in support of the link; dashed lines indicate that the link is speculative. Citations for links supported by empirical evidence are listed at the right.

Corbetta, M., & Shulman, G. L. (2002, March). Control of goal-directed and stimulus-driven attention in the brain. *Nature Review, Neuroscience, 3,* 201–218.

Deco, G., Jirsa, V. K., & McIntosh, A. R. (2011). Emerging concepts for the dynamical organization of resting-state activity in the brain. *Nature Reviews Neuroscience, 12*(1), 43–56.

Della Libera, C., & Chelazzi, L. (2009). Learning to attend and to ignore is a matter of gains and losses. *Psychological Science, 20*(6), 778–784.

Dichter, G., Damiano, C., & Allen, J. (2012). Reward circuitry dysfunction in psychiatric and neurodevelopmental disorders and genetic syndromes: Animal models and clinical findings. *Journal of Neurodevelopment Disorders, 4*(1), 19.

Elison, J., Paterson, S., Wolff, J., Reznick, S., Sasson, N. J., Gu, H., . . . Piven, J. (2013). White matter microstructure and atypical visual orienting in 7-month-olds at risk for autism. *American Journal of Psychiatry, 170*(8), 1–18.

Elsabbagh, M., Mercure, E., Hudry, K., Chandler, S., Pasco, G., Charman. T., . . . BASIS Team. (2012). Infant neural sensitivity to dynamic eye gaze is associated with later emerging autism. *Current Biology, 21,* 338–342.

Emberson, L. L., Richards, J. E., & Aslin, R. N. (2015). Top-down modulation in the infant brain: Learning-induced expectations rapidly affect the sensory cortex at 6 months. *Proceedings of the National Academy of Sciences of the USA, 112*(31), 9585–9590.

Emerson, R. W., Adams, C., Nishino, T., Hazlett, H. C., Wolff, J. J., Zwaigenbaum, L., . . . Piven, J. (2017, June). Functional neuroimaging of high-risk 6-month-old infants predicts a diagnosis of autism at 24 months of age. *Science Translational Medicine, 2882,* 1–8.

Estes, A., Zwaigenbaum, L., Gu, H., St. John, T., Paterson, S., Elison, J. T., . . . Piven, J. (2015). Behavioral, cognitive, and adaptive development in infants with autism spectrum disorder in the first 2 years of life. *Journal of Neurodevelopmental Disorders, 7*(1), 1–10.

Failing, M. F., & Theeuwes, J. (2014). Exogenous visual orienting by reward. *Journal of Vision, 14*(5), 6.

Finch, K. H., Seery, A. M., Talbott, M. R., Nelson, C. A., & Tager-Flusberg, H. (2017). Lateralization of ERPs to speech and handedness in the early development of autism spectrum disorder. *Journal of Neurodevelopmental Disorders, 9,* 1–14.

Fitzpatrick, P. (2018). The future of autism research: Dynamic and process-oriented approaches. *Journal of the American Academy of Child and Adolescent Psychiatry, 57*(1), 16–17.

Frazier, T. W., & Hardan, A. Y. (2010). A meta-analysis of the corpus callosum in autism. *Biological Psychiatry, 66*(10), 935–941.

Gao, W., Alcauter, S., Elton, A., Hernandez-Castillo, C. R., Smith, J. K., Ramirez, J., & Lin, W. (2015). Functional network development during the first year: Relative sequence and socioeconomic correlations. *Cerebral Cortex, 25*(9), 2919–2928.

Gao, W., Zhu, H., Giovanello, K. S., Smith, J. K., Shen, D., Gilmore, J. H., & Lin, W. (2009). Evidence on the emergence of the brain's default network from 2-week-old to 2-year-old healthy pediatric subjects. *Proceedings of the National Academy of Sciences of the USA, 106*(16), 6790–6795.

Green, J. J., Boehler, C. N., Roberts, K. C., Chen, L.-C., Krebs, R. M., Song, A. W., & Woldorff, M. G. (2017). Cortical and subcortical coordination of visual spatial attention revealed by simultaneous EEG–fMRI recording. *Journal of Neuroscience, 37*(33), 7803–7810.

Hardan, A. Y., Pabalan, M., Gupta, N., Bansal, R., Melhem, N., Fedorov, S., . . . Minshew, N. (2009). Corpus callosum volume in children with autism. *Psychiatry Research, 174*(1), 57–61.

Hazlett, H. C., Gu, H., Munsell, B. C., Kim, S. H., Styner, M., Wolff, J. J., . . . Gu, C. H. (2017). Early brain development in infants at high risk for autism spectrum disorder. *Nature, 542*(7641), 348–351.

Hermoye, L., Saint-Martin, C., Cosnard, G., Lee, S., Kim, J., Nassogne, M., . . . Mori, S. (2006). Pediatric diffusion tensor imaging: Normal database and observation of the white matter maturation in early childhood. *NeuroImage, 29,* 493–504.

Hickey, C., Chelazzi, L., & Theeuwes, J. (2010). Reward changes salience in human vision via the anterior cingulate. *Journal of Neuroscience, 30*(33), 11096–11103.

Holland, D., Chang, L., Ernst, T. M., Curran, M., Buchthal, S. D., Alicata, D., . . . Dale, A. M. (2014). Structural growth trajectories and rates of change in the first 3 months of infant brain development. *JAMA Neurology, 71*(10), 1266–1274.

Johnson, M. H. (2000). Functional brain development in infants: Elements of an interactive specialization framework. *Child Development, 71*(1), 75–81.

Johnson, M. H., Jones, E., & Gliga, T. (2015). Brain adaptation and alternative developmental trajectories. *Development and Psychopathology, 27*(2), 425–442.

Jones, W., & Klin, A. (2013). Attention to eyes is present but in decline in 2–6-month-old infants later diagnosed with autism. *Nature, 504*(7480), 427–431.

Kanner, L. (1943). Autistic disturbances of affective contact. *Nervous Child, 2,* 217–250.

Klin, A., Shultz, S., & Jones, W. (2015). Social visual engagement in infants and toddlers with autism: Early developmental transitions and a model of pathogenesis. *Neuroscience and Biobehavioral Reviews, 50,* 189–203.

Lainhart, J. E., Piven, J., Wzorek, M., Landa, R., Santangelo, S. L., Coon, H., & Folstein, S. E. (1997). Macrocephaly in children and adults with autism. *Journal of the American Academy of Child and Adolescent Psychiatry, 36*(2), 282–290.

LaMantia, A. S., & Rakic, P. (1990). Axon overproduction and elimination in the corpus callosum of the developing rhesus monkey. *Journal of Neuroscience, 10*(7), 2156–2175.

Lavelli, M., & Fogel, A. (2005). Developmental changes in the relationship between the infant's attention and emotion during early face-to-face communication: The 2-month transition. *Developmental Psychology, 41*(1), 265–280.

Leekam, S. R., Prior, M. R., & Uljarevic, M. (2011). Restricted and repetitive behaviors in autism spectrum disorders: A review of research in the last decade. *Psychological Bulletin, 137*(4), 562–593.

Levin, A. R., Varcin, K. J., O'Leary, H. M., Tager-Flusberg, H., & Nelson, C. A. (2017). EEG power at 3 months in infants at high familial risk for autism. *Journal of Neurodevelopmental Disorders, 9*(34).

Lewis, J. D., Evans, A. C., Pruett, J. R., Botteron, K. N., McKinstry, R. C., Zwaigenbaum, L., . . . Gu, H. (2017). The emergence of network inefficiencies in infants with autism spectrum disorder. *Biological Psychiatry, 82*(3), 176–185.

Lewis, J. D., Evans, A. C., Pruett, J. R., Botteron, K., Zwaigenbaum, L., Estes, A., . . . Piven, J. (2014). Network inefficiencies in autism spectrum disorder at 24 months. *Translational Psychiatry, 4*(5), e388.

Markant, J., & Amso, D. (2013). Selective memories: Infants' encoding is enhanced in selection via suppression. *Developmental Science, 16*(6), 926–940.

Markant, J., & Amso, D. (2016). The development of selective attention orienting is an agent of change in learning and memory efficacy. *Infancy, 21*(2), 154–176.

Markant, J. C., & Thomas, K. M. (2013). Postnatal brain development. In P. D. Zelazo

(Ed.), *The Oxford handbook of developmental psychology: Vol. 1. Brain and mind* (pp. 127–163). Oxford, UK: Oxford University Press.

Messinger, D. S., Young, G. S., Webb, S. J., Ozonoff, S., Bryson, S. E., Carter, A., . . . Zwaigenbaum, L. (2015). Early sex differences are not autism-specific: A Baby Siblings Research Consortium (BSRC) study. *Molecular Autism, 6*(1), 32.

Miller, M., Iosif, A.-M., Hill, M., Young, G. S., Schwichtenberg, A. J., & Ozonoff, S. (2017). Response to name in infants developing autism spectrum disorder: A prospective study. *Journal of Pediatrics, 183,* 1–7.

Mitra, A., Snyder, A. Z., Tagliazucchi, E., Laufs, H., Elison, J., Emerson, R. W., . . . Raichle, M. (2017). Resting-state fMRI in sleeping infants more closely resembles adult sleep than adult wakefulness. *PLOS ONE, 12*(11), 1–19.

Morton, J., & Johnson, M. H. (1991). CONSPEC and CONLERN: A two-process theory of infant face recognition. *Psychological Review, 98*(2), 164.

Nadig, A. S., Ozonoff, S., Young, G. S., Rozga, A., Sigman, M., & Rogers, S. J. (2007). A prospective study of response to name in infants at risk for autism. *Archives of Pediatrics and Adolescent Medicine, 161*(4), 378–383.

Newman, R. S. (2005). The cocktail party effect in infants revisited: Listening to one's name in noise. *Developmental Psychology, 41*(2), 352–362.

Niogi, S., Mukherjee, P., Ghajar, J., & McCandliss, B. (2010). Individual differences in distinct components of attention are linked to anatomical variations in distinct white matter tracts. *Frontiers in Neuroanatomy, 4,* 2.

Orekhova, E. V., Elsabbagh, M., Jones, E. J., Dawson, G., Charman, T., Johnson, M. H, & BASIS Team. (2014). EEG hyper-connectivity in high-risk infants is associated with later autism. *Journal of Neurodevelopmental Disorders, 6*(1), 40.

Ozonoff, S., Iosif, A.-M., Baguio, F., Cook, I. C., Moore Hill, M., Hutman, T., . . . Young, G. S. (2010). A prospective study of the emergence of early behavioral signs of autism. *Journal of the American Academy of Child and Adolescent Psychiatry, 49*(3), 256–266.

Ozonoff, S., Young, G. S., Carter, A., Messinger, D., Yirmiya, N., Zwaigenbaum, L., . . . Stone, W. L. (2011). Recurrence risk for autism spectrum disorders: A Baby Siblings Research Consortium study. *Pediatrics, 12*(3), e488–495.

Panizzon, M. S., Fennema-Notestine, C., Eyler, L. T., Jernigan, T. L., Prom-Wormley, E., Neale, M., . . . Kremen, W. S. (2009). Distinct genetic influences on cortical surface area and cortical thickness. *Cerebral Cortex, 19*(11), 2728–2735.

Piven, J., Arndt, S., Bailey, J., Havercamp, S., Andreasen, N. C., & Palmer, P. (1995). An MRI study of brain size in autism. *American Journal of Psychiatry, 152*(8), 1145–1149.

Piven, J., Bailey, J., Ranson, B. J., & Arndt, S. (1997). An MRI study of the corpus callosum in autism. *American Journal of Psychiatry, 154*(8), 1051–1056.

Piven, J., Elison, J. T., & Zylka, M. J. (2018). Toward a conceptual framework for early brain and behavior development in autism. *Molecular Psychiatry, 23*(1), 165.

Piven, J., Nehme, E., Simon, J., Barta, P., Pearlson, G., & Folstein, S. E. (1992). Magnetic resonance imaging in autism: Measurement of the cerebellum, pons, and fourth ventricle. *Biological Psychiatry, 31*(5), 491–504.

Posner, M. I., & Cohen, Y. (1984). Components of visual orienting. *Attention and Performance, 32,* 531–556.

Prigge, M. B. D., Lange, N., Bigler, E. D., Merkley, T. L., Shannon Neeley, E., Abildskov, T. J., . . . Lainhart, J. E. (2013). Corpus callosum area in children and adults with Autism. *Research in Autism Spectrum Disorders, 7*(2), 221–234.

Sadeghi, N., Prastawa, M., Fletcher, P. T., Wolff, J., Gilmore, J. H., & Gerig, G. N.

(2013). Regional characterization of longitudinal DT-MRI to study white matter maturation of the early developing brain. *NeuroImage, 68,* 236–247.

Sandin, S., Lichtenstein, P., Kuja-Halkola, R., Larsson, H., Hultman, C. M., & Reichenberg, A. (2014). The familial risk of autism. *JAMA, 311*(17), 1770.

Shen, M. D., Kim, S. H., McKinstry, R. C., Gu, H., Hazlett, H. C., Nordahl, C. W., . . . Gu, H. (2017). Increased extra-axial cerebrospinal fluid in high-risk infants who later develop autism. *Biological Psychiatry, 82,* 186–193.

Shen, M. D., Nordahl, C. W., Young, G. S., Wootton-Gorges, S. L., Lee, A., Liston, S. E., . . . Amaral, D. G. (2013). Early brain enlargement and elevated extra-axial fluid in infants who develop autism spectrum disorder. *Brain, 136*(9), 2825–2835.

Shic, F., Macari, S., & Chawarska, K. (2014). Speech disturbs faces scanning in 6-month-olds who develop autism spectrum disorder. *Biological Psychiatry, 75*(3), 231–237.

Simion, F., Di Giorgio, E., Leo, I., & Bardi, L. (2011). The processing of social stimuli in early infancy: From faces to biological motion perception. *Progress in Brain Research, 189*(April), 173–193.

Stevenson, R., Schroer, R., Skinner, C., Fender, D., & Simensen, R. J. (1997). Autism and macrocephaly. *The Lancet, 349*(9067), 1745–1746.

Summerfield, J. J., Rao, A., Garside, N., & Nobre, A. C. (2011). Biasing perception by spatial long-term memory. *Journal of Neuroscience, 31*(42), 14952–14960.

Swanson, M. R., Wolff, J. J., Elison, J. T., Gu, H., Hazlett, H. C., Botteron, K., . . . Gu, H. (2017). Splenium development and early spoken language in human infants. *Developmental Science, 20*(2), 1–13.

Tateuchi, T., Itoh, K., & Nakada, T. (2012). Neural mechanisms underlying the orienting response to subject's own name: An event-related potential study. *Psychophysiology, 49*(6), 786–791.

Theeuwes, J., & Belopolsky, A. V. (2012). Reward grabs the eye: Oculomotor capture by rewarding stimuli. *Vision Research, 74,* 80–85.

Tummeltshammer, K. S., Mareschal, D., & Kirkham, N. Z. (2014). Infants' selective attention to reliable visual cues in the presence of salient distractors. *Child Development, 85*(5), 1981–1984.

Wang, Q., DiNicola, L., Heymann, P., Hampson, M., & Chawarska, K. (2018). Impaired value learning for faces in preschoolers with autism spectrum disorder. *Journal of the American Academy of Child and Adolescent Psychiatry, 57*(1), 33–40.

Wass, S. V., Jones, E. J. H., Gliga, T., Smith, T. J., Charman, T., & Johnson, M. H. (2015). Shorter spontaneous fixation durations in infants with later emerging autism. *Scientific Reports, 5*(8284).

Wolff, J. J., Gerig, G., Lewis, J. D., Soda, T., Styner, M. A., Vachet, C., . . . Piven, J. (2015). Altered corpus callosum morphology associated with autism over the first 2 years of life. *Brain, 138*(7), 2046–2058.

Wolff, J. J., Gu, H., Gerig, G., Elison, J. T., Styner, M., Gouttard, S., . . . the IBIS Network. (2012). Differences in white matter fiber tract development present from 6 to 24 months in infants with autism. *American Journal of Psychiatry, 169*(6), 589–600.

Wolff, J. J., Swanson, M. R., Elison, J. T., Gerig, G., Pruett, J. R., Styner, M. A., . . . Piven, J. (2017). Neural circuitry at age 6 months associated with later repetitive behavior and sensory responsiveness in autism. *Molecular Autism, 8,* 8.

CHAPTER 7

• • • • • • •

Long-Term Outcomes of Infants at Risk for Autism Spectrum Disorder

Meghan Miller and Sally Ozonoff

For decades, since the pioneering twin and family studies of Folstein and Rutter (1977, 1988), empirical investigations have documented higher rates of a variety of difficulties in first-degree relatives of individuals with autism spectrum disorder (ASD) compared to relatives of individuals with dyslexia, Down syndrome, and other disorders (for a comprehensive review, see Sucksmith, Roth, & Hoekstra, 2011). Most notably, approximately 20% of younger siblings of children with ASD will go on to develop ASD themselves (Ozonoff et al., 2011). Yet more subtle group differences have also been reliably documented in first-degree family members. Bolton and colleagues (1994) coined the term *broader autism phenotype* (BAP) to describe subthreshold (nonclinical-level) differences seen in family members of children with ASD in the areas of reciprocal social interaction, social cognition, and pragmatic communication. While there is consensus in the field on the existence of such a broader phenotype, there is not yet agreement on what domains constitute it and there is substantial variation from study to study in how it is operationalized. For example, some studies limit use of the term *BAP* to behaviors that are qualitatively similar to the core symptom domains of ASD (e.g., social communication or repetitive behaviors), whereas others include psychiatric symptoms or diagnoses that are more prevalent in family members of individuals with ASD than in the general population (e.g., mood and anxiety disorders, attention-deficit/hyperactivity disorder [ADHD]). Thus, exactly what comprises the BAP remains an open question. In this chapter, we take a more inclusive approach, also reviewing studies of psychiatric outcomes in infant siblings of children with ASD.

The initial studies of the BAP focused on parents and older siblings of individuals with ASD. These studies found significantly higher rates of social challenges, deficits in theory of mind and other social cognitive abilities, executive dysfunction, and repetitive behaviors in family members of children with ASD than in family members of children with typical development or other disorders (Bailey, Palferman, Heavey, & LeCouteur, 1998; Bolton et al., 1994; see Sucksmith et al., 2011, for a comprehensive review). Elevated rates of mental health difficulties, particularly attention, mood, and anxiety symptoms, have also been found in many studies (Howlin, Moss, Savage, Bolton, & Rutter, 2015; Jokiranta-Olkoniemi et al., 2016; O'Neill & Murray, 2016; Shivers, Jackson, & McGregor, 2019). These studies laid the groundwork for the more recently employed infant sibling designs, which prospectively follow later-born siblings ascertained at very young ages, before parents have concerns about their development, and thus avoid ascertainment biases that may have inflated the rates of adverse outcomes.

Over the past decade, such investigations of infant siblings of children with ASD have proliferated. These studies have primarily focused on identifying early markers of ASD, with the hope that identification of such markers will aid in earlier and more reliable diagnosis. As described throughout this book (e.g., Chapters 5 and 6) and elsewhere (e.g., Jones, Gliga, Bedford, Charman, & Johnson, 2014; Szatmari et al., 2016), numerous insights have been gained from this work with respect to infant and toddler manifestations of emerging ASD. For example, research on infant siblings has demonstrated that behavioral signs of ASD begin to emerge late in the first year of life (e.g., Landa & Garrett-Mayer, 2006; Ozonoff et al., 2010). Unaffected (i.e., without ASD) siblings begin to demonstrate social communication, cognitive, and language challenges consistent with the BAP as early as 12 months of age (Macari et al., 2012; Ozonoff et al., 2014; Rowberry et al., 2015), and approximately 20–30% of siblings who do not develop ASD demonstrate these types of developmental concerns by age 3 (Messinger et al., 2013; Ozonoff et al., 2014).

Because few studies have yet followed these samples beyond the toddler/preschool years, it has been difficult to ascertain the longer-term outcomes of infants at risk for ASD. This chapter differs from the other chapters in this book in that we concentrate on developmental periods beyond infancy and toddlerhood, and we expand our focus to include familial aspects of ASD, reviewing the relatively small literature focused on longer-term outcomes of infant siblings of children with ASD. In this chapter, we describe how each individual study has conceptualized this "broader phenotype" rather than imposing our own definition. We conclude by highlighting important areas for future research.

Why Are Longer-Term Outcomes of Infant Siblings Relevant?

As described above, recent studies focused on infant sibling samples have indicated that a subset of these younger siblings who do not go on to develop ASD instead experience vulnerabilities in various developmental, social, and behavioral domains across both experimental (e.g., eye-tracking tasks of attention processing; Elsabbagh et al., 2013) and standardized measures (e.g., Mullen Scales of Early Learning; Messinger et al., 2013; Iverson et al., 2019). Yet, little is known about whether these challenges are time-limited or long-standing, and whether new challenges may emerge in middle childhood and beyond.

As stipulated in DSM-5 (American Psychiatric Association, 2013), ASD symptoms must be present "early in the developmental period," so why are later developmental stages relevant in research seeking to document the onset of ASD? The concept of multifinality is informative, whereby a common risk can result in a multitude of disparate outcomes across development (Hinshaw, 2013). Numerous population-based studies have shown that siblings of children with ASD are at elevated risk for other forms of psychopathology, including ADHD, learning disorders, conduct and oppositional disorders, and mood and anxiety disorders (Jokiranta-Olkoniemi et al., 2016). Moreover, new and increasing demands in later developmental periods may result in new challenges. Thus, a primary reason to be concerned about outcomes beyond age 3 is that the emergence of other challenges facing these high-risk siblings may not be fully apparent until they reach middle childhood and beyond. A more complete understanding of later outcomes may help identify additional domains to be screened and monitored earlier in life.

Longer-Term Follow-Up Studies of Infant Sibling Samples

Approaches to evaluating later outcomes in infant sibling samples have varied. Some studies focus on simple comparisons between siblings at familial high risk (HR) for ASD (hereafter, HR group) and low-risk (LR) groups (i.e., siblings of children with typical development), while others focus on the identification of subgroups within the HR sample (for example, those characterized by BAP traits). This may result, to some degree, in inconsistent findings. The impact of different methodological strategies on results is clearly demonstrated in the recent study of adult siblings of individuals with ASD (Howlin et al., 2015), which found that, when measured as a group, siblings were functioning in the average range across most domains. However, when subgroups were examined separately, those siblings who had been previously characterized by the BAP earlier in life showed difficulties as adults in social relationships and had significantly lower occupational attainment. Most striking was the high rate of significant mental health problems, including elevated symptoms of depression, anxiety, ADHD, and obsessive-compulsive behavior (Howlin et al., 2015). Another aspect of these studies around which there is methodological variation regards the composition of the samples themselves. Some longitudinal investigations include the siblings who go on to develop ASD (either combining them with the other HR children or examining them as a separate group), whereas others exclude the diagnosed children and instead focus on documenting outcomes of the non-ASD HR siblings. Thus, when evaluating the literature on longer-term outcomes of infant sibling samples, it is important to keep in mind the methodological approach employed, which we have specified in the review below.

The majority of previously conducted studies have concentrated on diagnostic outcomes, severity of social impairment, and language and cognitive delays. Given the literature reviewed above, however, this chapter also examines psychiatric functioning, a domain of functional relevance to the middle childhood period for which, admittedly, the literature base is much smaller. All of the studies described in this chapter and summarized in Table 7.1 (see pp. 236–238) rely on infant sibling samples recruited early in life and followed prospectively over time; most include both a HR group and a LR comparison group without known risk for ASD. Because these samples were originally ascertained in infancy, most follow-up studies do not specifically match on key demographic variables acquired at the later time point, instead having done so at time of initial study enrollment. Additionally, rather than matching on IQ, most have treated IQ as an outcome variable of interest.

Autism Symptoms and Diagnoses

In a sample of 37 HR and 22 LR 5-year-old siblings, Warren et al. (2012) examined behavioral and neurocognitive outcomes. The groups did not differ with respect to gender composition. The two children in the HR group diagnosed with ASD were not included in analyses. The authors examined Social Affect and Restricted and Repetitive Behavior scores on the Autism Diagnostic Observation Scale (ADOS; Lord et al., 2000) as well as parent- and teacher-reported Total Scores on the Social Responsiveness Scale (SRS; Constantino & Gruber, 2005). The two groups did not differ in the ADOS Social Affect domain, but the HR group exhibited significantly higher ADOS Restricted and Repetitive Behavior scores. Parent and teacher ratings on the SRS revealed no significant differences. Because of the small sample size, effect sizes were also examined, yielding a medium-sized effect for parent-reported SRS Total Scores. On the basis of this, the authors chose to examine parent-reported SRS subscale scores, finding a nonsignificant but medium-sized effect for the Social Cognition subscale. Overall, this small, initial study suggested that the siblings of children with ASD demonstrated vulnerabilities in social cognition and repetitive behavior.

Perhaps the largest school-age follow-up of an infant sibling sample included 139 participants (79 HR, 60 LR) between the ages of 5.5 and 9 years, none of whom had ASD diagnoses (Miller et al., 2016). This study examined a broad range of outcomes among HR and LR siblings, including ASD symptoms, cognitive and language functioning, and behavioral/psychiatric symptoms. Approximately 38% of the HR group was identified as having "clinical concerns" versus 13% of the LR group by clinically trained, expert examiners. Specific outcomes represented in the HR group included BAP (15.2%), ADHD Concerns (12.7%), Speech–Language Problems (5.1%), Learning Problems (3.8%), and Anxiety or Mood Problems (1.3%). These outcome ratings were not intended to map onto DSM diagnostic criteria but rather reflected examiners' clinical impressions (Ozonoff et al., 2014). The children who were classified by examiners as having clinical concerns had significantly more parent-reported ASD symptoms (SRS total scores) than the HR and LR typically developing (TD) children (Miller et al., 2016), but their SRS scores were, at a group level, still in the average range, indicating that these differences were likely not clinically significant. The findings from this study suggested continued vulnerability in a subgroup of school-age children and indicated that this population may benefit from continued screening and monitoring beyond early childhood.

Rather than examining dimensionally measured symptoms or traits, Brian and colleagues (2016) focused on the key question of stability and change in diagnosis among younger siblings of children with ASD from age 3 to middle childhood (mean age 9.5 years). A total of 67 children were evaluated by assessors unaware of their prior diagnoses or outcomes. In middle childhood, 17 of the 18 children (94%) diagnosed with ASD at age 3 retained the diagnosis, with one child no longer meeting DSM criteria for ASD. This single case with an unstable diagnosis was identified at age 9 as having intellectual delays and BAP traits (clinician-determined social communication difficulties, elevated ADOS score). In contrast, 6 of the 49 children (12%) who did not meet DSM criteria for ASD at age 3 were diagnosed with ASD in middle childhood (i.e., false negatives), all of whom evidenced some form of developmental concern at an earlier age. These data indicate the need for monitoring ASD symptoms in younger siblings into middle childhood, even if they do not meet diagnostic criteria as preschoolers and especially if they demonstrate other developmental concerns at earlier ages.

Shephard et al. (2017) took a multimethod approach, focusing on both diagnostic stability and dimensionally measured behaviors, including language, IQ, adaptive behavior, and symptoms of ASD, ADHD, and anxiety. A sample of 42 HR and 37 LR siblings was followed from infancy to age 7. When comparing ADOS, SRS, and Repetitive Behavior Scale—Revised (Bodfish, Symons, & Lewis, 1999) scores among three outcome groups (HR-ASD, HR non-ASD, and LR), as expected, the HR-ASD group had significantly higher scores than the other two groups on nearly all of these measures. The HR non-ASD group differed from the LR group only on the

Restricted and Repetitive Behavior domain of ADOS-2, exhibiting more symptoms than the comparison group, consistent with the findings of Warren et al. (2012). Of the 13 HR children who were diagnosed with ASD at age 3, 10 (76.9%) retained their diagnosis at the school-age follow-up, but 3 (23.1%) no longer met the diagnostic criteria for ASD. With respect to the HR children who did not receive an ASD diagnosis at age 3, 82.8% continued to fail to meet the criteria, but 5 (17.2%) were initially diagnosed at age 7. Of these 5, 3 demonstrated some social communication deficits at 36 months, while the other 2 seemed largely typical at age 3, as reported in a follow-up study (Ozonoff et al., 2018). Similar to the findings of Brian et al. (2016), this study demonstrates the need for monitoring ASD symptoms in younger siblings beyond age 3, given the rate of false negatives.

Overall, these studies demonstrate that younger siblings of children with ASD continue to exhibit vulnerabilities in social communication and repetitive behavior domains in school age. Diagnostic stability into middle childhood is relatively high (77–94% across two studies) and comparable with stability rates in noninfant siblings (Blumberg et al., 2016; Rondeau et al., 2011; Woolfenden, Sarkozy, Ridley, & Williams, 2012). Various explanations are possible for this interesting subgroup, from late symptom onset after age 3, to a protracted period of developmental unfolding of the phenotype, to an evolution of behaviors over time that are subthreshold in preschool but become more impairing once the environment exceeds the child's capacity (see Ozonoff et al., 2018, for further discussion). Ultimately, all these prospective longitudinal studies suggest that younger siblings should continue to be monitored into the school-age years.

Cognitive and Language Functioning

A number of studies have reported on the cognitive and language outcomes of infant sibling samples beyond the preschool period. The first was published by Gamliel, Yirmiya, Jaffe, Manor, and Sigman (2009), who studied 37 HR and 37 LR children (all without ASD outcomes) from infancy through age 7. The authors defined a BAP category based on parent-reported concerns and/or standardized scores of at least 1.5 standard deviations below average on any cognitive, language, or academic measure. Over twice as many HR siblings as LR siblings (39% vs. 16%) were classified as BAP. Notably, this study's definition of the BAP is broader than others described in this chapter, also including cognitive and academic delays, which likely accounts for the high BAP rates.

In 2011, Ben-Yizhak and colleagues published a follow-up containing a partially overlapping sample to that previously reported by Gamliel et al. (2009), when the children were between the ages of 9 and 12 years ($n = 35$ HR, $n = 42$ LR); children with ASD were excluded from analyses. At this time point, the authors found evidence of lower pragmatic language skills in the HR subgroup characterized by the BAP using a different definition than in the 2009 study. In particular, in contrast to the broad definition used in the earlier study, in the 2011 study, membership in the BAP subgroup had a very specific definition of ADOS scores ≥4 and not meeting the criteria for language delay, general developmental delay, or ASD. The measure of pragmatic language employed in the 2011 study was derived from the ADOS, which was also used (in part) to classify the group with BAP-related difficulties. This HR subgroup characterized by BAP-related difficulties showed no differences in school achievement (assessed via the Wide Range Achievement Test–III; Wilkinson, 1993) or reading/general linguistic abilities (Ben-Yizhak et al., 2011). It is difficult to determine how the findings from this study compare to the prior study (Gamliel et al., 2009) containing a partially overlapping sample due to methodological differences. For example, the original BAP subgroup was heterogeneous, with multiple ways of being classified as such. That is, low scores on *any* of the measures in the 2009 study could have resulted in a child meeting the criteria for the BAP subgroup. Thus, it is not clear how many children met "BAP" criteria by each individual measure.

With a primary goal of identifying early predictors of later language functioning, Gillespie-Lynch et al. (2015) reported on a sample of 63 siblings, recruited as infants, (*n* = 10 ASD, *n* = 30 HR non-ASD, *n* = 23 LR non-ASD) at an average age of 7 years. Using the Children's Communication Checklist—2nd Edition (CCC-2; Bishop, 2006) and Clinical Evaluation of Language Fundamentals (CELF-4; Semel, Wiig, & Secord, 2003), they found no differences in pragmatic and structural language measures between HR non-ASD and LR groups, consistent with Warren et al. (2012). Unsurprisingly, the ASD group demonstrated lower pragmatic and structural language relative to the other two groups.

Drumm, Bryson, Zwaigenbaum, and Brian (2015) evaluated language-related abilities in a small sample of younger siblings of children with ASD (*n* = 18) between the ages of 8 and 11 years, none of whom had ASD, by comparing their scores across a variety of standardized tests to the tests' normative samples. All of these children performed at or above the average range on the CELF-4 core language index, the Test of Pragmatic Language (TOPL-2; Phelps-Terasaki & Phelps-Gunn, 2007), an examiner-administered assessment of pragmatic language, and the Test of Word Reading Efficiency (TOWRE-2; Torgesen, Wagner, & Rashotte, 2012), a measure of single-word reading. On the parent-reported CCC-2 pragmatic language subscales, this HR sample performed significantly better than the normative sample. Given that pragmatic language deficits are commonly identified by comparing children's pragmatic language skills to their structural language skills, the authors also compared performance on the TOPL-2 to performance on the CELF-4, finding that the mean performance on the TOPL-2 (pragmatic language) was significantly lower than the mean performance on the CELF-4 (structural language), suggesting that, at a group level, this sample exhibited relative weakness in pragmatic language, despite performance being, on average, in the normative range. This sample also showed vulnerabilities in phonological memory and phonological awareness as compared to the normative samples of the Comprehensive Test of Phonological Processing (CTOPP-2; Wagner, Torgesen, Rashotte, & Pearson, 2013). A major limitation of this study is the fact that there was no LR control group for comparison, necessitating comparisons to the normative samples of standardized tests and limiting the generalizability of these findings. Notably, the measure on which the HR group performed better than the normative sample was parent-reported, whereas the measures demonstrating average or below-average functioning were directly assessed.

In a sample of 79 HR and 60 LR children (none of whom had ASD), those who were classified by examiners as having clinical concerns showed lower receptive and expressive language abilities on the CELF-4, but no differences in terms of nonverbal cognitive skills (as measured by the Differential Abilities Scale [DAS], relative to the HR- and LR-TD children, who did not differ from each other (Miller et al., 2016). As with several other measures, despite significant group differences in receptive and expressive language in this HR subgroup, group means were still within the average range.

Similar findings were obtained with respect to language functioning in a sample of prospectively followed siblings seen back at an average age of 5.7 years (Tsang, Gillespie-Lynch, & Hutman, 2016), who were classified into one of four groups: ASD ($n = 11$); HR non-TD ($n = 12$; comparable to the examiner-defined "clinical concerns" category utilized by Miller et al., 2016); HR-TD ($n = 24$); and LR-TD ($n = 22$). The ASD and HR non-TD groups demonstrated lower CELF-4 Core Language scores relative to the LR-TD group, which did not differ from the HR-TD group. This study also included an experimental theory of mind task, on which the same pattern was apparent. Lastly, parents reported on both cognitive and affective empathy in their children, with no significant differences emerging among the groups.

To assess potential differences in global cognitive functioning, Warren et al. (2012) compared 37 HR and 22 LR 5-year-old siblings, all without ASD, on the Differential Abilities Scale, 2nd Edition (DAS-II; Elliott, 2007), a measure of intelligence spanning both verbal and nonverbal functioning. They found a nonsignificant trend toward lower overall IQ (the Global Conceptual Ability score) in the HR group relative to the LR group, but with mean scores in both groups well within the average range. They also compared the groups on a composite of several executive functioning subscales from the NEPSY-II (Korkman, Kirk, & Kemp, 2007), finding significantly lower scores in the HR group compared to the

LR group; subsequent subscale comparisons revealed that this was largely driven by the Auditory Attention score. Group differences for the remaining NEPSY-II subscales were nonsignificant, although there was a trend toward lower scores on the Inhibition-Naming and Statue subscales in the HR group, with medium-sized effects. With respect to language functioning, the groups did not differ on either an examiner-administered measure of verbal ability, the CELF-4, or a parent-reported instrument, the CCC-2. Ultimately, this study demonstrated vulnerabilities in social cognition and executive functioning but intact language functioning in the HR group relative to the LR group.

In a sample of 7-year-old younger siblings, Shephard and colleagues (2017) found no significant differences in estimated Full Scale IQ on the Wechsler Abbreviated Scale of Intelligence (WASI-II; Wechsler, 2011), though the HR non-ASD group had marginally lower scores than the LR group. Similar to the findings of Miller et al. (2016), all group means were in the average range, but in contrast to that study, the groups did not differ in CELF expressive or receptive language scores. The discrepant findings are likely due to differences in study design, as Shephard et al. focused on HR versus LR comparisons, whereas Miller et al. examined an impaired subgroup of the HR sample.

In summary, given the mixed findings, sometimes limited sample sizes, and differences in methods across studies, it remains unclear whether younger siblings of children with ASD experience cognitive and language problems by middle childhood. Overall, based on the small literature, HR siblings without ASD appear to perform similarly to LR siblings in terms of intellectual functioning. Substantial variability in study findings exists with respect to language functioning, including pragmatics, with the studies focused on identifying impaired subgroups (whether defined by low cross-domain standardized test scores or by examiner clinical judgment) being the ones most likely to find evidence of group differences. Vulnerabilities in executive functioning were apparent in the one study that examined this domain.

Psychiatric Functioning and Behavior Problems

Several studies have examined psychiatric functioning and behavior problems in infant sibling samples, using broadband psychopathology instruments that measure internalizing problems (e.g., anxiety, depression), externalizing problems (e.g., aggressive/disruptive behavior), and ADHD-related symptoms (i.e., inattention/hyperactive–impulsive behavior). In their sample of 5-year-old siblings, Warren and colleagues (2012) examined group differences on a broadband parent-rated measure of common childhood behavior problems, the Child Behavior Checklist (CBCL; Achenbach & Rescorla, 2001), finding no differences on the Total Problems subscale.

They also found no differences on the Teacher Report Form (TRF; Achenbach & Rescorla, 2001), the parallel version of the CBCL rated by teachers. The authors did not examine Internalizing and Externalizing scores or specific DSM-based subscale scores that may provide more useful information than the less commonly used Total Score.

Another school-age follow-up study (Miller et al., 2016) found that the children who were classified by examiners as having clinical concerns showed elevated scores on the CBCL Withdrawn/Depressed, Attention Problems, Aggressive Behavior, and Rule-Breaking Behavior subscales relative to the comparison groups. As with many other findings reported in this chapter, T-scores were, at a group level, still in the average range for all groups, suggesting that the significant group differences may not translate into clinically meaningful problems.

In contrast to this broadband approach to measuring psychopathology, Shephard and colleagues (2017) took a more targeted approach focused on ADHD and anxiety symptoms in a sample of 7-year-olds. They found significant differences in Hyperactive/Impulsive and Inattentive scores on the Conners 3 (Conners, 2008), with the HR-ASD group having higher scores on both subscales than the LR group, but there were no differences between the HR non-ASD group and either of the other two groups. The Spence Children's Anxiety Scale (SCAS; Spence, 1998) showed that the HR ASD group also had higher scores than the LR group on multiple anxiety subscales (separation anxiety, obsessive-compulsive, panic/agoraphobia, generalized anxiety, total anxiety) and higher panic/agoraphobia scores than the HR non-ASD group. The HR non-ASD group had higher separation anxiety scores compared to the LR group.

In another infant sibling follow-up sample, Miller and colleagues (2018) applied DSM-5 criteria for ADHD to 34 HR and 23 LR siblings, none of whom were diagnosed with ASD, between the ages of 8 and 10 years. They found that 42% ($n = 14$) of the HR sample met full diagnostic criteria for ADHD by middle childhood versus 13% ($n = 3$) of the LR group. Although the possibility that the high rates of ADHD in this sample are due to retention biases cannot be ruled out, the retained sample was not more impaired than the nonretained sample at 36 months of age on any measure evaluated, making such an explanation less likely. Moreover, the rate of ADHD in the LR group was similar to recent estimates of the Centers for Disease Control and Prevention (11%; Visser et al., 2014), and two of the three LR infants who developed ADHD had family histories of ADHD or learning disorder, potentially increasing their risk for ADHD. Ultimately, given the small sample and ascertainment methods, firm conclusions regarding the prevalence of ADHD among younger-born siblings of children with ASD cannot be drawn from this study. However, a more recent medical records-based investigation examined recurrence risk and rates of ADHD among later-born siblings of children diagnosed with ASD,

TABLE 7.1. Summary of School-Age Follow-Up Studies of Infant Sibling Samples

Authors (year)	Sample size	Method of comparison	ASD symptoms and diagnoses	Cognitive and language functioning	Psychiatric functioning and behavior problems
				Symptom/functional domain	
Gamliel et al. (2009)	HR n = 37; LR n = 37	HR vs. LR	Higher proportion of HR group (40.54%) demonstrating parent concerns and/or broad-based elevated/impaired scores (cognitive, language, academic) relative to LR group (16.22%).		—
Ben-Yizhak et al. (2011)	HR n = 35; LR n = 42	HR-BAP subgroup (algorithmically defined) vs. HR-TD vs. LR-TD	—	Lower pragmatic language skills in HR-BAP subgroup relative to other two groups, but no differences in school achievement or reading/linguistic ability.	
Warren et al. (2012)	HR n = 37; LR n = 22	HR vs. LR	HR siblings demonstrated vulnerabilities in repetitive behaviors compared to LR.	HR siblings demonstrated vulnerabilities in executive functioning and social cognition compared to LR.	No differences between HR and LR groups.
Gillespie-Lynch et al. (2015)	HR n = 40 (10 with ASD); LR n = 23	ASD vs. HR-non-ASD vs. HR vs. LR	—	No differences in pragmatic and structural language measures between the HR-non-ASD and LR groups. ASD group demonstrated lower language skills relative to the non-ASD groups.	—

236

Study	Sample	Comparison			
Drumm et al. (2015)	HR n = 18	HR vs. standardized test normative samples		HR group exhibited poorer performance in phonological memory and awareness. No differences in word-level reading or pragmatic language. Pragmatic performance relatively weaker than structural language performance.	—
Brian et al. (2016)	HR n = 67	ASD vs. non-ASD	ASD stability of 94% from age 3 to middle childhood; 12% who did not receive ASD diagnosis at age 3 met criteria in middle childhood.	—	—
Miller et al. (2016)	HR n = 79; LR n = 60	HR "clinical concerns" (examiner-defined) vs. HR-TD vs. LR	Higher SRS scores in HR "clinical concerns" subgroup compared to HR-TD and LR	Lower receptive and expressive language scores in HR "clinical concerns" subgroup compared to other two groups. No differences in nonverbal cognitive skills.	Higher scores on CBCL Withdrawn/Depressed, Attention Problems, Aggressive Behavior, and Rule-Breaking Behavior subscales in HR "clinical concerns" subgroup compared to other two groups.
Miller et al. (2018)	HR n = 34; LR n = 23	HR vs. LR	—	—	Higher rate of DSM-5 ADHD diagnoses in HR (42%) vs. LR (13%).

(continued)

TABLE 7.1. *(continued)*

| Authors (year) | Sample size | Method of comparison | ASD symptoms and diagnoses | Symptom/functional domain | | Psychiatric functioning and behavior problems |
				Cognitive and language functioning		
Tsang et al. (2016)	ASD *n* = 11 (9 HR, 2 LR); HR-non-ASD *n* = 36; LR-TD *n* = 22	ASD vs. HR-non-TD (examiner-defined) vs. HR-TD vs. LR-TD	—	No differences between HR-TD and LR-TD. ASD and HR-non-TD had lower CELF-4 Core Language scores and lower scores on a theory-of-mind task relative to the LR-TD group. No differences on empathy measures.		—
Shephard et al. (2017)	HR *n* = 42 (15 with ASD); LR *n* = 37	HR-ASD vs. HR-non-ASD vs. LR	HR-ASD group demonstrated elevations on ASD symptom measures compared to non-ASD groups. HR-non-ASD siblings exhibited vulnerabilities in repetitive behaviors relative to LR siblings.	No differences in estimated FSIQ or receptive/expressive language ability.		Elevated ADHD and broad-based anxiety symptoms in HR-ASD group compared to non-ASD groups. HR-non-ASD group demonstrated higher separation anxiety compared to LR group.

Note. FSIQ = Full Scale IQ; HR = high risk; LR = low risk; TD = typically developing. Unless otherwise specified, all studies excluded children with ASD from the HR group.

238

finding that younger siblings of children with ASD were at elevated risk not only for ASD, but also for ADHD (Miller et al., 2019).

Overall, the few studies of psychiatric functioning and behavior problems beyond age 3 consistently report mental health and/or behavioral challenges in a subset of infant siblings and, as such, replicate earlier studies using noninfant sibling samples (Howlin et al., 2015; Jokiranta-Olkoniemi et al., 2016; O'Neill & Murray, 2016; Shivers et al., 2019). Studies using broadband measures such as the CBCL found significant group differences, but scores were generally still in the nonclinical range, whereas studies using specific measures of psychopathology have revealed more clinically significant findings.

Summary

The relatively sparse literature focused on longer-term outcomes of infants at risk for ASD suggests that the stability of ASD diagnoses is high between age 3 and middle childhood in prospective samples, comparable to stability rates in samples who are not at familial risk for ASD (Blumberg et al., 2016; Rondeau et al., 2011; Woolfenden et al., 2012). Although the stability overall is high, rates of children receiving first diagnoses of ASD after age 5 are higher than expected, as summarized in a recent multisite study (Ozonoff et al., 2018). This body of work also indicates that a variety of difficulties—spanning social communication, language, certain aspects of neurocognitive functioning (e.g., executive function), and psychiatric functioning—may emerge for a subgroup of infants at risk for ASD by the time they reach 5–12 years of age. Collectively, this work suggests that younger siblings of children with ASD would benefit from having their behavior and development monitored well beyond age 3.

Although many of the studies reviewed in this chapter consist of relatively small samples and employ diverse methodological approaches, they do provide several new insights. In the area of social communication and autism symptoms, the studies find evidence of the BAP in many siblings. These studies contribute to what is known about continuity, at the group level, between the early twin and family studies (Bailey et al., 1998; Bolton et al., 1994; Bolton, Pickles, Murphy, & Rutter, 1998; Folstein & Rutter, 1977, 1988) and the more recent infant sibling studies of children younger than age 3 (e.g., Macari et al., 2012; Ozonoff et al., 2014; Rowberry et al., 2015). Too few studies have been done to examine longitudinal continuity in symptoms and to know how often clinical concerns identified in infancy are followed by BAP-like challenges in school-age individuals. In the areas of cognition and language, the findings are more ambiguous, with the best evidence for pragmatic communication difficulties in school age, but showing limited consistency with respect to other aspects of language and cognitive functioning. Finally, in the area of psychiatric symptoms, although few studies have sought to probe these domains in later follow-up investigations of infant siblings, there is emerging evidence that attention and activity level concerns are prominent and may be one of the more common later outcomes of siblings of children with ASD. The high rate of ADHD outcomes (Miller et al., 2018) is consistent with other studies demonstrating that, despite having conceptually distinct behavioral phenotypes, ASD and ADHD co-occur at rates well above chance (Rommelse, Geurts, Franke, Buitelaar, & Hartman, 2011) and share overlapping genetic underpinnings (Rommelse, Franke, Geurts, Hartman, & Buitelaar, 2010; Ronald, Simonoff, Kuntsi, Asherson, & Plomin, 2008) and familial transmission (Musser et al., 2014; Miller et al., 2019; also reviewed by Johnson, Gliga, Jones, & Charman, 2015). This area deserves further investigation.

Because methodological approaches vary across these follow-up studies, it is somewhat difficult to make direct comparisons among them. However, a pattern has emerged, suggesting that those studies focused on identifying subgroups of children within the HR samples are more likely to report group differences in cognitive, language, academic, social, and psychiatric functioning. Thus, we conclude that it is critical to examine subgroups of HR siblings who do not develop ASD but who may exhibit atypical development in other domains, and to follow infant siblings long enough to pass through the windows of risk for all of the domains previously identified as potential vulnerability areas via prior family studies. Simply focusing on comparisons of group means between HR and LR samples may mask the vulnerabilities of subgroups of children within these samples. It is likely that consistent use of such approaches at later ages—including the development of algorithmically defined nontypically developing outcomes, as has been done across multiple studies focused on 36-month outcome data—will begin to resolve some of the inconsistencies in the literature. Moreover, by obtaining diagnostic outcomes across a range of conditions (e.g., learning disorders, anxiety disorders, ADHD), more specific subgroups can be formed that meet the diagnostic thresholds of impairment. Lastly, this literature has suffered from small samples and would benefit from pooling data across sites with common measures and follow-up time points, as has been done with data collected at earlier ages by the Baby Siblings Research Consortium.

Ultimately, the literature focused on long-term outcomes of infants at risk for ASD suggests that at least a subgroup of these children will benefit from continued screening and monitoring into the school-age years. It is important, however, to also avoid overpathologizing. Although multiple studies have reported significant group differences across various domains of functioning, most HR siblings still appear to perform within the normative range, and the magnitude of between-group differences is typically small to moderate and of unclear clinical significance. This highlights the point that group differences in mean scores on individual measures do not necessarily equate to, or fully capture, impairment (see Lee, Lahey, Owens, & Hinshaw, 2008), necessitating the use of additional approaches to understanding long-term functioning in infant sibling samples. Indeed, a central debate in the literature is whether the BAP—which is not a diagnostic category and which is defined by *subclinical* traits—is associated with functional impairment. Studies have established that there are group differences between siblings of children with and without ASD in multiple domains, but it is not clear if these differences negatively impact daily life. Recent findings of elevated rates of psychopathology and functional impairment in adulthood (Howlin et al., 2015; O'Neill & Murray, 2016) suggest that they do indeed have long-term impact. This is important to determine, but few samples have been followed long enough or with the intent to ascertain actual diagnoses (including meeting impairment criteria), rather than assess average scores on dimensional symptom measures, particularly not in prospectively collected samples. Additionally, further follow-up of the HR children identified as TD may provide a unique opportunity to focus on identifying not only early predictors of later impairment, which has obvious implications for early intervention (see Chapters 4 and 8), but also early predictors of and mechanisms underlying later competence, with wide-reaching implications for the fields of developmental and clinical science.

Future Directions

The incorporation of additional measurements of functional domains appropriate to these later developmental periods will be critical, including peer processes, learning problems, and more thorough and in-depth assessments of psychiatric symptoms and diagnoses. It will also be imperative to examine processes underlying skill acquisition—as predictors, mediators, and outcomes—to determine whether infants at risk for ASD who do not develop ASD themselves rely on typical underlying developmental mechanisms to achieve "normative" functioning versus compensatory mechanisms. Infant sibling researchers have greatly benefited over the years from the ability to pool infant and toddler data across sites through organizations such as the Baby Siblings Research Consortium. As these samples age, it becomes increasingly important for investigators to rely on, in part, a common set of measures. This is why we intentionally highlight the measures used throughout this chapter in hopes that future infant sibling researchers might utilize this information to select measures for their protocols that allow direct comparison to, and perhaps integration with, the data from previously collected samples to address these questions.

As these samples age, it is also important to consider the other potential uses of these vast amounts of data beyond ASD and even beyond the BAP. Such datasets allow for the potential to identify early predictors of a wider range of outcomes beyond ASD, given the known elevated risk for a variety of challenges among HR siblings. Based on the literature reviewed above, which illustrates the wide range of phenotypic variation and elevated rates of atypical outcomes characterizing HR infant sibling samples, we propose that such samples could be leveraged to investigate the early emergence of a broader range of clinical outcomes. Indeed, infant sibling samples may provide an unprecedented opportunity to study the earliest manifestations of significant clinical phenomena affecting children who are traditionally not diagnosed until the school-age years.

For example, as described above, we recently published a study drawing from our own infant sibling follow-up data suggesting that earlier detection of ADHD risk may be possible. This was the first study to evaluate prospectively collected infant predictors of verified DSM-5 diagnoses of ADHD in middle childhood, and the first ASD infant sibling study to leverage the vast amounts of longitudinal data collected in these study designs to identify early predictors of other forms of psychopathology. Our findings suggested that it may be possible to detect a signal for ADHD early in life and, as noted previously, that many younger siblings of children with ASD meet criteria for ADHD by school age, emphasizing that continued follow-up of infant sibling samples beyond age 3 is critical (Miller et al., 2018). This example demonstrates how these datasets, enriched with a wide range of phenotypic variation, may be leveraged far beyond their initial purpose of studying ASD to better understand the emergence of other, traditionally later-diagnosed forms of psychopathology, subsequently providing a foundation for future prospective studies of these disorders.

Lastly, the prospective infant sibling design is well suited to investigations of developmental mechanisms, given the reliance on repeated assessments over time. Future studies should aim to capitalize on these unprecedented samples of children followed from infancy by seeking to identify early predictors of school-age outcomes—including determining which factors very early in life predict competence and which factors predict persistent difficulty—and testing theoretically based mediation models that may provide further insights into mechanisms underlying longer-term outcomes. For example, one might hypothesize that communication difficulties underlie the expression of higher levels of psychopathology symptoms or behavioral problems among HR siblings as they enter middle childhood. Similarly, difficulties with executive function might mediate the higher rates of psychopathology at school age. Longer-term follow-up within infant sibling designs can address these critical questions that may have applications far beyond ASD.

REFERENCES

Achenbach, T. M., & Rescorla, L. A. (2001). *Manual for the ASEBA school-age forms and profiles*. Burlington: University of Vermont, Research Center for Children, Youth, and Families.

American Psychiatric Association. (2013). *Diagnostic and statistical manual of mental disorders* (5th ed.). Arlington, VA: Author.

Bailey, A., Palferman, S., Heavey, L., & LeCouteur, A. (1998). Autism: The phenotype in relatives. *Journal of Autism and Developmental Disorders, 28*, 369–392.

Ben-Yizhak, N., Yirmiya, N., Seidman, I., Alon, R., Lord, C., & Sigman, M. (2011). Pragmatic language and school related linguistic abilities in siblings of children with autism. *Journal of Autism and Developmental Disorders, 41*, 750–760.

Bishop, D. V. M. (2006). *The Children's Communication Checklist–2, United States Edition*. San Antonio, TX: Harcourt Assessment.

Blumberg, S. J., Zablotsky, B., Avila, R. M., Colpe, L. J., Pringle, B. A., & Kogan, M. D. (2016). Diagnosis lost: Differences between children who had and who currently have an autism spectrum disorder diagnosis. *Autism, 20*, 783–795.

Bodfish, J., Symons, F., & Lewis, M. (1999). *The repetitive behavior scale*. Morganton, NC: Western Carolina Center.

Bolton, P., Macdonald, H., Pickles, A., Rios, P., Goode, S., Crowson, M., . . . Rutter, M. (1994). A case-control family history study of autism. *Journal of Child Psychology and Psychiatry, 35*, 877–900.

Bolton, P. F., Pickles, A., Murphy, M., & Rutter, M. (1998). Autism, affective and other psychiatric disorders: Patterns of familial aggregation. *Psychological Medicine, 28*, 385–395.

Brian, J., Bryson, S. E., Smith, I. M., Roberts, W., Roncadin, C., Szatmari, P., & Zwaigenbaum, L. (2016). Stability and change in autism spectrum disorder from age 3 to middle childhood in a high-risk sibling cohort. *Autism, 20*, 888–892.

Conners, K. (2008). *Conners 3rd Edition* (Conners-3). Toronto, Canada: Multi-Health Systems.

Constantino, J. N., & Gruber, C. P. (2005). *The Social Responsiveness Scale Manual*. Los Angeles: Western Psychological Services.

Drumm, E., Bryson, S., Zwaigenbaum, L., & Brian, J. (2015). Language-related abilities in "unaffected" school-aged siblings of children with ASD. *Research in Autism Spectrum Disorders, 18*, 83–96.

Elliott, C. D. (2007). *Differential Ability Scales* (2nd ed.). San Antonio, TX: Harcourt Assessment.

Elsabbagh, M., Fernandes, J., Webb, S. J., Dawson, G., Charman, T., Johnson, M. H., & BASIS Team. (2013). Disengagement of visual attention in infancy is associated with emerging autism in toddlerhood. *Biological Psychiatry, 74*, 189–194.

Folstein, S. E., & Rutter, M. L. (1977). Infantile autism: A genetic study of 21 twin pairs. *Journal of Child Psychology and Psychiatry, 18*, 297–321.

Folstein, S. E., & Rutter, M. L. (1988). Autism: Familial aggregation and genetic implications. *Journal of Autism and Developmental Disorders, 18*, 3–30.

Gamliel, I., Yirmiya, N., Jaffe, D. H., Manor, O., & Sigman, M. (2009). Developmental trajectories in siblings of children with autism: Cognition and language from 4 months to 7 years. *Journal of Autism and Developmental Disorders, 39*, 1131–1144.

Gillespie-Lynch, K., Khalulyan, A., del Rosario, M., McCarthy, B., Gomez, L., Sigman,

M., & Hutman, T. (2015). Is early joint attention associated with school-age pragmatic language? *Autism, 19,* 168–177.

Hinshaw, S. P. (2013). Developmental psychopathology as a scientific discipline: Rationale, principles, and advances. In T. P. Beauchaine & S. P. Hinshaw, *Child and adolescent psychopathology* (2nd ed., pp. 3–32). Hoboken, NJ: Wiley.

Howlin, P., Moss, P., Savage, S., Bolton, P., & Rutter, M. (2015). Outcomes in adult life among siblings of individuals with autism. *Journal of Autism and Developmental Disorders, 45,* 707–718.

Iverson, J. M., Shic, F., Wall, C. A., Chawarska, K., Curtin, S., Estes, A., . . . Young, G. S. (2019). Early motor abilities in infants at heightened versus low risk for ASD: A Baby Siblings Research Consortium (BSRC) study. *Journal of Abnormal Psychology, 128,* 69–80.

Johnson, M. H., Gliga, T., Jones, E., & Charman, T. (2015). Annual research review: Infant development, autism, and ADHD—early pathways to emerging disorders. *Journal of Child Psychology and Psychiatry, 56,* 228–247.

Jokiranta-Olkoniemi, E., Cheslack-Postava, K., Sucksdorff, D., Suominen, A., Gyllenberg, D., Chudal, R., . . . Sourander, A. (2016). Risk of psychiatric and neurodevelopmental disorders among siblings of probands with autism spectrum disorders. *Journal of the American Medical Association, 73,* 622–629.

Jones, E. J. H., Gliga, T., Bedford, R., Charman, T., & Johnson, M. H. (2014). Developmental pathways to autism: A review of prospective studies of infants at risk. *Neuroscience and Biobehavioral Reviews, 39,* 1–33.

Korkman, M., Kirk, U., & Kemp, S. (2007). *The NEPSY-II.* San Antonio, TX: Harcourt.

Landa, R., & Garrett-Mayer, E. (2006). Development in infants with autism spectrum disorders: A prospective study. *Journal of Child Psychology and Psychiatry, 47,* 629–638.

Lee, S. S., Lahey, B. B., Owens, E. B., & Hinshaw, S. P. (2008). Few preschool boys and girls with ADHD are well-adjusted during adolescence. *Journal of Abnormal Child Psychology, 36,* 373–383.

Lord, C., Risi, S., Lambrecht, L., Cook, E., Leventhal, B., DiLavore, P., . . . Rutter, M. (2000). The Autism Diagnostic Observation Schedule—Generic: A standard measure of social and communication deficits associated with spectrum of autism. *Journal of Autism and Developmental Disorders, 18,* 505–524.

Macari, S. L., Campbell, D., Gengoux, G. W., Saulnier, C. A., Klin, A. J., & Chawarska, K. (2012). Predicting developmental status from 12 to 24 months in infants at risk for autism spectrum disorder: A preliminary report. *Journal of Autism and Developmental Disorders, 42,* 2636–2647.

Messinger, D., Young, G. S., Ozonoff, S., Dobkins, K., Carter, A., Zwaigenbaum, L., . . . Sigman, M. (2013). Beyond autism: A Baby Siblings Research Consortium study of high-risk children at three years of age. *Journal of the American Academy of Child and Adolescent Psychiatry, 52,* 300–308.

Miller, M., Iosif, A. M., Young, G. S., Hill, M., & Ozonoff, S. (2018). Early detection of ADHD: Insights from infant siblings of children with autism. *Journal of Clinical Child and Adolescent Psychology, 47*(5), 737–744.

Miller, M., Iosif, A. M., Young, G. S., Hill, M., Phelps-Hanzel, E., Hutman, T., . . . Ozonoff, S. (2016). School-age outcomes of infants at risk for autism spectrum disorder. *Autism Research, 9,* 632–642.

Miller, M., Musser, E. D., Young, G. S., Olson, B., Steiner, R. D., & Nigg, J. T. (2019).

Sibling recurrence risk and cross-aggregation of attention-deficit/hyperactivity disorder and autism spectrum disorder. *JAMA Pediatrics, 173,* 147–152.

Musser, E. D., Hawkey, E., Kachan-Liu, S. S., Lees, P., Roullet, J. B., Goddard, K., . . . Nigg, J. T. (2014). Shared familial transmission of autism spectrum and attention-deficit/hyperactivity disorders. *Journal of Child Psychology and Psychiatry, 55,* 819–827.

O'Neill, L. P., & Murray, L. E. (2016). Anxiety and depression symptomatology in adult siblings of individuals with different developmental disability diagnoses. *Research in Developmental Disabilities, 52,* 116–125.

Ozonoff, S., Iosif, A. M., Baguio, F., Cook, I. C., Hill, M. M., Hutman, T., . . . Young, G. S. (2010). A prospective study of the emergence of early behavioral signs of autism. *Journal of the American Academy of Child and Adolescent Psychiatry, 49,* 256–266.

Ozonoff, S., Young, G. S., Belding, A., Hill, M., Hill, A., Hutman, T., . . . Iosif, A. M. (2014). The broader autism phenotype in infancy: When does it emerge? *Journal of the American Academy of Child and Adolescent Psychiatry, 53,* 398–407.

Ozonoff, S., Young, G. S., Brian, J., Charman, T., Shephard, E., Solish, A., & Zwaigenbaum, L. (2018). Diagnosis of autism spectrum disorder after age 5 in children evaluated longitudinally since infancy. *Journal of the American Academy of Child and Adolescent Psychiatry, 57,* 849–857.

Ozonoff, S., Young, G. S., Carter, A., Messinger, D., Yirmiya, N., Zwaigenbaum, L., . . . Stone, W. L. (2011). Recurrence risk for autism spectrum disorders: A Baby Siblings Research Consortium study. *Pediatrics, 128,* e488–e495.

Phelps-Terasaki, D., & Phelps-Gunn, T. (2007). *Test of pragmatic language, 2nd edition.* East Moline, IL: Linguisystems.

Rommelse, N. N., Franke, B., Geurts, H. M., Hartman, C. A., & Buitelaar, J. K. (2010). Shared heritability of attention-deficit/hyperactivity disorder and autism spectrum disorder. *European Child and Adolescent Psychiatry, 19,* 281–295.

Rommelse, N. N., Geurts, H. M., Franke, B., Buitelaar, J. K., & Hartman, C. A. (2011). A review on cognitive and brain endophenotypes that may be common in autism spectrum disorder and attention-deficit/hyperactivity disorder and facilitate the search for pleiotropic genes. *Neuroscience and Biobehavioral Reviews, 35,* 1363–1396.

Ronald, A., Simonoff, E., Kuntsi, J., Asherson, P., & Plomin, R. (2008). Evidence for overlapping genetic influences on autistic and ADHD behaviours in a community twin sample. *Journal of Child Psychology and Psychiatry, 49,* 535–542.

Rondeau, E., Klein, L. S., Masse, A., Bodeau, N., Cohen, D., & Guile, J. M. (2011). Is pervasive developmental disorder not otherwise specified less stable than autistic disorder?: A meta-analysis. *Journal of Autism and Developmental Disorders, 41,* 1267–1276.

Rowberry, J., Macari, S., Chen, G., Campbell, D., Leventhal, J. M., Weitzman, C., & Chawarska, K. (2015). Screening for autism spectrum disorders in 12-month-old high-risk siblings by parental report. *Journal of Autism and Developmental Disorders, 45,* 221–229.

Semel, E., Wiig, E. H., & Secord, W. (2003). *Clinical evaluation of language fundamentals* (4th ed.). San Antonio, TX: Psychological Corporation.

Shephard, E., Milosavljevic, B., Pasco, G., Jones, E. J. H., Gliga, T., Happé, F., . . . BASIS Team. (2017). Mid-childhood outcomes of infant siblings at familial high-risk of autism spectrum disorder. *Autism Research, 10,* 546–557.

Shivers, C. M., Jackson, J. B., & McGregor, C. M. (2019). Functioning among typically developing siblings of individuals with autism spectrum disorder: A meta-analysis. *Clinical Child and Family Psychology Review, 22*(2), 172–196.

Spence, S. H. (1998). A measure of anxiety symptoms among children. *Behaviour Research and Therapy, 36,* 545–566.

Sucksmith, E., Roth, I., & Hoekstra, R. A. (2011). Autistic traits below the clinical threshold: Re-examining the broader autism phenotype in the 21st century. *Neuropsychology Review, 21,* 360–389.

Szatmari, P., Chawarska, K., Dawson, G., Georgiades, S., Landa, R., Lord, C., . . . Halladay, A. (2016). Prospective longitudinal studies of infant siblings of children with autism: Lessons learned and future directions. *Journal of the American Academy of Child and Adolescent Psychiatry, 55,* 179–187.

Torgesen, J. K., Wagner, R. K., & Rashotte, C. A. (2012). *Test of word reading efficiency, 2nd edition.* Austin, TX: PRO-ED.

Tsang, T., Gillespie-Lynch, K., & Hutman, T. (2016). Theory of mind indexes the broader autism phenotype in siblings of children with autism at school age. *Autism Research and Treatment.* [Epub ahead of print]

Visser, S. N., Danielson, M. L., Bitsko, R. H., Holbrook, J. R., Kogan, M. D., Ghandour, R. M., . . . Blumburg, S. J. (2014). Trends in the parent-report of health care provider-diagnosed and medicated attention-deficit/hyperactivity disorder in the United States, 2003–2011. *Journal of the American Academy of Child and Adolescent Psychiatry, 53,* 34–46.

Wagner, R., Torgesen, J., Rashotte, C., & Pearson, N. A. (2013). *Comprehensive test of phonological processing* (2nd ed.). Austin, TX: PRO-ED.

Warren, Z. E., Foss-Feig, J. H., Malesa, E. E., Lee, E. B., Taylor, J. L., Newsom, C. R., . . . Stone, W. L. (2012). Neurocognitive and behavioral outcomes of younger siblings of children with autism spectrum disorder at age five. *Journal of Autism and Developmental Disorders, 42,* 409–418.

Wechsler, D. (2011). *WASI-II: Wechsler Abbreviated Scale of Intelligence.* New York: Psychological Corporation.

Wilkinson, G. (1993). *The Wide Range Achievement Test (WRAT-III)* (3rd ed.). Wilmington, DE: Wide Range.

Woolfenden, S., Sarkozy, V., Ridley, G., & Williams, K. (2012). A systematic review of the diagnostic stability of autism spectrum disorder. *Research in Autism Spectrum Disorders, 6,* 345–354.

CHAPTER 8

• • • • • • •

Intervention during the Prodromal Stages of Autism Spectrum Disorder

Jonathan Green

Preemptive Intervention

The "arrival of preemptive psychiatry," announced by Tom Insel more than a decade ago (Insel, 2007), aimed to alter the focus of intervention from reactive to anticipatory. Insel bemoaned the lack of ambition of much existing therapeutics in mental health and offered a vision that intervention in the early phases of an evolving condition might hold out the best hope of moderating its evolution into a chronic and disabling course. He held up the example of coronary artery disease, where prediction of risk based on family history and lipid profiles, early detection, and preemptive treatment had hugely reduced mortality. He later went further in the context of developmental disorder by suggesting that the treatment focus be shifted from the current behaviorally defined syndrome clusters to early neurodevelopmental trajectories. In doing so, he made the core point that, generally in neurodevelopmental and brain disorders, the currently defining behavioral symptoms are but late manifestations of underlying neurodevelopmental and other processes (Insel, 2014a). This same thinking parallels the launch of the National Institutes of Health Research Domain Criteria project (RDoC; *www.nimh.nih.gov/research-priorities/rdoc/index.shtml*), which aimed to produce an organizing framework for identifying and understanding the developmental mechanisms underpinning behavioral outcomes (Insel, 2014b).

Insel may have announced their arrival, but these ideas have long roots in prevention thinking, both within mental health (Mrazek & Haggerty, 1994) and within biomedicine, where the search for precursor mechanisms has largely been cast in the language of "biomarkers." Frank and Hargreaves (2003) identified a simple, useful classification of biomarkers: *natural history* markers of risk for later disorder from longitudinal observation studies; *treatment biomarkers,* which reflect the biological effects of intervention relevant to outcome; and, most strongly, *surrogate endpoints,* which are so closely linked to the outcome disorder that their change on intervention can substitute for a change in the downstream outcome itself and thus simplify and shorten trial testing (Prentice, 1989). Examples of each of these biomarkers are highlighted in the text below in relation to developmental disorders. The Institute of Medicine's Continuum of Care Model (Mrazek & Haggerty, 1994; see Table 8.1) in turn identifies three kinds of prevention intervention: universal, selective, and indicated. While the prevalence rates for autism preclude the feasibility of "universal" prevention (at least in our current state of etiological understanding), both *selective* intervention, based on the identification of known "at-risk" groups, and *indicated* intervention, based on the identification and intervention of early signs of disorder, are not only feasible but timely.

Insel (2007) further understood that the term *prevention* might have inappropriate connotations in a neurodevelopmental disorder such as autism (the increased sensitivity around this idea will be discussed later in this chapter). Instead, he suggested the term *preemptive intervention* to define an early response to the at-risk or prodromal symptom state, focused on optimizing early prodromal trajectories rather than "preventing" a condition. For that reason, I have adopted this term in this chapter.

Opportunities in the Autism Prodrome

The autism prodrome can be defined as the period of development prior to consolidation of early symptoms into a diagnosable behavioral phenotype of autism spectrum disorder (ASD). The time frame of the prodrome will

---

TABLE 8.1. Definitions of Universal, Selective, and Indicated Prevention Intervention

- *Universal* prevention is defined as those interventions that are targeted at the general public or to a whole population group that has not been identified on the basis of increased risk.

- *Selective* prevention targets individuals or subgroups of the population whose risk of developing a mental disorder is significantly higher than average, as evidenced by biological, psychological, or social risk factors.

- *Indicated* prevention targets high-risk people who are identified as having minimal but detectable signs or symptoms foreshadowing mental disorder or biological markers indicating predisposition for mental disorder but who do not meet diagnostic criteria for disorder at that time.

Note. Based on Hosman, Jane-Llopis, and Saxena (2004, after Mrazek & Haggerty, 1994).

vary by child but will usually last until at least 18–24 months of age—that is, ASD is not thought to be reliably diagnosable until at least that time. Identification of cases in the prodrome can use selective or indicated strategies. A decade and more of prospective studies of infant siblings at increased familial likelihood of developing autism (a selective identification strategy) and of work on identifying early atypicality in the general population (an indicated strategy) have provided a science that speaks to all the themes in the previous section. Through investigation of its emerging mechanisms, it has begun to revolutionize our approach to the psychopathology of autism. Important progress has been made in identifying *natural history markers* of risk in the first year or two of life and showing how they may act together to form prodromal trajectories toward ASD emergence at 2–3 years and thereafter (Johnson, Gliga, Jones, & Charman, 2015; Szatmari et al., 2016). Identification of such early markers and trajectories naturally leads to a rationale for preemptive intervention, in targeting these early markers and processes so as to, in theory, mitigate or even prevent risk outcomes. In the context of neurodevelopmental disorders such as autism, there is the added hope that intervening in these early stages of the disorder may benefit from the potential plasticity of early social brain networks to altered input and experience. Moreover, well-designed experimental tests of prevention interventions can make an excellent contribution to developmental science itself by providing a unique way to elucidate "treatment biomarkers" and causal relationships between complex developmental phenomena (Green & Dunn, 2008; Howe, Reiss, & Yuh, 2002). Longitudinal observational designs in themselves can struggle to identify clear causal relationships beyond associations, whereas observation of the downstream developmental effects from intervention-sensitive biomarker change can confirm truly causal dependences. Identification of such target endpoint markers linked to later autism will help accelerate adoption of Insel's idea of replacing behavioral syndrome definitions by developmental trajectory modeling.

These possibilities for intervention in the prodrome of autism, though highly appealing, currently are based in little substantive evidence. We do not yet know whether preemptive intervention of this kind may indeed give more added value over reactive intervention with diagnosed cases. Thus, given the sense of momentum toward Insel's vision resulting from recent science in the field, this chapter is a timely review of how preemptive intervention science itself is developing. To what extent do prodromal intervention approaches that have been tested reflect understanding of current developmental science? How successful have these approaches been? And has any progress been made toward the identification of treatment-responsive markers and how they might in turn illuminate basic developmental science?

Ethical Issues

The emergence of a real sense of progress in this area has been accompanied by the rise of a counternarrative from some members of the autism community. The autism phenotype is sometimes asserted to be a core identity, therefore leading to challenge of any intervention approach that impacts these early developmental processes (indeed, as preemptive intervention intends to do). There are other potential issues common to any preemptive program in health—for instance, the accuracy of any screening or identification process, or the potential negative impact of identification or treatment on those identified who may not develop the disorder. This chapter will end with some thoughts from my own perspective as a clinical scientist; arguing for an emerging and necessary dialogue among interventionists, ethicists, and members of the autism community.

The Nature of Preemptive Intervention

To capitalize on the promise of prodromal understanding in autism, preemptive interventions in the spirit described above will need to be truly developmental. That is, they will need to be theoretically conceptualized on, and targeted to influence, natural history markers of increased autism risk or related developmental processes identified within the developmental science. Their success will be determined first by their impact on these prodromal risk trajectories and processes, but then crucially though their longer-term downstream impact on autism behavioral symptoms and developmental adaptation. Such is the likely complexity of cumulative risk profiles in the autism prodrome that a single "surrogate treatment endpoint" for autism is very unlikely to be found; rather, the aim will be the modification of specific risk trajectories in relationship to phenotypic outcome. In what follows we will see evidence for a number of "natural history" biomarkers in the prodrome of autism, although how they may interact together to produce cumulative risk is still unclear. We will also see evidence of the existence of "treatment-responsive biomarkers." We are as yet far from identifying anything that might be a "surrogate endpoint." There is no intervention yet that has shown the ability to affect the emergence of a behavioral syndrome at the categorical level, although there is one intervention to be discussed that has succeeded in altering prodromal autism symptom trajectories in an apparently sustained way.

Nondevelopmental Approaches

Alternative approaches to intervention could essentially be what I would call "nondevelopmental." That is, simply applying into the prodrome intervention methods developed for use with older children who have a diagnosis of autism. These approaches would not follow the developmental science logic described above, but they might of course still be effective (many interventions in health have been serendipitous and were not developed from prior theory). However, to be convincing, they would still need to be tested as above using rigorous analysis of downstream effects.

Treatment Targets:
Natural History Markers within the RDoC Matrix

The call to use RDoC domains as substitutes for behavioral syndrome definition is an aspiration rather than something that is viable in the current state of knowledge (Peterson, 2015). However, there is an emerging empirical base from high-risk (HR) infancy studies, as well as theory from extensive work within neurotypical development, which suggests rational targets for prodromal intervention prior to the emergence of behavioral symptoms. The nature of these targets is summarized next, framed in the context of current RDoC domains.

Infant Social Attention

Clearly, the social communication construct of the RDoC matrix is likely to be core to prodromal ASD. One of the earliest sets of natural history markers for later ASD to be reported concerns elements of social perception. Thus, in a number of independent studies, infant siblings at risk who later develop ASD at 3 years of age ("HR-ASD" siblings) show evidence of altered visual social processing compared to at-risk siblings who do not develop ASD. As early as 6 months, they show altered regulation of attention to complex social scenes and less attention to faces (Chawarska, Macari, & Shic, 2013; Shic, Macari, & Chawarska, 2014). They also show less differentiation of visual event-related potentials (ERPs) in response to distinguishing direct gaze versus averted gaze (Elsabbagh et al., 2015). Later HR-ASD siblings show disruption of gaze following, with reduced sustained gaze to reference objects (Bedford et al., 2012), and when studied in naturalistic real-time dyadic interaction rather than in experimental settings, they show less infant positive affect and infant attentiveness to parents during parent–child interaction (PCI; Wan et al., 2013). This and other similar evidence during the latter part of the child's first year therefore suggests escalating atypicalities in social perception at linked neurophysiological and behavioral levels, which then seem continuous with emergent social atypicalities in naturalistic settings. The timing of this emergence is coincident with, among other things, observed structural brain changes at this time (Hazlett et al., 2017).

Parent–Infant Interaction

RDoC also emphasizes the dynamic quality of social communication and shows how it is distinguishable from other cognitive systems by the fact that it particularly involves interaction with conspecifics. Further, it emphasizes that the underlying substrates are complex, involving receptive and expressive aspects. Much research in neurotypical development suggests that aspects of parental behavior can affect both social communicative learning and the development of executive function (Johnson et al., 2015). Thus, this could in principle be relevant to key aspects of the autism syndrome. For instance, a social pragmatic model of early child communication in neurotypical development emphasizes the early foundations of social as well as communicative competency in the infant's experience of parental attunement and reciprocity (Sameroff, 2009; Tomasello, 2008); enhanced parental attention cues (Walton & Ingersoll, 2015); or developmentally appropriate contingent comments and reciprocal social engagement (Siller, Hutman, & Sigman, 2013) during early parent–infant social interaction. It is an important empirical question as to whether such findings may be relevant in the "atypical" developmental context of autism.

A recent systematic review (Wan, Green, & Scott, 2019) identifies 15 studies of naturalistic parent–infant interaction dynamics in infants at higher risk for ASD versus low-risk (LR) controls. Overall findings are that trajectories of PCI in infants who will go on to develop ASD do show emerging differences from neurotypical trajectories in the latter months of the infant's first year. The strongest overall evidence related to eventual ASD is early delay in preverbal infant dyadic communication, including gesture use, prelinguistic vocalization, and vocal–gesture coordination; these mirror trajectories reported in the wider HR literature based on experimenter-led structured testing and can be more sensitive indicators than generally observed early social behavior. Importantly, parental dyadic responses themselves are not generally found to differentiate ASD outcomes, although the review does identify a distinction between parental provision of positive "social scaffolding" for their infants and a more "directive" style that can inhibit early sociocommunicative response.

Independent of the differentiation of ASD outcomes, however, some prospective studies have found early-emerging group differences in parental interaction style between HR dyads and LR controls, and these may be relevant in considering targets for prodromal intervention. Wan et al. (2012) found reduced parental responsiveness and increased directiveness at 7 months in a sibling at-risk group ($n = 45$) compared to LR controls ($n = 47$), with early findings that alterations in these parental response behaviors were associated with concurrent atypicality in ERP to dynamic eye gaze in their infants (Elsabbagh et al., 2015), suggesting the reciprocal effect might be related to infant neurodevelopment. Harker, Ibañez,

Nguyen, Messinger, & Stone (2016) report increased parental directiveness in a similar way at 9 months. At 13 months, Wan et al. (2013) found that the relatively reduced parental responsiveness and increased directiveness continued, but now also with alterations in infant attentiveness to parent, affect sharing, and mutuality. It was these changes in *infant* dyadic behavior that predicted the ASD outcome for those children at 3 years of age (Wan et al., 2013). Steiner, Gengoux, Smith, and Chawarska (2018) reported that parents of 12-month HR siblings (*n* = 27) showed higher "synchrony-demanding" parental reactions compared to LR controls (*n* = 14), reactions associated with parental perception of infant affective distress. However, in a large prospective study of 152 infants using an outcome design similar to the one presented by Wan et al. (2013), Schwichtenberg, Kellerman, Young, Miller, and Ozonoff (2019) failed to replicate these findings, with no PCI differences found between HR and LR infants at 6, 9, or 12 months and no prediction to ASD diagnostic outcomes. Although many aspects of this prospective design were similar to those of the Wan et al. study, the PCI observational protocol was rather different in focus and method, being based on a 3-minute free-play observation of social behavior with event counting rather than the 6-minute observation using a global rating scheme focused on interaction quality (Wan, Brooks, Green, Abel, & Elmadih, 2016). Such measure differences may be important for replication across studies, and future work would benefit from convergence in PCI measurement for both observational and intervention research. (Event-count and global ratings are complementary. Wan et al. [2019] found that global ratings are generally more sensitive to effects; concern that they may be more prone to rating bias needs to be counteracted by rigorous blinding in research design.)

Study of PCI in prodromal ASD is notable in applying normative developmental theory to the dynamics of early prodromal parent–infant interaction. Current evidence supports infant interactions within PCI as a natural history marker for later ASD development, and there is also evidence of group differences in parent dyadic responses. There may be an important distinction between parental positive "social scaffolding" for their infants and a more "directive" style, and this will need to be discriminated in measurement. This basic science in the prodrome is important, since targeting PCI perturbations (explicitly or implicitly) has provided the theory and target for many social communication interventions in the prodrome (see below).

Attention Disengagement

Alterations in the quality of attention are well described and among the most predictive in the prodrome. Of particular note is a decrease in attentional disengagement, forming so-called sticky attention, whereas in normative development, the speed and flexibility of attentional disengagement and shifting increase in the last part of the first year of life. Slowing attentional visual disengagement in the latter part of the first year is associated with later ASD (Elison et al., 2013; Elsabbagh et al., 2013; Zwaigenbaum et al., 2015) and is also seen in the context of response to name (Johnson et al., 2015). The timing of its emergence coincides with the emergence of the PCI and neurophysiological perturbations described above. Just as social perception difficulties provide striking potential links to later social communication impairments, so these attentional difficulties may suggest possible heterotypic continuity with later autistic rigidity and inflexibility, as well as difficulties in executive functioning. Therefore, attentional rigidity reasonably constitutes another natural history marker and a logical target for discrete attention-training models or, given caregiving contributions to executive functioning development (Cuevas et al., 2014), a PCI approach. An example of the latter will be seen below in the iBASIS trial.

Sensory Processes and Motor Control

In the latter part of the first year, infants who go on to develop ASD are more likely to show atypicalities in individual engagement with objects and more reactiveness to sensory stimulation (Clifford et al., 2013). Difficulties in motor control are identified as some of the earliest signals related to later ASD outcome. However, they are perhaps less specific as a risk indicator, being present across a number of developmental disabilities, including intellectual disability (Parlade & Iverson, 2015). Both of these areas provide further potential treatment targets, although the work in these treatment areas is less advanced.

Areas Not Affected

Also worth considering are aspects of development noted in the RDoC that are *not* systematically affected in autism. As an example, the affiliation attachment system, despite being an interpersonal social system that one might a priori expect to be affected in ASD, does not seem to be so affected. Specifically, attachment patterns formally assessed in toddlerhood in ASD show a normal range of autistic child attachment styles to parents, when the ascertainment method (for instance, in the Strange Situation Procedure or autism-specific Q Sort) is adjusted for the specifics of autism behavior (Koren-Karie, Oppenheim, Dolev, & Yirmiya, 2009; van IJzendoorn et al., 2007). More child attachment insecurity has been associated with higher levels of autism severity and intellectual disability in some studies (Rutgers, Bakermans-Kranenburg, van IJzendoorn, & van Berckelaer-Onnes, 2004), but not in others (Koren-Karie et al., 2009; Willemsen-Swinkels, Bakermans-Kranenburg, Buitelaar, van IJzendoorn,

& van Engeland, 2000). This disconnect in autism between abnormalities present in the social communication domain, yet not in the attachment affiliation domain, is in itself a fascinating and potentially highly informative developmental finding. This aspect has been insufficiently studied or discussed but could throw light on key processes in both attachment and social interaction within autism and more broadly (Green, 2009). It also implies that autism is not a disorder of early attachment, nor is there logic for early therapies in autism that specifically target attachment processes, all of which is important to note in the historical context of autism theory.

Current Prodromal Intervention Studies and Their Targets

The literature has been searched within Web of Science, PubMed, PsychNet, Google Scholar, and Wiley Online Library, using the search terms *autism, intervention, infancy, infants, prodromal, early intervention, randomized controlled trial (RCT), treatment,* and *social intervention.* Reviews and secondary sources have also been used. Early work consisted of reports on small case series, whose value lies in their delineation of details of the intervention method and feasibility of evaluation design rather than any inference about efficacy. Although it is often thought that all early interventions in ASD are rather similar, in fact they often differ markedly in their theoretical background and hypothesized mechanism. Since clarity on this issue is critical to a mechanistic approach to intervention science, attention has been paid to it in the review that follows.

Two reports used pivotal response training (PRT), an intervention approach whose theory of intervention effect is rooted in principles of applied behavior analysis (see also Pizzano and Kasari, Chapter 4, this volume). PRT targets "pivotal" areas that are thought likely, from theory and case-level work with diagnosed older children with autism, to impact broad areas of functioning in development, usually including social motivation as a key factor. Therefore, neither study used explicit natural history targets identified from prodromal research, which is an important distinction within early intervention methods. The first report, *Steiner, Gengoux, Klin, and Chawarska (2013)*, used PRT in three children sampled from an ongoing longitudinal infant sibling study (infant siblings at familial risk) and selected regardless of developmental concern (thus, a "selective" intervention design). The infants were selected for intervention at 12 months and studied using a multiple-baseline, across-participants design. The intervention included 10 hourly parent education sessions at weekly intervals over 3 months. Clinicians modeled the procedures with the child for the parent and provided opportunities for parents to practice with constructive feedback. The intervention used principles of behavioral learning as mechanism of change, applied in a low-intensity fashion to developmental targets in order to reinforce desired motivational and social behaviors. The dependent outcome was child functional communication within the dyadic therapy interaction context, operationally defined and measured with a time-sampling technique during 10-minute probe observations at every session. The study shows that PRT-type techniques can be applied to children in the early months of the second year and that a parent-directed approach is acceptable; parents demonstrated implementation of the therapy techniques.

The second report, *Koegel, Singh, Koegel, Hollingsworth, and Bradshaw (2014)*, presented a case series using recruitment based on social concerns—in effect, observed early signs of difficulty in relation to affect, social interest, eye contact avoidance, or response. They used an adaptation of PRT with three children, using a multiple-baseline design. Children were ages 4, 7, and 9 months at the beginning of therapy, making this the earliest prodromal report of intervention in the literature. Intervention was through therapy modeling and coaching of the parent. Initial observation of free play identified naturally occurring activities in which the infant was more responsive to the parent, compared to "neutral activities" that elicited no response. The parent was then asked to present just the "preferred" activities to the child for a 5- to 7-minute period, with a new stimulus every 5 seconds. The method therefore applied a classical conditioning paradigm to improve infant responsiveness. Coding was undertaken by blinded raters of 10-minute PCIs at each session, using a Likert-type scale coding of items that mirrored the aim of the intervention. "Training to the test" confounds within such study designs are thus likely. The results suggested that parents could learn to correctly implement the intervention. There were descriptions of increases in infant social engagement in these individual infants, observed at 2- and 6-month follow-up.

Three further reports concern the Early Start Denver Model (ESDM). All used an "indicated" at-risk recruitment design, identifying infants and toddlers showing early atypicalities assumed to be precursor markers for ASD and using a developmentally focused behavioral learning intervention.

Rogers et al. (2014) identified infants (*n* = 7) showing six specific risk indices in the "latter part of the first year," derived from developmental research (Bryson, Zwaigenbaum, McDermott, Rombough, & Brian, 2008; Johnson et al., 2015): (1) unusual visual examination and fixations; (2) unusual repetitive patterns of object exploration; (3) lack of intentional communicative acts; (4) lack of age-appropriate phonemic development; (5) lack of coordinated gaze, affect, and voice in reciprocal social communicative interaction; and (6) decreased eye contact, social interest, and engagement. For each child, five to six measurable learning and behavioral change targets were agreed to between professional and parent at baseline, along with specific interventions for other delays. The treatment of these symptoms consisted of 12 consecutive weekly 1-hour clinic sessions of an adapted therapist-delivered ESDM therapy plus parental coaching. The treatment involved therapist-observed parent–child play, followed by coaching, reflection, and written materials. The parent was encouraged to use daily home practice between sessions. The therapeutic mechanism within ESDM needed to achieve change derives from generic applied behavioral analysis principles. This is in contrast to some other interventions discussed below that target specific putative etiological developmental processes, themselves identified from prodromal research. The infants were individually matched to members of three comparison groups: HR infants who developed autism; HR infants who did not develop autism; and LR infants, plus four infants who met entry criteria but declined intervention. The report does not clarify how the seven children varied across the presenting target symptoms, but the intervention group had significantly more symptoms than the other groups at baseline. It proved difficult to identify the required number of "symptomatic" infants at this age and more difficult still to enroll families in the intervention study. Most of the children were at the upper end of the age range (i.e., more than 1 year) by the time treatment started. Perhaps the main lesson from this case series is the difficulty in identification and recruitment of behaviorally symptomatic infants in the first year, although Koegel et al. (2014) seemed to manage this with more ease.

Rogers et al. (2012) was a related opportunistic RCT of a parent-coaching version of ESDM (p-ESDM) delivered from a mean age baseline of 21 months during the wait-list period before a three-site therapist-delivered ESDM program trial. Ninety-eight children were randomized to p-ESDM or the wait list. The children included met the clinical cutoff on the ADOS-T; thus, this sits on the border of an indicated and postdiagnostic selection. The intervention combined therapist modeling and live parent feedback on intervention procedures, plus a self-instructional manual for home practice. The results reported that p-ESDM improved the parent-rated working alliance with their therapist over control. However, no treatment effect was found on child outcomes, including language, socialization, or development quotient (DQ), and there was no evidence of moderation of effect by baseline social orientating or imitation level. A subsequent smaller RCT (n = 45; *Rogers et al., 2019*) tested p-ESDM against an "enhanced" version; doubling the "dosage" to two sessions per week, with a home-based session; widened coaching modalities, including video capture of home behavior; and motivational interviewing for parent engagement. The enhanced model did result in increased parent fidelity to the delivery model (though with the caveat that the fidelity measure used to test this showed relatively low reliability at ICC [intraclass correlation] 0.47), but it did not enhance child behavior or development over the original. Therefore, given the results of the 2012 trial, it must be concluded that this form of parent-coached ESDM has not yet shown evidence of effectiveness on parent or child outcomes.

Kasari et al. (2014) conducted a selective preemptive study of 66 HR children (mean age 22.37 months). These children were defined as being at risk of developing autism through positive screening on the Modified Checklist for Autism in Toddlers (M-CHAT) and follow-up interview and one standard deviation below the mean on the Communication and Symbolic Behavior Scale (CSBS). The intervention was the *Focused Playtime Intervention,* a parent education program with 12 in-home training sessions (one per week for 12 weeks) on eight topics. The initial interactive play session between parent and child was videotaped with modeled strategies from the therapist and specific feedback in real time. In the second part of the session, the therapist worked with the parent using video feedback of the taped interaction and conventional teaching with a workbook. Outcomes were parent–child play using video interaction, the Early Social Communication Scale (ESCS), and Mullen; at 1-year follow-up, the children were assessed on the ADOS module 1. There was 20% dropout at the endpoint follow-up. Within the parent–child dyad, level of parent responsiveness was conceptualized as a response to the child play acts and was defined as the proportion of times the parent responded to the child within a 10-minute parent–child play session (e.g., responsiveness was coded if the parent showed follow-in engagement with their child's actions). This was compared to directive (i.e., intrusive) or ignoring responses. The analysis was based on the percentage of time the parent spent in each response mode. The study showed a treatment effect to increase the proportion of parental responsiveness. There was, however, no associated effect either on child variables (language scores, joint attention from Mullen or ESCS) or on diagnostic outcome; 27/32 in the intervention group and 29/34 in the nonintervention were above the ASD threshold on 3-year ADOS. Across the whole cohort, there was no relationship between parental responsiveness and child outcome language and joint attention. Nor was there moderation of outcome by parent variables. Thus, this study shows an intervention effect on independently rated parent responsiveness during the intervention.

Carter et al. (2011) conducted an RCT of Hanen's More Than Words, a group parent training program against usual care. It used an indicated sampling, with 62 children recruited at mean age 20 months having met at-risk criteria for ASD on the screening tool for autism, Screening Tool for Autism in Two-Year-Olds (STAT; Stone, Coonrod, & Ousley, 2000) plus expert judgment. The 3.5-month intervention comprised eight group sessions and three in-home individualized sessions, with the latter utilizing some video feedback. Outcomes were measured at 5 and 9 months after randomization and consisted of a video parent–child free-play procedure, a developmental play assessment, and early social communication scales, along with cognitive and developmental measures. The internal validity of the study was compromised by a high level of data missing for unexplained reasons (e.g., the central free-play measure was missing at baseline in one-third of the interventions and one-fifth of controls, at primary endpoint on just under one-fifth of interventions and one-third of controls). Consequently, they used a "partial intent to treat" analysis. During the first 5 months, the authors reported an intervention effect on parental responsivity, with a substantive point estimate but a confidence interval that just crossed the null: 0.71 (−0.01, 1.44). At 9 months, the effect had diminished. There were no overall outcome effects on child variables but in non-planned secondary analysis, initial low levels of object interest in baseline play moderated better outcome on child measures, including joint attention and communication.

The 16 children in a preliminary trial conducted by *Baranek et al. (2015)* were randomized on a 2:1 ratio (11 active intervention vs. 5 controls). The authors used an Adapted Responsiveness Teaching (ART) group, a 6-month relationship-focused home-based intervention aimed at improving parental responsiveness and child developmental outcomes based on the responsive teaching curriculum. Parents were taught responsive strategies such as following the child's lead, imitating, or taking one turn and waiting. The intervention employed modeling and coaching in order to encourage parents to use responsive strategies. Responsive teaching strategies were also taught to parents for use during daily routines, along with family action plans. The targeted intervention dose was 33 therapist–family contacts, with the highest number occurring at the beginning and then fading over the intervention course. The families were followed for 20 months, and a 6-month follow-up took place after treatment. The intervention phase was associated with significant changes in parent interactive style toward less directiveness, and increased child sensory responsiveness and adaptive behavior. However, these intervention-related effects were not shown at 6-month postintervention follow-up.

Green et al.'s (2015, 2017) Intervention within the British Autism Study of Infant Siblings (iBASIS) was a preemptive trial for infants at familial autism risk, located within a U.K. "babysibs" longitudinal study, the British Autism Study of Infant Siblings (BASIS; *basisnetwork.org*). The timing of the intervention was set between the 8- and 14-month assessment time points in BASIS, when developmental science suggests that the early atypicalities at brain and cognitive level first emerge (Jones, Gliga, Bedford, Charman, & Johnson, 2014; Szatmari et al., 2016); when PCI is central to infant social development; and when independent study suggests early emergence of interactional perturbation in parent–infant social communication. The target of intervention was this parent–child dyadic natural history marker. As above, the basic research into early parent–infant interaction conducted within BASIS found specific early perturbation in this interaction, first identified at the risk-group level at 8 months and then amplified at 14 months (Wan et al., 2012, 2013). Evidence that the 7-month effects were associated with altered neurophysiological visual social processing in the infant (Elsabbagh et al., 2015) and that infant rather than parent interactional behaviors predicted later ASD emergence supported the idea that these observed interactional cycles are initially evoked by an atypical infant development, but can then feed back to alter the infant's further social learning and amplify preexisting vulnerability. This does not imply primary parenting difficulties, but rather indicates that contingent responses are more challenging for parents in the context of infant with atypical development (Slonims & McConachie, 2006). The specific goal of the iBASIS intervention was to reverse such disrupted patterns of early parent–infant interaction based on the hypothesis that as a result there would be positive effects on other infant developmental markers and emerging prodromal autism symptom trajectories.

Building on an initial case-series feasibility study (*n* = 7; *Green et al., 2013*), the study tested the efficacy of the time-limited (5-month), parent-mediated intervention for 8- to 10-month-old infants (mean 8.4 months) at familial high risk of autism in a two-site two-arm RCT of iBASIS against usual care (*n* = 54). The endpoint results of the 15-month treatment (Green et al., 2015) showed wide effect size (ES) confidence intervals (CIs), in keeping with the modest sample size. There was significant increase in parent nondirectiveness, the proximal target of the parent-mediated intervention. Infant measures of attentiveness to parent, autism-related behavior, and child attention disengagement all showed point estimates of effect with CIs crossing the null. Follow-up was at 27 and 39 months (12 months and 24 months, respectively, after the end of treatment), with prodromal or emerging autism symptoms measured with AOSI and ADOS as the primary outcome, prior to phenotypic classification at 39 months. In contrast to endpoint-only analysis, analysis of repeated measures over the course of the intervention and follow-up period (Green et al., 2017) revealed a significant treatment effect on emerging autism symptom severity (ES = 0.32; 95% CI 0.04, 0.60; *p* = .026; Figure 8.1), as well as in parent nondirectiveness/synchrony (ES = 0.33; 95% CI 0.04, 0.63; *p* = .013) and child attentiveness/communication initiation (ES = 0.36; 95% CI 0.04, 0.68; *p* = .015) (Figure 8.1). There was no effect on categorical diagnostic outcome or formal language or other developmental measures. Analyzing outcomes using repeated measures through development thus reveals intervention effects not seen at endpoint alone and suggests a sustained treatment effect in development following treatment end.

A recent RCT testing the same intervention with the same design and outcome measures on a larger, indicated referral sample (*n* = 103, mean age 12.39 months) has now reported endpoint data (*Whitehouse et al., 2019*). The pattern of results on AOSI and PCI measures are somewhat similar to the Green et al. (2015) endpoint, with relevant point estimates having CIs crossing the null. Unblinded parent report of child communication (MCDI/VABS) showed positive treatment effect. A planned repeated

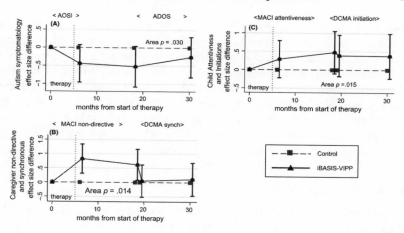

FIGURE 8.1. Time profile of treatment effects on autism symptoms and caregiver–child interaction ("area" = area between curves estimation). The effect size difference is shown by holding treatment as usual (TAU) as zero. (A) Primary outcome, autism prodromal symptoms (the negative effect size reflects a reduction in symptom severity in iBASIS-VIPP relative to TAU); (B) parental dyadic social interaction; (C) child dyadic social interaction. From Green et al. (2017). Reprinted by permission.

measures follow-up analysis will test whether the treatment effects on emergent developmental trajectories seen in Green et al. (2017) are replicated in this cohort.

   Watson et al. (2017) used an indicated sampling of 13-month-old children identified by community mailshot of a screening questionnaire (First Year Inventory), which in other studies had been reported to have a positive predictive value of 0.31 for a later diagnosis of ASD and of 0.85 for any developmental disorder. A 6-month ART (described above under Baranek et al., 2015) provided parental coaching designed to modify the key pivotal behaviors identified as problematic in each child. The trial was well conducted and was reported with low attrition; analysis of multiple (14) primary outcomes used adjusted significance levels. No intervention effects were found on the multiple-child outcomes tested. There was an identified treatment effect on parent responsiveness, which showed some mediation of child outcomes in a separate mediation analysis.

   Descriptive data on these three moderate to substantial RCT cohorts from three continents (Green et al., 2015; Watson et al., 2017; Whitehouse et al., 2019) reported in Whitehouse et al. (2019; supplementary table 11) provide a useful preliminary opportunity to compare the results of selective vs. indicated sampling in infancy, a substantive matter for the future preemptive intervention field. Selective sampling here identifies infants younger than currently possible in indicated sampling (mean 8.91 months in Green et al. compared to 13.75 and 12.39 months in the two indicated cohorts); it identifies a more equal gender balance compared to a male predominance in the clinical ascertainment, higher MSEL T scores (mean nonverbal composite 55.5 against 46.3 and 48.8 in the indicated samples), and broadly equivalent autism signs on AOSI despite the younger selective sampling age. While perhaps not surprising given their recruitment origins, these different sampling frames nevertheless need to be taken into account in interpreting different intervention studies, while providing the field with opportunities for greater representative breadth in study cohorts.

Electrophysiological Targets

EEG and habituation responses to social stimuli have been linked to underlying social processing and social attention and can be some of the earliest identified atypicalities in infants at risk who go on to develop ASD (Johnson et al., 2015; Szatmari et al., 2016). *Jones, Dawson, Kelly, Estes, & Webb (2017)* reported on the EEG outcomes within an RCT of parent-delivered psychosocial Promoting First Relationships (PFR) interventions designed to facilitate parent–infant interaction and delivered between 9 and 11 months of infant age, against usual care control. Sampling was selective, within a longitudinal infant–sibling developmental study. There was an increase in social habituation to faces versus objects, and in addition, there was a greater increase in frontal EEG theta power at 12 months and 18 months compared to control. The analyzed sample was small, with valid data available from 15 or less in the PFR group and 10 or less in the control group over the range of assessments. However, the study is the first covering this age to suggest that a targeted psychosocial intervention can affect neurophysiological markers. No behavioral outcomes from this trial have yet been published, so it is unclear how the electrophysiological changes link to behavior.

Summary of Intervention Studies Reviewed

The developmental science of the autism prodrome has made great strides but is still in its early stages, and it is thus not surprising that prodromal intervention science is also just beginning. In this chapter, I have reviewed thirteen studies (see Table 8.2) that could be considered prodromal interventions (although three of these are borderline). There are four small case series composed of three to seven patients that provide initial information on theoretical approaches and feasibility, and nine effectiveness RCTs of various sizes.

We do not have evidence suggesting an effectiveness preference for selective versus indicated sampling or for age at intervention. However, we have seen that the profile of cases sampled by each approach is likely to be

TABLE 8.2. Preemptive Intervention Studies

Authors (year)	Design/population	Intervention/ comparator	Intervention target/ mechanism of action	Results	Comments
			Case series		
Steiner et al. (2013)	Case series; $n = 3$, infants @ 12 months	PRT	"Pivotal interaction behaviors"—using learning theory	Reported improvements	
Koegel et al. (2014)	Case series; $n = 3$, infants @ 4–9 months	PRT	Ditto	Reported improvements	
Rogers et al. (2014)	Case series; $n = 7$, infants 12 months onward	ESDM	Assessed areas of developmental impairment—behavioral learning	Reported improvements	
Green et al. (2013)	Case series; $n = 7$, infants from 8 months	iBASIS-VIPP	Autism prodromal symptoms; through change in parental synchronous responses		Paper considered outcomes not reportable in a case series
			RCT		
Carter et al. (2011)	RCT; $n = 62$ infants, mean age 20 months; indicated sampling meeting criteria on STAT	3.5-month Hanan More Than Words group intervention versus usual care	Parent training program; support, education, and practical skills structuring routines and responding to child communication	No effect on child variables; trend toward nonsignificant effect on parent responsiveness	Analysis used "partial ITT" due to very high levels of missing data

(continued)

TABLE 8.2. *(continued)*

Authors (year)	Design/population	Intervention/ comparator	Intervention target/ mechanism of action	Results	Comments
Rogers et al. (2012)	RCT, *n* = 98, mean age 21 months	3 months parent-delivered Early Start Denver Model (p-ESDM)	Assessed areas of developmental need—therapist–parent coaching and therapist modeling	No effect on parent or child variables	
Rogers et al. (2019)	RCT *n* = 45 @ 2.1 years; indicated/postdiagnostic sampling using ADOS-T clinical cutoff	p-ESDM versus "Enhanced" p-ESDM; enhanced with double dose (2 sessions/week), enriched learning modalities, motivational interviewing for parents	As above	Enhanced version produces improved parent fidelity to the ESDM intervention model but no improvement in proximal or distal child outcomes	Small RCT subject to significant attrition but analyzed by ITT; primary outcome fidelity measure showed poor interrater reliability (ICC 0.47)
Kasari et al. (2014)	RCT; selective sampling after positive screen; *n* = 66, mean age 22.4 months	12 weeks focused Playtime Intervention versus usual care	Mutual shared attention	Increase parental responsiveness; no effect on child variables (language scores, joint attention from Mullen or ESCS) or diagnostic outcome	No relation between parental responsiveness and child outcome
Baranek et al. (2015)	Small pilot RCT; indicated sampling of *n* = 16 @ 12 months; 6-month follow-up assessment	6-month ART group versus usual care	Parent responsiveness, child development outcomes	Increased parent responsiveness, child adaptive behavior at endpoint, not sustained at follow-up	Small pilot trial for Watson et al. (2017)

264

Study	Design and sample	Intervention/comparison	Outcomes measured	Results	Comments
Green et al. (2015, 2017)	RCT; $n = 54$ @ mean age 9 months; endpoint 15 months; follow-up @ 39 months	iBASIS-VIPP versus usual care (as in the Green et al., 2013, case series)	Autism prodromal symptoms; using parent-mediated video-feedback methods to optimize parental synchronous interactions	Reduced autism prodromal symptom severity, parent synchrony, child attentiveness/communication initiation sustained from intervention period through to 39 months	The only trial to have included longer-term follow-up assessment of development
Jones et al. (2017)	RCT; $n = 33$ @ 9–11 months	Promoting First Relationships (PFR)	Habituation times to face versus object stimuli; frontal EEG theta power; P400 response to faces and objects	Greater reduction in habituation times; greater increase in frontal EEG theta power; more comparable P400 response	Valid data available from 15 or less in the PFR group and 10 or less in the control group over the range of assessments; thus, small study
Watson et al. (2017)	RCT; $n = 87$ @ 13.75 months; indicated community sampling using the First-Year Inventory screen	ART versus monitoring (as in the Baranek et al., 2015, pilot)	Parent responsiveness and child development outcomes—through parent coaching of selected pivotal behaviors related to social communication and sensory regulation	Improved parent responsiveness, no effect on child outcomes	Multiple primary outcomes but included adjustment for multiple testing
Whitehouse et al. (2019)	RCT; $n = 103$ @ mean age 12.39 months; indicated referral sampling using the SACS (Social Attention and Communication Surveillance; Barbaro & Dissanayake, 2013); 6 month endpoint results	iBASIS-VIPP versus usual care	Autism prodromal symptoms; using parent-mediated video-feedback methods to optimize parental synchronous interactions	No effect on child dyadic prodromal symptoms, social attention, developmental indices including language or parent synchrony; significant treatment effect on parent-reported receptive and expressive language and functional language use	Similar design to Green et al. (2017) but indicated rather than selective sampling; 3-year developmental follow-up to be reported later

different, since the current selective strategy is based on familial risk and indicated strategy on community screening or clinical referral. Green et al. (2015) and Jones et al. (2017) successfully used a selective strategy within the context of infant–sibling developmental studies. Watson et al. (2017) and Whitehouse et al. (2019) have shown that successful community screening is possible as early as 12–13 months, but the profile of these cases is likely to be slightly different to selective strategy cohorts. Before 12 months, Koegel et al. (2014) were able to identify three very young infants at least on the basis of "social concerns," but Rogers et al. (2012) found community recruitment and parental acceptance of intervention to be challenging. All studies in the second year are on indicated samples, and because syndrome trajectories rapidly firm up in the second and third years and the science of early identification is progressing, the distinction between truly prodromal and early reactive intervention paradigms becomes increasingly blurred.

Prospective at-risk sibling studies have identified a number of *treatment-responsive risk markers* for later development of autism. Of these, the most explicitly targeted to date by intervention has been the early perturbation in parent–infant interactions between infant autism siblings and their parents (Wan et al., 2019)—perturbations specifically targeted by iBASIS (Green et al., 2015) but also related to other aspects of PCI targeted by Baranek et al. (2015), Kasari et al. (2014), and Carter et al. (2011). This risk marker has shown itself to be reliably treatment responsive: all these studies (bar Carter et al., which is borderline) suggest effective alteration of PCI in the targeted direction during the treatment period, and the Green et al. study suggests some sustained change during follow-up. *Early atypical behavior,* as another natural history risk marker, has shown mixed results. Interventions that use a naturalistic parent-mediated approach to the process of change have shown infant behavior effects, either during the treatment phase (Baranek et al., 2015) or during follow-up after end of treatment (Green et al., 2015, 2017). But early endpoint results from Whitehouse et al. (2019) are less convincing, and an ESDM intervention using a behavioral learning approach to generating change showed no effects (Rogers et al., 2019). The third risk marker to have shown the potential impact of intervention is *attentional disengagement.* The one study that targeted this directly produced evidence of a trend of intervention effect measured at 14 months, a time during which potential inflexibility is associated with later ASD outcomes. This result is interesting because it represents a "cross-domain" effect from a PCI-focused intervention (see the section "Treatment Targets" above). A final risk marker targeted has been *EEG and habituation responses to social stimuli,* with one study finding preliminary evidence of treatment effects on these markers in a selective high-likelihood sample in infancy (Jones et al., 2017).

No studies to date have been powered enough to undertake detailed mediation process analyses, which would begin to help us understand how interventions impact the dynamics of early development in the prodrome and what we could learn from them about this development. Also, only one study so far has conducted a systematic repeated measures follow-up. There has indeed been a general lack of measurement of downstream or developmentally independent outcomes, and many of the studies report as "outcome" what is in reality a measure of a process closely tied to the intervention; this cannot then exclude "training to the test." Therefore, larger samples and improved methods have enormous potential. The early data suggest the importance of developmental follow-up after intervention end and the potential of analyses of emerging developmental trajectories rather than single endpoints. In this, the direction of the data echoes Tom Insel's ambition for a "preemptive" developmental perspective on intervention development and testing that began this chapter. It is an exciting prospect that the field may slowly be building an evidence base toward this end, but there is much work still to do.

What Can We Learn from Intervention Studies about Developmental Science?

Just as intervention strategies are informed by developmental theory, so controlled intervention studies, especially those with mechanism testing, can illuminate developmental science.

1. *Parental interactive behaviors relevant to autism are identifiable and responsive to therapy.* Across the range of age, social class, education, and ability, there are identifiable parental dyadic behaviors that are shown in therapy to be relevant to child autism functioning and development. These parental behaviors can reliably be optimized (at least in the short-term) with a range of therapies, ranging from developmental social communication to behavioral learning (Green & Garg, 2018). The most replicated effects have come from therapies that incorporate, as a central or partial component, parent video feedback (VF; Green et al., 2015; Kasari et al., 2014). Since this is also found in work using VF on autism at later ages (e.g., Aldred, Green, & Adams, 2004; Green et al., 2010; Pickles et al., 2016; Poslawsky et al., 2014; Rahman et al., 2016) and in nonautism (Juffer, Bakermans-Kranenburg, & van IJzendoorn, 2008), VF seems to be at least one core effective component of therapy designed to impact parental behaviors. There is general evidence of washout of such therapeutic parent effects after treatment ends (Baranek et al., 2015; Carter et al., 2011; Green et al., 2017; Kasari et al., 2014), although trajectory analysis over time in the latter study does nevertheless suggest an overall significant treatment effect on parental responsiveness over a 2-year postintervention follow-up period.

2. *Specific alterations in parental dyadic behavior can improve child social functioning in the dyad.* Well-designed intervention studies are invaluable for demonstrating directions of effect within early developmental interaction. Transaction between parental and child behavior is a well-established feature of neurotypical development, and early prodromal intervention science supports this being also true in autistic development (Kasari et al., 2014; Baranek et al., 2015; Green et al., 2017; as well as indications from the Koegel et al., 2014, and Steiner et al., 2013, case series). No studies in the prodrome have yet done causal mediation analysis to confirm the *direction* of such effects, but those that have been done in diagnosed cases in later childhood (Gulsrud, Hellemann, Shire, & Kasari, 2016; Pickles et al., 2016) find that targeted alteration in parental dyadic behavior does alter child social interaction in the dyad. This has implications for developmental science because it suggests that autistic development can share similar underlying developmental processes in this regard to neurotypical development.

3. *Can change in child dyadic social functioning generalize into the rest of development?* This is a key question for developmental science. Generalization of acquired or learned skills across person or context has always been considered to be very difficult for autistic individuals and a key limitation in their development. Intervention experiments can potentially offer rigorous investigation as to whether and how this could happen, although the majority of reported studies to date define endpoints that are too "proximal" in time or context for such inferences to be made (Green & Garg, 2018). Studies are, however, increasingly including both follow-up and contextually distinct outcomes. One prodromal study here does suggest such sustained effects for 2 years after intervention ends and beyond a time when the effect on parental synchrony itself appears to be diminishing. A similar pattern was shown in another social communication intervention delivered in the preschool period after diagnosis, extending 6 years after treatment end (Pickles et al., 2016). These findings suggest that improvements in social competency in the child may take on a momentum of their own in development, relatively independent of contingent interaction, although the mechanism by which this may happen is not yet clear.

Ultimate Aims and Ethics

What are the ultimate aims of preemptive intervention? The answer might seem obvious: the aim of prevention is to prevent, and the aim of preemption is to mitigate the level of autism severity. Many parent groups and others in the autism community would support this view. However, for other commentators and adult-oriented advocates within the autism community, this can feel like an attack on identity, and this should give intervention-ists pause for thought. Extreme forms of this latter argument imply a form of genetic determinism ("I was born autistic and always have been from conception") that is at variance with how we understand the development generally of personality, identity, and well-being. Nevertheless, key questions regarding the ethics of preemptive intervention need to be addressed.

One starting point can be the intent and theoretical background of an intervention. Some interventions are understood to act as if their goal was to "eliminate" atypical behaviors and replace them with "normal" behaviors. Applied behavior analysis (ABA) and early intensive behavioral intervention (EIBI) methods have received criticism in this regard (e.g., Milton, 2014). However, an account of prodromal intervention informed by modern developmental science is likely to have a different intent and theory background. The early prodromal perspective is useful here. Plotting the emergence of autism symptoms from their earliest neurophysiological beginnings into identifiable behavioral trajectories suggests not "predestination" but "process." A transactional account of development, which implicitly underpins much of the intervention work described in this chapter, will see the emergence of positive developmental outcomes such as positive social relationships, social engagement and integration, and emotional and family well-being, as the result of reciprocal processes between an individual organism and environment, often simplified by the term *goodness of fit* (Sameroff, 2009). The exact meaning of each of these terms could be contested. Nevertheless, the developmental account given above suggests that autism should not be seen as so literally atypical as to constitute a "parallel version" of development, but rather as a form of individual difference as understood within the developmental research tradition. In turn, the autism situation understood as individual difference needs a particular kind of considered environmental response in order to create good transactional outcomes. In the prodrome, the "environment" in question is that of formative early caregiver–child interaction (in the same way as, later, the environment may constitute an adapted school classroom or social space). Thus, prodromal interventions for autism of this kind (naturalistic or developmental interventions) take the form of an adapted environmental response to autism difference based on what we know about the processes behind the development of autism, but using the same rationale as early intervention in "neurotypical" contexts.

Much normative developmental theory leads us to believe that optimizing early reciprocal interaction will benefit a spectrum of later outcomes ranging from *relationship quality* to *positive social functioning, relationship formation, emotional well-being,* and *mental health.* These, then, could be the kind of outcomes that preemptive intervention can aspire to. The paradox of autism is that success in those outcomes may well also impact the level of autism symptoms as we define them; and these "symptoms" can seem to some to be coincident with autism identity. When we measure autism symptoms using ADOS, are we measuring autism identity or autism outcomes? Certainly, we assume that reducing the severity of autism symptom as a positive goal will improve aspects of social functioning in autism. The idea is to support strengths and well-being rather than challenge identity, but one has to recognize a subtle paradox and some complexity here in terms of intervening in the early processes of development.

Insel advocated the four P's in relation to early intervention. These are probably key to the way forward for this aspect of the field: (1) *participatory*, in that experts-by-experience of autism should join with interventionists in thinking about the most beneficial intervention outcomes; (2) *personalized*, in that there should be informed participation in the treatment process but also that the intervention offered should be tailored to the needs of the individual; (3) *predictive*, in that the intervention should be followed downstream and be shown to change things that are theoretically important for developmental science—but also for families and individuals; and (4) *preemptive* in the timeliness of such intervention at a point in development where it may do most benefit. This, however, is not the end of a dialogue between parents and families, ethicists, and interventionists to plot a way forward for autism intervention. No one has a monopoly on wisdom here. Autism advocates are unlikely to speak for many families struggling with very disadvantaged children; interventionists may carry assumptions that need challenging. The fact that this dialogue has added urgency now is a testament to the advances that have been made in developing potentially effective interventions; this success necessitates dialogue but can also have real promise for the developmental outcomes of children with autism.

Conclusion

In conclusion, many different interventions can show immediately proximal outcomes tied to the intervention context, but intervention outcomes distal and downstream in time have been less commonly shown (although this review suggests that evidence in this regard is emerging). For the future, truly prodromal intervention studies will need to be larger and more focused on mechanism and process analysis, and take a targeted approach to what are known to be emerging developmental processes. They should build on what has proved to be successful in this current generation of early studies, and they should be adventurous in tackling other targets suggested by developmental science. We await whether more biological interventions may be mounted and whether they will be considered ethically acceptable. More cognitive training-type approaches are also expected, and at least one of these approaches in relation to attention training is in process. Above all, prodromal intervention should not be tied to legacy theories of the past. It needs to be responsive to the emerging results from basic science, leading to a more profound understanding of early developmental processes and the best ways of intervening in it. These are encouraging signs for what could be accomplished in the future.

A crucial parallel task is to engage with the autism community, advocates, ethicists, and other stakeholders in answering the social questions of what constitutes the desired outcomes for early autism intervention. In the future, if they are to carry this field forward successfully, it will be necessary for clinical intervention scientists to hold together a combination of detailed robust and sophisticated science with profound social engagement. For more information about treatment in young children with ASD, see Pizzano and Kasari (Chapter 4, this volume).

REFERENCES

Aldred, C., Green, J., & Adams, C. (2004). A new social communication intervention for children with autism: Pilot randomised controlled treatment study suggesting effectiveness. *Journal of Child Psychology and Psychiatry, 45*(8), 1420–1430.

Baranek, G. T., Watson, L. R., Turner-Brown, L., Field, S. H., Crais, E. R., Wakeford, L., . . . Reznick, J. S. (2015). Preliminary efficacy of adapted responsive teaching for infants at risk of autism spectrum disorder in a community sample. *Autism Research and Treatment*, Article ID 386951.

Barbaro, J., & Dissanayake, C. (2013). Early markers of autism spectrum disorders in infants and toddlers prospectively identified in the Social Attention and Communication Study. *Autism, 17*(1), 64–86.

Bedford, R., Elsabbagh, M., Gliga, T., Pickles, A., Senju, A., Charman, T., . . . BASIS Team. (2012). Precursors to social and communication difficulties in infants at-risk for autism: Gaze following and attentional engagement. *Journal of Autism and Developmental Disorders, 42*(10), 2208–2218.

Bryson, S. E., Zwaigenbaum, L., McDermott, C., Rombough, V., & Brian, J. (2008). The Autism Observation Scale for Infants: Scale development and reliability data. *Journal of Autism and Developmental Disorders, 38*(4), 731–738.

Carter, A. S., Messinger, D. S., Stone, W. L., Celimli, S., Nahmias, A. S., & Yoder, P. (2011). A randomized controlled trial of Hanen's "More Than Words" in toddlers with early autism symptoms. *Journal of Child Psychology and Psychiatry, 52*(7), 741–752.

Chawarska, K., Macari, S., & Shic, F. (2013). Decreased spontaneous attention to social scenes in 6-month-old infants later diagnosed with autism spectrum disorders. *Biological Psychiatry, 74*(3), 195–203.

Clifford, S. M., Hudry, K., Elsabbagh, M., Charman, T., Johnson, M. H., & BASIS Team. (2013). Temperament in the first 2 years of life in infants at high-risk for autism spectrum disorders. *Journal of Autism and Developmental Disorders, 43*(3), 673–686.

Cuevas, K., Deater-Deckard, K., Kim-Spoon, J., Watson, A. J., Morasch, K. C., & Bell, M. A. (2014). What's mom got to do with it?: Contributions of maternal executive function and caregiving to the development of executive function across early childhood. *Developmental Science, 17,* 224–238.

Elison, J. T., Paterson, S. J., Wolff, J. J., Reznick, J. S., Sasson, N. J., Gu, H., . . . IBIS Network. (2013). White matter microstructure and atypical visual orienting in 7-month-olds at risk for autism. *American Journal of Psychiatry, 170,* 899–908.

Elsabbagh, M., Bruno, R., Wan, M. W., Charman, T., Johnson, M. H., Green, J., & BASIS Team. (2015). Infant neural sensitivity to dynamic eye gaze relates to quality of parent–infant interaction at 7-months in infants at risk for autism. *Journal of Autism and Developmental Disorders, 45*(2), 283–291.

Elsabbagh, M., Fernandes, J., Webb, S. J., Dawson, G., Charman, T., Johnson, M. H., & BASIS Team. (2013). Disengagement of visual attention in infancy is associated with emerging autism in toddlerhood. *Biological Psychiatry, 74*(3), 189–194.

Frank, R., & Hargreaves, R. (2003). Clinical biomarkers in drug discovery and development. *Nature Reviews Drug Discovery, 2*(7), 566–580.

Green, J. (2009). Attachment and social impairment in development. *ACAMH Occasional Papers No. 29: Attachment: Current Focus and Future Directions,* 25–36.

Green, J., Charman, T., McConachie, H., Aldred, C., Slonims, V., Howlin, P., . . . PACT Consortium. (2010). Parent-mediated communication-focused treatment in children with autism (PACT): A randomised controlled trial. *The Lancet, 375*(9732), 2152–2160.

Green, J., Charman, T., Pickles, A., Wan, M. W., Elsabbagh, M., Slonims, V., . . . BASIS Team. (2015). Parent-mediated intervention versus no intervention for infants at high risk of autism: A parallel, single-blind, randomised trial. *The Lancet Psychiatry, 2*(2), 133–140.

Green, J., & Dunn, G. (2008). Using intervention trials in developmental psychiatry to illuminate basic science. *British Journal of Psychiatry, 192*(5), 323–325.

Green, J., & Garg, S. (2018). The state of autism intervention science: Process, target psychological and biological mechanisms and future prospects. *Journal of Child Psychology and Psychiatry and Allied Disciplines, 59*(4), 424–443.

Green, J., Pickles, A., Pasco, G., Bedford, R., Wan, M. W., Elsabbagh, M., . . . BASIS team. (2017). Randomised trial of a parent-mediated intervention for infants at high risk for autism: Longitudinal outcomes to age 3 years. *Journal of Child Psychology and Psychiatry, 58*(12), 1330–1340.

Green, J., Wan, M. W., Guiraud, J., Holsgrove, S., McNally, J., Slonims, V., . . . BASIS team. (2013). Intervention for infants at risk of developing autism: A case series. *Journal of Autism and Developmental Disorders, 43*(11), 2502–2514.

Gulsrud, A. C., Hellemann, G., Shire, S., & Kasari, C. (2016). Isolating active ingredients in a parent-mediated social communication intervention for toddlers with autism spectrum disorder. *Journal of Child Psychology and Psychiatry, 57,* 606–613.

Harker, C. M., Ibañez, L. V., Nguyen, T. P., Messinger, D. S., & Stone, W. L. (2016) The effect of parenting style on social smiling in infants at high and low risk for ASD. *Journal of Autism and Developmental Disorders, 46*(7), 2399–2407.

Hazlett, H. C., Gu, H., Munsell, B. C., Kim, S. H., Styner, M., Wolff, J. J., . . . IBIS Network. (2017). Early brain development in infants at high risk for autism spectrum disorder. *Nature, 542,* 348–351.

Hosman, C. M. H., Jane-Llopis, E., & Saxena, S. (Eds.). (2004). *Prevention of mental disorders: Effective interventions and policy options: Summary report.* Oxford, UK: Oxford University Press.

Howe, G. W., Reiss, D., & Yuh, J. (2002). Can prevention trials test theories of etiology? *Development and Psychopathology, 14*(4), 673–694.

Insel, T. R. (2007). The arrival of pre-emptive psychiatry. *Early Intervention in Psychiatry, 1*(1), 5–6.

Insel, T. R. (2014a). Mental disorders in childhood: Shifting the focus from behavioral symptoms to neurodevelopmental trajectories. *Journal of the American Medical Association, 311*(17), 1727–1728.

Insel, T. R. (2014b). The NIMH Research Domain Criteria (RDoC) project: Precision medicine for psychiatry. *American Journal of Psychiatry, 171*(4), 395–397.

Johnson, M. H., Gliga, T., Jones, E., & Charman, T. (2015). Annual Research Review: Infant development, autism, and ADHD–Early pathways to emerging disorders. *Journal of Child Psychology and Psychiatry, 56*(3), 228–247.

Jones, E. J. H., Dawson, G., Kelly, J., Estes, A., & Webb, S. J. (2017). Parent-delivered early intervention in infants at risk for ASD: Effects on electrophysiological and habituation measures of social attention. *Autism Research, 10*, 961–972.

Jones, E. J., Gliga, T., Bedford, R., Charman, T., & Johnson, M. H. (2014). Developmental pathways to autism: A review of prospective studies of infants at risk. *Neuroscience and Biobehavioral Reviews, 39*, 1–33.

Juffer, F., Bakermans-Kranenburg, M. J., & van IJzendoorn, M. H. (Eds.). (2008). *Promoting positive parenting: An attachment-based intervention.* New York: Taylor & Francis.

Kasari, C., Siller, M., Huynh, L. N., Shih, W., Swanson, M., Hellemann, G. S., & Sugar, C. A. (2014). Randomized controlled trial of parental responsiveness intervention for toddlers at high risk for autism. *Infant Behavior and Development, 37*(4), 711–721.

Koegel, L. K., Singh, A. K., Koegel, R. L., Hollingsworth, J. R., & Bradshaw, J. (2014). Assessing and improving early social engagement in infants. *Journal of Positive Behavior Interventions, 16*(2), 69–80.

Koren-Karie, N., Oppenheim, D., Dolev, S., & Yirmiya, N. (2009). Mothers of securely attached children with autism spectrum disorder are more sensitive than mothers of insecurely attached children. *Journal of Child Psychology and Psychiatry, 50*(5), 643–650.

Milton, D. (2014). So what exactly are autism interventions intervening with? *Good Autism Practice, 15*(2), 6–14.

Mrazek, P. J., & Haggerty, R. J. (Eds.). (1994). *Reducing risks for mental disorders: Frontiers for preventive intervention research.* Washington, DC: National Academies Press.

Parlade, M. V., & Iverson, J. M. (2015). The development of coordinated communication in infants at heightened risk for autism spectrum disorder. *Journal of Autism and Developmental Disorders, 45*(7), 2218–2234.

Peterson, B. S. (2015). Editorial: Research Domain Criteria (RDoC): A new psychiatric nosology whose time has not yet come. *Journal of Child Psychology and Psychiatry, 56*(7), 719–722.

Pickles, A., Le Couteur, A., Leadbitter, K., Salomone, E., Cole-Fletcher, R., Tobin, H., . . . Green, J. (2016). Parent-mediated social communication therapy for young children with autism (PACT): Long-term follow-up of a randomised controlled trial. *The Lancet, 388*(10059), 2501–2509.

Poslawsky, I. E., Naber, F. B., Bakermans-Kranenburg, M. J., van Daalen, E., van Engeland, H., & van IJzendoorn, M. H. (2014). Video-feedback Intervention to promote Positive Parenting adapted to Autism (VIPP-AUTI): A randomized controlled trial. *Autism, 19*(5), 588–603.

Prentice, R. L. (1989). Surrogate endpoints in clinical trials: Definition and operational criteria. *Statistics in Medicine, 8*(4), 431–440.

Rahman, A., Divan, G., Hamdani, S. U., Vajaratkar, V., Taylor, C., Leadbitter, K., . . . Green, J. (2016). Effectiveness of the parent-mediated intervention for children with autism spectrum disorder in South Asia in India and Pakistan (PASS): A randomised controlled trial. *The Lancet Psychiatry, 3*(2), 128–136.

Rogers, S. J., Estes, A., Lord, C., Vismara, L., Winter, J., Fitzpatrick, A., . . . Dawson, G. (2012). Effects of a brief Early Start Denver Model (ESDM)-based parent intervention on toddlers at risk for autism spectrum disorders: A randomized controlled trial. *Journal of the American Academy of Child and Adolescent Psychiatry, 51*(10), 1052–1065.

Rogers, S. J., Estes, A., Vismara, L., Munson, J., Zierhut, C., Greenson, J., . . . Talbott, M. (2019). Enhancing low-intensity coaching in parent implemented Early Start Denver Model intervention for early autism: A randomized comparison treatment trial. *Journal of Autism and Developmental Disorders, 49,* 632–646.

Rogers, S. J., Vismara, L., Wagner, A. L., McCormick, C., Young, G., & Ozonoff, S. (2014). Autism treatment in the first year of life: A pilot study of infant start, a parent-implemented intervention for symptomatic infants. *Journal of Autism and Developmental Disorders, 44*(12), 2981–2995.

Rutgers, A. H., Bakermans-Kranenburg, M. J., van IJzendoorn, M. H., & van Berckelaer-Onnes, I. A. (2004). Autism and attachment: A meta-analytic review. *Journal of Child Psychology and Psychiatry, 45*(6), 1123–1134.

Sameroff, A. J. (2009). The transactional model. In A. J. Sameroff (Ed.), *The transactional model of development: How children and contexts shape each other* (pp. 3–21). Washington, DC: American Psychological Association.

Schwichtenberg, A. J., Kellerman, A. M., Young, G. S., Miller, M., & Ozonoff, S. (2019). Mothers of children with autism spectrum disorders: Play behaviors with infant siblings and social responsiveness. *Autism, 23*(4), 821–833.

Shic, F., Macari, S., & Chawarska, K. (2014). Speech disturbs face scanning in 6-month-old infants who develop autism spectrum disorder. *Biological Psychiatry, 75*(3), 231–237.

Siller, M., Hutman, T., & Sigman, M. (2013). A parent-mediated intervention to increase responsive parental behaviors and child communication in children with ASD: A randomized clinical trial. *Journal of Autism and Developmental Disorders, 43*(3), 540–555.

Slonims, V., & McConachie, H. (2006). Analysis of mother–infant interaction in infants with Down syndrome and typically developing infants. *American Journal on Mental Retardation, 111*(4), 273–289.

Steiner, A. M., Gengoux, G. W., Klin, A., & Chawarska, K. (2013). Pivotal response treatment for infants at-risk for autism spectrum disorders: A pilot study. *Journal of Autism and Developmental Disorders, 43*(1), 91–102.

Steiner, A. M., Gengoux, G. W., Smith, A., & Chawarska, K. (2018). Parent–child interaction synchrony for infants at-risk for autism spectrum disorder. *Journal of Autism and Developmental Disorders, 48,* 3562.

Stone, W. L., Coonrod, E. E., & Ousley, O. Y. (2000). Brief report: Screening Tool for Autism in Two-Year-Olds (STAT): Development and preliminary data. *Journal of Autism and Developmental Disorders, 30*(6), 607–612.

Szatmari, P., Chawarska, K., Dawson, G., Georgiades, S., Landa, R., Lord, C., . . .

Halladay, A. (2016). Prospective longitudinal studies of infant siblings of children with autism: Lessons learned and future directions. *Journal of the American Academy of Child and Adolescent Psychiatry, 55*(3), 179–187.

Tomasello, M. (2008). *Origins of human communication.* Cambridge, MA: MIT Press.

van IJzendoorn, M. H., Rutgers, A. H., Bakermans-Kranenburg, M. J., Swinkels, S. H. N., van Daalen, E., Dietz, C., . . . van Engeland, H. (2007). Parental sensitivity and attachment in children with autism spectrum disorder: Comparison with children with mental retardation, with language delays, and with typical development. *Child Development, 78*(2), 597–608.

Walton, K. M., & Ingersoll, B. R. (2015). The influence of maternal language responsiveness on the expressive speech production of children with autism spectrum disorders: A microanalysis of mother–child play interactions. *Autism, 19*(4), 421–432.

Wan, M. W., Brooks, A., Green, J., Abel, K., & Elmadih, A. (2016). Psychometrics and validation of a brief rating measure of parent–infant interaction: Manchester Assessment of Caregiver-Infant Interaction. *International Journal of Behavioral Development, 41*(4), 542–549.

Wan, M. W., Green, J., Elsabbagh, M., Johnson, M., Charman, T., Plummer, F., & BASIS Team. (2012). Parent–infant interaction in infant siblings at risk of autism. *Research in Developmental Disabilities, 33*(3), 924–932.

Wan, M. W., Green, J., Elsabbagh, M., Johnson, M., Charman, T., Plummer, F., & BASIS Team. (2013). Quality of interaction between at-risk infants and caregiver at 12–15 months is associated with 3 year autism outcome. *Journal of Child Psychology and Psychiatry, 54*(7), 763–771.

Wan, M. W., Green, J., & Scott, J. (2019). A systematic review of parent–infant interaction in infants at risk of autism. *Autism, 23*(4), 811–820.

Watson, L. R., Crais, E. R., Baranek, G. T., Turner-Brown, L., Sideris, J., Wakeford, L., . . . Nowell, S. W. (2017). Parent-mediated intervention for one-year-olds screened as at-risk for autism spectrum disorder: A randomized controlled trial. *Journal of Autism and Developmental Disorders, 47*(11), 3520–3540.

Whitehouse, A., Varcin, K., Alvares, G., Barbaro, J., Bent, C., Boutrus, M., . . . Hudry, K. (2019). Pre-emptive intervention versus treatment as usual for infants showing early behavioural risk signs of autism spectrum disorder: A single-blind, randomised controlled trial. *The Lancet Child and Adolescent Health, 3*(9), 605–615.

Willemsen-Swinkels, S. H. N., Bakermans-Kranenburg, M. J., Buitelaar, J. K., van IJzendoorn, M. H., & van Engeland, H. (2000). Insecure and disorganised attachment in children with a pervasive developmental disorder: Relationship with social interaction and heart rate. *Journal of Child Psychology and Psychiatry and Allied Disciplines, 41*(6), 759–767.

Zwaigenbaum, L,, Bauman, M. L., Stone, W. L., Yirmiya, N., Estes, A., Hansen, R. L., . . . Wetherby, A. (2015). Early identification of autism spectrum disorder: Recommendations for practice and research. *Pediatrics, 136*(Suppl. 1), S10–S40.

CHAPTER 9

· · · · · · · ·

Providing Medical Care to Young Children with Autism Spectrum Disorder

Fred R. Volkmar, Roald A. Øien, and Lisa Wiesner

The provision of high-quality health care to young children with autism spectrum disorder (ASD) necessitates looking at multiple issues: (1) case detection and diagnosis, (2) awareness of potentially associated medical conditions, and (3) awareness of approaches to care that will facilitate long-term engagement of the child and family. Each is reviewed in detail in this chapter. In this context, prevention of problems is important, for example, through awareness of potential safety concerns and ongoing regular well-child visits. As we have discussed elsewhere (Volkmar & Wiesner, 2017), children with autism/ASD can have deficits in communication and social interaction that complicate interaction with health care providers. For example, the child with minimal verbal ability might have a significant problem that results in pain but cannot communicate this problem effectively, which instead presents clinically as irritability or some other change in behavior. For others, changes in sleeping or eating habits may signal some emerging condition. For pediatricians and other health care providers, the impairment of understanding and social interaction in individuals with ASD may complicate physical examination because the patient may find the examimation physically and psychologically disturbing, leading to noncompliant behavior.

There have been important changes in approaches to medical care for children with ASD. With the advent of electronic medical records, some aspects of care have been improved (e.g., in terms of access to the medical [but not other] records). On the other hand, the sheer number of medical visits per clinician has increased, and therefore, this very fast pace of medical care can be a challenge. We will discuss some of the accommodations that can be made to facilitate child and parental engagement and satisfaction and the role of the "medical home" in optimizing care.

Regular well-child visits are particularly important for the child with autism. They give the child and family a chance to get to know the pediatrician or other care provider without the burden of associated illness. When the care provider takes an active role in coordination of services (as we will discuss subsequently), overall care is improved, and parents rely less on resources such as emergency visits or walk-in clinics (Lin, Margolis, Yu, & Adirim, 2014). When emergency services are needed, the emergency department presents other challenges in terms of care coordination and service (see Volkmar & Wiesner, 2017). Our increasingly complex health care system presents other barriers for families, such as finding specialists and coordinating care with school as well as intervention programs (Volkmar & Wiesner, 2017).

Early Detection and Diagnosis

As discussed elsewhere in this volume, there has been an explosion of research on the nature of autism in young children, and new approaches to detection and treatment have been presented. For children of all ages, obtaining an accurate diagnosis of ASD is of importance in establishing eligibility for services and in guiding the services provided. The primary care provider may be the first to suspect the presence of an ASD or some other problem, even though the definitive (or at least provisional) diagnosis may be established by specialists. In the United States, eligibility for services can be established for children under 3 with provision of needed services before the child turns 3 even before a definitive diagnosis is made. After the age of 3, the child becomes eligible for school-based services/programs. There is often a dichotomy between the medical/mental health providers who give a diagnosis and those who deliver the intervention. This is not unique to the United States; indeed, it is relatively typical around the world.

It is imperative that primary care providers look for warning signs or red flags for autism *and* carefully listen to parental concerns. This is particularly important around the first birthday and soon after. As children pass 12 months of age and are not yet speaking, the number of potential warning signs increases (Chawarska, Macari, Volkmar, Kim, & Shic, 2014a). Even though diagnostic stability becomes much greater after age 3 (Chawarska et al., 2014a; Lord & Schopler, 1988), eligibility for special services from state and other agencies can be based on risk (Volkmar & Wiesner, 2017). Fortunately, the age of first diagnosis has decreased over time, but delays in diagnosis do sometimes occur for various reasons, such as heterogeneity in time of onset and symptom patterns (Volkmar & Wiesner, 2017; Øien et al., 2018).

Screening and Diagnosis

In making a diagnosis of autism, clinicians typically rely on observation and history. Although a number of guidelines, rating scales, and checklists have been developed and may help in the process (Ibañez, Stone, & Coonrod, 2014; Lord, Corsello, & Grzadzinski, 2014; McClure, 2014; Volkmar et al., 2014b), these should never replace thoughtful clinical judgment. As discussed in Chapter 1 (Volkmar and Øien, this volume), there have been a number of changes in how both categorical and dimensional approaches to autism have evolved over time.

The use of diagnostic criteria (i.e., in the current DSM-5 approach; American Psychiatric Association, 2013) has presented some complexities for the early identification process as some studies (e.g., Barton, Robins, Jashar, Brennan, & Fein, 2013) have raised serious concerns about the limitations of this approach for the more cognitively able younger child (see also Smith, Reichow, & Volkmar, 2015, for a meta-analysis confirming this as a general concern). As Volkmar and Øien noted in Chapter 1, this volume, it is somewhat paradoxical that with the advent of the autism spectrum concept in DSM-5, the actual criteria are more appropriate to the narrower "Kanner's autism" (Smith et al., 2015).

Care providers should also be aware of potential risk factors for autism—particularly genetic ones. It is clear that having one child with autism substantially raises the risk for subsequent children with a 10 to 20% recurrence risk (Ozonoff et al., 2011; Rutter & Thapar, 2014). There is also some suggestion that obstetric and neonatal complications can increase risk—possibly in interaction with genetic vulnerabilities—but this topic remains somewhat controversial (Gardener, Spiegelman, & Buka, 2009). There are clear associations of autism with several genetic conditions, such as fragile X syndrome and tuberous sclerosis; therefore, a detailed family history should be completed, and as we discuss subsequently, an awareness of these associations may guide physical exam and laboratory studies. Some data suggests that increased parental age, especially paternal age, may be a risk factor (Cantor, Yoon, Furr, & Lajonchere, 2007). Though of considerable interest to date, the association of autism with specific environmental risk factors has been controversial (Lyall, Schmidt, & Hertz-Picciotto, 2014).

Over the past two decades, general population screening for autism has been recommended for all children at 18 months of age, with followup at 24 months (Committee on Practice and Ambulatory Medicine and Bright Futures Steering Committee, 2007; Bright Futures Steering Committee, 2006; Committee on Practice and Ambulatory Medicine Bright Futures Periodicity Schedule Workgroup, 2016; Johnson, Myers, & American Academy of Pediatrics Council on Children with Disabilities, 2007). However, whether or not general population screening should be recommended remains controversial (Siu et al., 2016). The recommendation of general population screening for ASD is founded on early identification to implement early interventions, ultimately improving outcome for children with ASD (Howlin, 2014). Chawarska and colleagues (2014a) revealed that parental concern is present at a mean toddler age of 15 months, though with great variance. This is in contrast to a mean age of 4.5 years of age for diagnosis in the United States (Baio, 2014), and only 43% of the children with ASD receive evaluations by 3 years of age. The primary aim of screening for ASD is to identify all children, those both with and without early parental concern, to maximize opportunities of early diagnosis and interventions. The various screening instruments are often designed as brief parental-endorsed questionnaires or assessments, whereas a positive screen should lead to a referral for autism-specific assessment. In terms of performance, a sensitivity (SE) of .80 and specificity (SP) above .80 is regarded as recommendable (Ibañez et al., 2014). Positive predictive value (PPV) and negative predictive value (NPV) are largely affected by the prevalence of the disorder. Thus, PPV is most often higher in a high-risk clinical sample than in a general population. According to Cicchetti and colleagues, a PPV above .70 is recommended as acceptable (Cicchetti, Volkmar, Klin, & Showalter, 1995). Next we will address the different dimensions of screening, current knowledge on the performance of early general population screening, and implications for future research and clinical practice.

There is a distinction between Level 1 screening (i.e., screening in unselected general populations) and Level 2 screening (i.e., screening children already showing developmental concern to differentiate children with a possible ASD diagnosis from other developmental disorders; Ibañez et al., 2014). Level 1 screening instruments are often designed to be completed by parents at pediatric well visits and are not restricted to the ASD-specific screening instruments. Level 2 screening instruments are often used in subspecialized clinics to determine if a child should be referred for ASD-specific assessment, and they often combine clinician observation and parent report. The most frequently used Level 1 screening instrument for ASD in young children is the Modified Checklist for Autism in Toddlers (M-CHAT; Ibañez et al., 2014; Robins et al., 2014; Robins, Fein, Barton, & Green, 2001). This 23-item parent-reported questionnaire is designed to be completed in a primary care provider setting (Robins et al., 2001), for example, at pediatric well visits. In 2014, a revision of the M-CHAT, M-CHAT-R/F, was released (Robins et al., 2014). The M-CHAT-R/F introduced new cutoffs, with the aim of reducing false positives (Robins et al., 2014). However, it is still not known if the M-CHAT-R/F reduces false negatives. It has been recommended for use in toddlers at 18 months of age, with follow-up at 24 months of age (Committee on Practice and Ambulatory Medicine Bright Futures Periodicity Schedule Workgroup, 2016; Council on Children with Disabilities et al., 2006). Concerning Level 2 screeners, a wide range of instruments are available. Among the most frequently used are the Childhood Autism Rating Scale (CARS/CARS-2; Schopler, Van Bourgondian, Wellman, & Love, 2010); the Social Communication Questionnaire (SCQ; Rutter, Bailey, & Lord, 2003); the Autism Mental Status Exam (AMSE; Grodberg, Siper, Jamison, Buxbaum, & Kolevzon,

2016; Øien, Siper, Kolevzon, & Grodberg, 2016); and the Screening Tool for Autism in Toddlers (STAT; Stone, Coonrod, Turner, & Pozdol, 2004). While most Level 1 screening instruments are intended to screen for ASD in toddlers and young children under the age of 30 months, Level 2 screening instruments are, besides the STAT, often designed to screen for ASD in a wider age range of children already determined to be at risk for ASD (Ibañez et al., 2014). Furthermore, Level 1 screening instruments in most cases rely on parent report, while Level 2 screening instruments more often also utilize clinician observation.

Currently, most studies using general population screening are conducted in selected populations. The debate with regard to screening in unselected general population samples frequently questions whether ASD-specific screening instruments have sufficiently high specificity and positive predictive value (McPheeters et al., 2016; U.K. National Screening Committee, 2012). As most studies are conducted utilizing selected populations, where screen-positives are invited for clinical assessment, little information exists on screen-negative cases that later receive an ASD diagnosis (Øien et al., 2018). Considering the substantial heterogeneity in the onset of recognizable symptoms (Ozonoff et al., 2010) and the patterns of symptom expression (Chawarska, Klin, Paul, & Volkmar, 2007; Chawarska et al., 2014b), symptoms of ASD may be recognizable at different ages owing to variance in social demand. There is also some uncertainty in regard to how parents understand questions and various grading options, as well as to which degree the design on concurrent screening instruments affects the responses. However, a recent study by Macari and colleagues (2018) revealed good concurrence between clinicians and parents on the rating of autism-related symptoms on the First Year Inventory (FYI).

In terms of performance, the validation study of the M-CHAT (Robins et al., 2001) yielded an SE of .97, an SP of .95, and a PPV of .36 (NPV .99) before a follow-up was conducted. The follow-up raised SP to .99 and PPV to .68. Although these numbers seemed to be excellent, it is important to note that the sample consisted of both low-risk (unselected) and high-risk (selected) toddlers, and only three children from the unselected population ultimately received an ASD diagnosis. A follow-up study conducted by Kleinman and colleagues (Kleinman et al., 2008) revealed a PPV of .36, which is in line with the validation study of the M-CHAT (Robins et al., 2001). However, as in the validation study, performance in low-risk (unselected) children was low (PPV .11; Kleinman et al., 2008). Later studies conducted based on the Norwegian Mother and Child Cohort (MoBa; Magnus et al., 2016), a prospective unselected population study with linkage to the Norwegian Patient Registry, revealed a PPV of 1.5% for the 23-item criterion and 3.3% for the six-critical-item criterion (Stenberg et al., 2014) conducted without follow-up. More importantly, Stenberg (2015) revealed that 65.3% of children later diagnosed were false screen negative cases, that is, children who would not meet cutoff for a follow-up. Furthermore, it was revealed that the M-CHAT first and foremost identified later-diagnosed ASD children with cognitive and language disabilities (Stenberg, 2015). A recent study by Øien and colleagues reported that 76.8% of all children later diagnosed with ASD were screened negative on the six-critical-item criterion (false negatives; Øien et al., 2018), highlighting the need to focus efforts also on children screened negative. The latter also indicated that, even if these children did not meet cutoff on the ASD-specific measures of the M-CHAT, utilizing other developmental measures showed significant developmental delays compared to true negatives and true positives. Regarding Level 2 screening instruments, most of the mentioned instruments (STAT, SCQ, AMSE, and CARS/CARS-2) show excellent psychometric properties when applied in children determined to be at risk in community settings. While an experienced clinician may eliminate the need for Level 2 screening instruments, the instruments can provide valuable information for clinical judgment in subspecialized settings when referring children to ASD-specific assessment and can be of great use in determining strengths and difficulties for individual children.

While identifying all children with a later diagnosis of ASD might be impossible since onset patterns might differ between children, the aim should be to identify all children with a later diagnosis of ASD. The present chapter highlights the difficulties of screening in unselected populations, while it acknowledges that screening for ASD might also benefit children with developmental delay and other disorders. However, studies have revealed that most children with a later diagnosis of ASD are missed at 18 months, a fact that questions the efficiency (Siu et al., 2016) and cost effectiveness (Yuen, Carter, Szatmari, & Ungar, 2018) of universal screening. The issue of false negatives is not solved by modifying cutoff scores of current instruments and should encourage clinicians to rely not only on the screening instrument itself but also on good clinical judgment, parental concern, and surveillance of developmental milestones (Øien et al., 2018). Future research should emphasize learning more about children that are being missed at 18-months screening and should assess if there are limitations to the design of current screening instruments that cause them to perform poorly in unselected general populations at 18 months. It should also be examined whether or not there is a great improvement in identification at 24 months, as recommended by the American Academy of Pediatrics (AAP). One hypothesis is that utilizing only one instrument to screen children for ASD might be insufficient in unselected populations due to the heterogeneity in symptoms, time, and pattern of onset. Furthermore, instruments measuring developmental milestones such as social communication, motor skills, and communication skills could provide additional valuable information. It is also important to note that parents of children not meeting actionable concern at 18 or 24 months of age might not recognize or understand the behaviors that concurrent screening instruments probe for, further complicating the screening process. Broder-Fingert and colleagues asked whether it is time for something new, given that later studies utilize prospective general population cohorts (Broder-Fingert, Feinberg, & Silverstein, 2018). While this question remains unanswered, it is clear that more research is needed.

Comprehensive Diagnostic Assessments

Often, initial evaluations following a positive screen or parental/provider concern are relatively brief and limited to an assessment of eligibility and initial needs. Practices vary from country to country and sometimes within country. A more comprehensive assessment is sought for other purposes, such as clarifying the child's complete cognitive profile (to identify strengths and weaknesses for intervention planning) and associated medical conditions (e.g., genetic problems, seizures), and addressing any diagnostic uncertainty. Many symptoms are not specific to ASD, but also are present in other developmental disorders and in children with significant developmental delays. As Volkmar and Øien note in Chapter 1, this volume, definite diagnosis is often made after age 3, as diagnostic instruments become more accurate and as the clinical picture is more clearly established. In the United States, it is at 3 years that schools become mandated to provide educational service and may conduct their own assessments.

A number of specialists and specialties are involved in the initial confirmatory diagnosis assessment and in subsequent follow-up assessments. It is important for the primary care provider to be sure that assessment results are integrated in the service plan. Sometimes specialists operate individually although the team approach is often most helpful if it can provide an integrated picture of the child's developmental status, diagnosis, and intervention needs (Volkmar, Booth, McPartland, & Wiesner, 2014a). The primary care provider must take an active role in this process and is aware of local and regional resources. University-based medical schools or clinics or children's hospitals will often have such programs, and some parent organizations can provide information as well.

Typically, a comprehensive assessment will use various components such as gathering a detailed history; psychological testing, including diagnostic-specific instruments (to establish developmental/intellectual levels, areas of strength and weakness, and to address issues of diagnosis); adaptive skills (generalization of abilities or real-world contexts); communication (not limited simply to vocabulary but taking a broader view of communication abilities); and sometimes occupational and/or physical therapy assessments.

The primary care provider has a special role in coordinating medical professionals and assessments—typically neurology and genetics. As noted by Volkmar and Øien in Chapter 1, this volume, a number of diagnostic instruments have now been developed, some of which focus more specifically on younger children with autism. These instruments can be based on structured history from parents and/or observation/assessment of the child. For school-age children, teacher-oriented screeners and instruments are available (see Lord et al., 2014). Although these instruments can be helpful, they should not replace informed clinical judgment. For primary care providers less familiar with standardized assessment and autism-specific instruments, resources are available (Volkmar & Wiesner, 2017).

Medical Evaluations

Once the issue of possible autism has been raised, it is important to also conduct a comprehensive medical assessment. This assessment should include a careful developmental history, with a review of the pregnancy, labor and delivery, and early development and developmental milestones. Any history of possible regression or unusual behaviors suggesting seizure disorder should be noted. Given that screeners are well known to pick up developmental problems other than autism, the primary care provider also needs to be able to follow up with appropriate testing and referral for all potential conditions associated with positive screening. Guidelines and practice parameters are available and summarize procedures in detail (McClure, 2014; Volkmar et al., 2014b; Wilson et al., 2014).

Conditions often confused with autism include other developmental disorders (e.g., language disorder, intellectual disability), sensory impairments, and potentially associated medical conditions (e.g., seizure disorders, fragile X syndrome, and tuberous sclerosis). For children with a history of prenatal exposure to drugs or alcohol, their presentation may be complicated if the child has received suboptimal care (Volkmar & Wiesner, 2017). Usually, children with developmental delay without autism will have social abilities that are on a par with overall intellectual skills. Young children with developmental language disorders often will attempt to compensate for their language difficulty through, among other means, sign, gesture, or other nonverbal tools. Stereotyped movement is frequently present in autism (particularly as infants move into the toddler phase and beyond), but they are also common with more significant intellectual disability and, as single diagnostic features, they are not necessarily predictive of autism. As such, careful and comprehensive diagnostic assessment is needed.

It is important to emphasize that service provision should not be delayed if there are clear targets for intervention, even if the specific diagnosis remains unclear. Some children who have traits of autism as young children outgrow them, while others experience regression in development. A history of regression in development should be noted and may prompt additional testing.

Medical evaluations can be conducted at the same time as the comprehensive diagnostic assessment is in process. As noted above, there are various guidelines, and usually these specify the need for physical examination, a hearing screen, and, when language is delayed, a full audiological assessment (Volkmar & Wiesner, 2017). During the physical exam and history, the clinician should be alert to findings such as staring spells or possible seizure-like activity, unusual movements, and dysmorphic features.

Given the increased risk for seizure disorders (of all types but usually major motor seizures), the clinician should be aware of any reports on the child's history or observation suggesting potential seizures. If the patient has a history of seizures, major motor seizures, or other types of seizures, neurological consultation should be obtained. In the absence of specific indications, the yield of "routine" EEG is relatively low, although nonspecific EEG abnormalities are frequent (Volkmar & Wiesner, 2017).

A history of loss of skills should particularly prompt a thorough medical assessment (Volkmar & Wiesner, 2017). In a large sample of children with autism, parents report some aspect of regression in about 20% of cases. However, upon further examination, the child may often demonstrate early delays (Siperstein & Volkmar, 2004). This is a complication for interpreting much of the work done on the topic (where sometimes parent report is equated with true regression). When you think about it, of course, it is understandable that sometimes parents become worried only as skills fail to develop. At other times, the child's history, EEG results, or language regression may suggest a specific diagnosis such as Landau–Klefner syndrome (acquired aphasia with epilepsy), which can be verified on EEG (Deonna & Roulet-Perez, 2010).

Guidelines for genetic testing have been evolving over the past decade and have moved from the older karyotype analysis to much more sophisticated tests. The American College of Human Genetics has provided a series of recommendations (Schaefer, Mendelsohn, & Professional Practice and Guidelines Committee, 2013), and these are periodically updated. The current guidelines indicate that all children with ASD should undergo basic or "first-tier" testing, with more complex testing if indicated. At present, the positive yield of such testing is on the order of 10–15% of cases (Tammimies et al., 2015). Referral for genetic counseling should be prompted by family history, physical examination (e.g., specific findings suggest a known syndrome, dysmorphic features, etc.), and developmental and medical history.

The advent of more sophisticated genetic testing has begun to reveal previously unrecognized associations. The geneticist should carefully discuss the significance of positive findings for the child and/or for siblings and future pregnancies with the families. An MRI may be needed if seizures, regression, microcephaly, macrocephaly, or other relevant findings on history or examination suggest it; it need not be routinely done, however. In one study of patients with general developmental delay referred for neurological assessment, the positive "yield" of medical testing was over 50% (Majnemer & Shevell, 1995). Medical evaluation procedures are summarized in Table 9.1.

TABLE 9.1. Evaluation Procedures for Autism and Pervasive Developmental Disorders

1. Historical information
   a. Early development and characteristics of development
   b. Age and nature of onset
   c. Medical and family history (especially for autism)

2. Psychological/communicative examination
   a. Estimate(s) of intellectual level (particularly nonverbal IQ)
   b. Communicative assessment (receptive and expressive language, use of nonverbal communication, pragmatic use of language)
   c. Adaptive behavior (how the child copes with the real world)
   d. Social and communicative skills evaluation relative to nonverbal intellectual abilities

3. Psychiatric examination
   a. Nature of social relatedness (eye contact, attachment behaviors)
   b. Behavioral features (stereotypy/self-stimulation, resistance to change, unusual sensitivities to the environment, etc.)
   c. Play skills (nonfunctional use of play materials, developmental level of play activities) and communication
   d. Various rating scales, checklists, and instruments specific to autism may be used

4. Medical evaluation
   a. Search for any associated medical conditions (infectious, genetic, pre- and perinatal risk factors, etc.)
   b. Genetic testing (first tier, including chromosomal microarray and fragile X testing) with more specialized testing if these are negative
   c. Hearing test (usually indicated and not limited to simple three-tone screening)
   d. Other tests and consultations as indicated by history and current examination (e.g., EEG, CT/MRI scan) if unusual features are present (seizures, physical anomalies, microcephaly, regression)

5. Additional consultations
   a. Occupational or physical therapy, as needed
   b. Respiratory therapy and/or orthopedic specialists (Rett syndrome)

Note. Based on Volkmar et al. (2014a).

Preventive Care

For children with autism, regular well-child visits are particularly important. They help the child and parents become familiar with the physical setting, office staff, and procedures. As we note below, some accommodations on the part of the practice for children with autism can be very helpful. These visits provide parents the opportunity to discuss the child's development, evaluation feedback, and progress in treatment, as well as any concerns about the child. They not only give care providers the opportunity to present important information to parents about resources, but they also focus on practical problems typical for children with autism. As will be further discussed in this chapter, care providers should also include a discussion of child safety. Preventive dental care is also important since simple interventions (learning to tolerate a toothbrush, use of fluoridated water, and so forth) can have tremendous benefit (see Green & Flanagan, 2008; Marshall, Sheller, Williams, Mancl, & Cowan, 2007; Lai, Milano, Roberts, & Hooper, 2012). A number of strategies have been developed to help children tolerate dental visits (Volkmar & Wiesner, 2017). Several excellent resources for training primary care providers are available (Kobak et al., 2011; Warren, Stone, & Humberd, 2009).

Immunizations

Historically, until the advent of modern antibiotics, the leading cause of death among children was infection. Over the past century, the development of immunizations for illnesses such as measles, mumps, diphtheria, and tetanus have led to the prevention of these illnesses. A paper subsequently withdrawn from the medical journal *The Lancet* led to major concerns that perhaps immunizations caused or contributed to the onset of autism (Wakefield, 1999). Concerns spread rapidly, even though it quickly became apparent that there were major problems with this paper. Many parents worried that either the measles shot or a mercury-containing compound called thimerosal might cause autism and so immunization rates began to fall. A plethora of studies have now been conducted and have debunked this theory that vaccines cause autism. Even so, many parents continue to have concerns, and as a result, communicable diseases such as mumps and measles have reemerged (see Fombonne & Chakrabarti, 2001; Offit, 2008; Mrozek-Budzyn, Kieltyka, & Majewska, 2010; Institute of Medicine, 2004). Unfortunately, the major news coverage given to the original paper and subsequent reporting likely contributed to heightened parental concerns (Smith, Ellenberg, Bell, & Rubin, 2008).

It is important that primary care providers encourage immunization and educate parents about the serious implications of being unvaccinated. Lower rates of immunization increase the risk of the return of the epidemics of communicable diseases seen in the past century. It is important that care providers help parents understand the real (rare but real) risks of immunization as well as the very real risks of illnesses such as measles.

Safety

Accidental injury is the leading cause of death in children in general as it is for children with autism, albeit at perhaps double the rate of the typical population (Shavelle & Strauss, 1998). Several factors likely contribute to these increased rates. Children with ASD are more likely to have associated problems such as seizures, which may contribute to this risk (Bilder et al., 2013; Gillberg, Billstedt, Sundh, & Gillberg, 2010). For the developing child with autism problems with impulsivity, lack of judgement, and delays in communication can contribute to risk (Volkmar & Wiesner, 2017). For example, the younger child with ASD may be less likely to engage in joint attention and social referencing and hence will not learn from parents about situations or common risks such as open flames. Similarly, unusual sensitivities and interests in smell may lead to accidental ingestion of dangerous substances. The problem is compounded when, as is often the case, motor development is not yet delayed. Drowning is a common cause of death, and interest in water without an appreciation of its dangers likely contributes to incidents of drowning, as do associated problems such as seizures.

Primary care providers routinely address issues surrounding child safety during well-child visits. It is particularly important to discuss these issues with parents of children with autism and to help them become aware of safety issues not only at home but in the community; for example, as a child becomes older, learning to cross the street becomes important (Goldsmith, 2009). Given the dangers of drowning, teaching swimming skills is indicated. Parents should of course also be aware of local "attractive" dangers, such as houses under construction, a neighbor's swimming pool, and unfriendly dogs (Volkmar & Wiesner, 2017).

A number of steps can be taken, including a review of household safety and safety proofing the house, awareness of common danger areas, and use of audio and visual monitoring. As children become more mobile, tracking devices can help; these can now be essentially embedded in the child's clothing. This becomes particularly true for children with autism as they move more frequently since many (perhaps 50% or more) will wander or bolt (Solomon & Lawlor, 2013). This increases risks for accidental injury and death (Anderson et al., 2012). Issues of safety also include community and school settings—playgrounds can be particularly risky places for the child who is socially isolated and unaware of the movements and activities of others. As young children become older, they should be explicitly taught about dangerous situations such as responding to strangers.

Eating and Feeding Issues

Young children with ASD can present with various issues relative to eating/feeding and associated gastrointestinal (GI) problems (Volkmar & Wiesner, 2017). These problems can include unusual food preferences and sensitivities as well as pica—the last-named increasing risks of lead poisoning (Volkmar & Wiesner, 2017). Most often, these issues become more problematic in toddlers (Volkmar & Wiesner, 2017). Although occasional issues in early feeding/nursing are reported, rarely do children with autism have a history of failure to thrive (Volkmar & Wiesner, 2017). Occasionally, as children become older, they have pronounced sensitivities to certain tastes or have preferences in terms of smells or even colors of food (Bennetto, Kuschner, & Hyman, 2007). They may become highly selective as to what they eat, thus raising issues about nutrition (Volkmar & Wiesner, 2017). Sometimes these issues first arise as solid foods are introduced (Volkmar & Wiesner, 2017).

Of course, even typically developing toddlers can have struggles with their parents concerning food. Unfortunately, some of the things that can help the typical child to cope (e.g., parental praise or interest in modeling siblings' behavior) will not be so successful for the child with autism. As one might imagine, these issues become greatly magnified when parents are trying complementary dietary treatments that may severely limit the kind of foods served.

Dealing with eating/feeding issues can be a challenge for parents and care providers alike. Often the assistance of others, notably occupational, speech–language, and/or behavioral therapists, can help. As discussed elsewhere (Volkmar & Wiesner, 2017), a range of strategies can be employed. These can include very gradual introduction of new foods and attempts to work within the child's food preferences (e.g., if smooth foods are desired, many things can be put in the blender). As children get older, it may be helpful to involve them in food preparation in some way.

Eating nonfood substances (pica) is sometimes observed and is more prevalent in children with developmental delays (Chaidez, Hansen, & Hertz-Picciotto, 2014). This can take the form of eating dirt, paint chips, string, or even clothing. Sometimes these items are only chewed, but sometimes they are also swallowed. Potential toxins are a major concern, and if pica is observed, special attention should be paid, for example, to lead levels. Strategies that help include both behavioral (Piazza et al., 1998) and, potentially, pharmacological interventions (Lerner, 2008).

The issue of associated gastrointestinal problems in children with ASD has attracted increased attention over the years. However, several studies have found no solid data suggesting that these problems have actually increased (e.g., Kuddo & Nelson, 2003). Constipation and/or diarrhea are among the most frequently reported gastrointestinal symptoms (Chaidez et al., 2014; Wang, Tancredi, & Thomas, 2011), but they are not clearly related to severity of autism (Chandler et al., 2013). Restricted eating patterns reduce social (and thus motor) engagement, and complementary diets may also contribute (Volkmar & Wiesner, 2017). Establishing healthy eating habits early on is important, given what appears to be a significant risk for obesity as children with ASD become older (Volkmar & Wiesner, 2017).

Sleep and Sleep Problems

Over half of children with ASD are estimated to experience some sleep issue during their development, and these problems vary over the course of development (Goldman, Richdale, Clemons, & Malow, 2012; Park et al., 2012). Some children with ASD develop sleep problems during toddlerhood, including difficulty falling asleep, need to have a parent sleep with them, early awakening, and unusual sleep–wake cycles (Goldman et al., 2012; Park et al., 2012). Some toddlers and young children will adapt complicated routines/rituals that have to be followed. Lack of sleep can be increasingly disruptive to the lives of parents (Volkmar & Wiesner, 2017).

Fortunately, an increasing body of research on sleep problems is now available (for a summary, see Volkmar & Wiesner, 2017). This work has tended to show that when detailed records are kept, sleep problems are even more common than parents report.

Parents can take several steps to help the practioner understand the nature of the problem, including keeping a sleep diary for several weeks to document the sleep patterns. For parents, decreasing daytime sleep, avoiding overly energizing activities in the evening, encouraging use of a specific pattern or routine to introduce the child to falling asleep at the beginning of the night, and so forth are recommended (see Durand, 2008; Volkmar & Wiesner, 2017). Pharmacological interventions, including use of over-the-counter melatonin, are also available (see Volkmar & Wiesner, 2017). One study found the use of melatonin helpful and well tolerated (Malow et al., 2012). Severe sleep problems may require the help of a sleep specialist and sometimes sleep studies as well.

Ensuring Successful Medical Visits

Parents and office staff can make efforts to improve the experience of going to the doctor for children with autism. It is important that regular visits go well to ensure that sick visits also go well. Various strategies can be used to make visits successful, and they include preparation of the child as well as thoughtful scheduling and mechanics of visits. Picture books and, for older children, social stories about doctor visits can be used, along with actual photographs of the building, staff, exam room, and so forth. Parents should bring activities that the child can engage in before the visit. Office staff should be thoughtful about the schedule—for example, at the very beginning of the morning or afternoon, they can minimize wait time and give extra time for the visit (for an extended review, see Volkmar & Wiesner, 2017). For the health care provider, starting with a relatively quiet period with the parents is often helpful, followed by conducting the less intrusive aspects of the physical exam. Giving extra time and being deliberate, predictable, and consistent are recommended. Being direct with the child and keeping language simple are also helpful, as is ending on a positive note whenever possible (Volkmar & Wiesner, 2017). Some of these approaches are summarized in Table 9.2.

TABLE 9.2. Making Medical Visits Successful

Prepare the parents for the visit.

- There should be a prenatal visit with the health care provider.
- It is important to emphasize that well-child visits are particularly important.
- Educate parents about resources and supports.
- Facilitate referral after positive screen (and follow-up with parents).
- Health care providers should take an important role in coordination of information.

Prepare the child for the visit.

- As children become older (but even as toddlers), picture books, visual schedules, or even the various computer applications available for autism (e.g., showing a schedule, the physical office, pictures of the staff and doctor) may be helpful.

Schedule

- Schedule appointments early in the morning or afternoon—minimize waiting time.
- If possible, have a quiet (separate) waiting area.
- If possible, have staff who know (or come to know) the child well.

Activities

- If possible, parents should have favorite activities available for the child.
- As children become older, you can effectively use the phone/iPad to keep the child occupied, potentially showing information to help the child familiarize himself/herself with what will happen.

Examination

- Give the child extra time for processing.
- Keep language simple as children become older.
- Encourage (reinforce) cooperation and compliance.
- When conducting the physical exam, be deliberate, predictable, consistent, and thoughtful; do more intrusive things at the end of the exam.
- Try to end on a positive note (for both parents and child).

Note. Based on Volkmar and Wiesner (2017).

The Medical Home

Primary care providers have an increasingly important role in coordinating medical services in all health care. For young children with autism, they can also have an important role as liaison and can coordinate with all the various service providers involved with the child and family. Primary care providers can also help with the transition from preschool to school-based programs (Volkmar & Wiesner, 2017). The new model of care, the medical home, is increasingly being recognized as a best practice health care approach. The concept was originally developed within the American Academy of Pediatrics (2002) to encompass preventive, acute, and chronic care. The coordination of care with specialists and other service providers is family centered and should include consideration of cultural issues. This model of care is particularly effective for children with special needs; it both improves care for the child and increases parental satisfaction (Brachlow, Ness, McPheeters, & Gurney, 2007; Carbone, Behl, Azor, & Murphy, 2010; Cheak-Zamora & Farmer, 2015; Farmer et al., 2014; Golnik, Scal, Wey, & Gaillard, 2012; Hyman & Johnson, 2012; Knapp et al., 2013). Conversely, children who are seen in more traditional care models have greater difficulty in accessing specialty care and sources of parental support.

The medical home model improves health and reduces the financial burden to parents (Cheak-Zamora & Farmer, 2015; Golnik et al., 2012). It is also associated with reduced use of the emergency room (Lin et al., 2014). The functions of a medical home that are central to health care for children with ASD include developmental screening to identify signs and symptoms at the earliest point in time; referral for more comprehensive evaluation and intervention; coordination of care with specialists and all other agencies and professionals involved; ongoing monitoring and management of ASD and coexisting medical problems; medication management and support; education for families in seeking interventions, including complementary and alternative medicine; and transition to adult services. For the young child with autism, the medical home may include an individualized care plan, coordination of care and access (e.g., dentists), as well as educational materials and tools for parents (and practioners) to make visits go more successfully (Golnik et al., 2012; Carbone et al., 2010).

Practice Guidelines and Evidence-Based Practice

In medicine and psychology, and increasingly in education, evidence-based treatments have become important (Reichow & Barton, 2014). A growing body of work has now shown many model programs and an even greater number of specific educational/intervention techniques to be evidence based (see National Research Council, 2001; Odom, Boyd, Hall, & Hume, 2014; Paul & Fahim, 2015; Warren et al., 2011). For the primary care provider, several sets of practice guidelines are available that, in varying ways, adopt specific standards for what can and cannot be regarded as evidence based (see Isaksen et al., 2013; McClure, 2014; Volkmar et al., 2014b). Several reviews have also summarized the literature on associated medical problems (Coury, 2010; Levy et al., 2010).

The very influential initial report on the effectiveness of early intervention in autism from the National Research Council (2001) summarized the then-existing evidence for various treatment approaches and noted many similarities and a few differences. At that early stage, the standards for including programs, that is, having at least one peer-reviewed report supporting the treatment, would now be regarded as insufficient. The various practice guidelines and reviews adopt varying standards for what can be regarded as established (e.g., several independent well-controlled studies, multiple locations, or one or more meta-analyses). It is important to realize how central the preliminary decisions on study selection are in interpreting results and recommendations—for example, treatments that are shown to be effective based on independent observation versus treatments whose results are based primarily or solely on parent reports. Depending on the way these treatments are formulated, it may be difficult to adequately evaluate some of them. For example, there are thousands of single-case studies showing the effectiveness of applied behavior analyses in autism, but there is no randomized controlled study. Sometimes it is unethical to conduct the rigorous kinds of studies that would show that treatment works. All these complexities must be considered when one is developing the treatment program for the child as assessment results are translated into an intervention program (see Volkmar et al. [2014a] for a more detailed discussion). In some cases, for example, the statewide division, Treatment and Education of Autistic and Related Communication Handicapped Children (TEACCH) program in North Carolina, aspects of the program may be regarded as well established and evidence based, but it is impossible to perform double-blind controlled studies. In some cases, treatments may have some, but relatively minimal, supporting evidence, which are often termed *emerging treatments* (see Paul & Fahim, 2015). In other instances, the supporting evidence is based on word of mouth, the Internet, case reports, and so forth; this kind of support should be regarded as minimal at best. Some countries, for example, Australia, have adopted national guidelines on diagnosis (Whitehouse, Evans, Eapen, & Wray, 2018), and more general practice guidelines are available as well (McClure, 2014).

Parents of very young children appear to be most likely to engage in the use of complementary treatments (those used in addition to established or alternative treatments; i.e., those used in place of such effective treatments) (see Smith, Oakes, & Selver, 2014). The latter of course is the most complicated situation, as parents may expend considerable amounts of their time and resources at a time when intervention may be most effective in pursuing unproven treatments. Parents who go on the Internet for information will find over 100 million hits on Google, and if they search for autism and treatment, about 30 million hits. Unfortunately, some work has shown that even among the top 100 websites (regardless of search engine), there are a significant number of offers for treatments that have little or no empirical basis (Reichow et al., 2012a; Reichow, Naples, Steinhoff, Halpern, & Volkmar, 2012b).

The primary care provider can be an important source of guidance to parents as they evaluate their treatment options. He or she should help parents be informed consumers. By their very nature, nonestablished treatments have little in the way of scientific research (with some notable exceptions such as facilitated communication). Several resources can be helpful to providers and parents alike (Levy & Hyman, 2003; Smith et al., 2014; Volkmar & Wiesner, 2017). It should be noted that some treatments may actually be dangerous to the child, and thus practioners should be particularly alert to them (Volkmar & Wiesner, 2017).

Conclusions

In this chapter, we have reviewed some of the issues and complexities involved in providing medical care for young children with ASD. This care is best provided in the context of an overall model of care, the medical home, which is now recognized as a best practice approach. Health care providers can play an important role in early detection of risk for autism and referral for additional evaluations. They can also search for potential associated medical conditions and problems, as well as make referrals to specialists in neurology, genetics, and other fields, as clinically indicated. They also serve an important function in helping parents obtain initial services and ensuring that these are of high quality and have a good evidence base. For children on the autism spectrum, preventive care is very important—this includes well-child visits, immunizations, awareness of safety concerns, and available, appropriate dental care. Both parents and practitioners can take several steps to ensure that visits go well. The overarching goal is to establish a long-term collaborative relationship with parents and child.

REFERENCES

American Academy of Pediatrics. (2002, July). Policy statement: Medical home. *Pediatrics, 110*(1), 184–186.

American Psychiatric Association. (2013). *Diagnostic and statistical manual of mental disorders* (5th ed.). Arlington, VA: Author.

Anderson, C., Law, J. K., Daniels, A., Rice, C., Mandell, D. S., Hagopian, L., & Law, P. A. (2012). Occurrence and family impact of elopement in children with autism spectrum disorders. *Pediatrics, 130*(5), 870–877.

Baio, S. (2014). Prevalence of autism spectrum disorder among children aged 8 years— Autism and Developmental Disabilities Monitoring Network, 11 Sites, United

States, 2010. *Morbidity and Mortality Weekly Report Surveillance Summaries 2010, 63*(No. SS-02), 1–21.

Barton, M. L., Robins, D. L., Jashar, D., Brennan, L., & Fein, D. (2013). Sensitivity and specificity of proposed DSM-5 criteria for autism spectrum disorder in toddlers. *Journal of Autism and Developmental Disorders, 43*(5), 1184–1195.

Bennetto, L., Kuschner, E. S., & Hyman, S. L. (2007). Olfaction and taste processing in autism. *Biological Psychiatry, 62*(9), 1015–1021.

Bilder, D., Botts, E. L., Smith, K. R., Pimentel, R., Farley, M., Viskochil, J., . . . Coon, H. (2013). Excess mortality and causes of death in autism spectrum disorders: A follow up of the 1980s Utah/UCLA autism epidemiologic study. *Journal of Autism and Developmental Disorders, 43*(5), 1196–1204.

Brachlow, A. E., Ness, K. K., McPheeters, M. L., & Gurney, J. G. (2007). Comparison of indicators for a primary care medical home between children with autism or asthma and other special health care needs: National Survey of Children's Health. *Archives of Pediatrics and Adolescent Medicine, 61*(4), 399–405.

Broder-Fingert, S., Feinberg, E., & Silverstein, M. (2018). Improving screening for autism spectrum disorder: Is it time for something new? *Pediatrics, 141*(6), e20180965.

Cantor, R. M., Yoon, J. L., Furr, J., & Lajonchere, C. M. (2007). Paternal age and autism are associated in a family-based sample. *Molecular Psychiatry, 12*(5), 419–421.

Carbone, P. S., Behl, D. D., Azor, V. A., & Murphy, N. A. (2010). The medical home for children with autism spectrum disorders: Parent and pediatrician perspectives. *Journal of Autism and Developmental Disorders, 40*(3), 317–324.

Chaidez, V., Hansen, R. L., & Hertz-Picciotto, I. (2014). Gastrointestinal problems in children with autism, developmental delays or typical development. *Journal of Autism and Developmental Disorders, 44*(5), 1117–1127.

Chandler, S., Carcani-Rathwell, I., Charman, T., Pickles, A., Loucas, T., Meldrum, D., . . . Baird, G. (2013). Parent-reported gastro-intestinal symptoms in children with autism spectrum disorders. *Journal of Autism and Developmental Disorders, 43*(12), 2737–2747.

Chawarska, K., Klin, A., Paul, R., & Volkmar, F. (2007). Autism spectrum disorder in the second year: Stability and change in syndrome expression. *Journal of Child Psychology and Psychiatry, 48*(2), 128–138.

Chawarska, K., Macari, S., Volkmar, F. R., Kim, S. H., & Shic, F. (2014a). ASD in infants and toddlers. *Handbook of autism and pervasive developmental disorders: Diagnosis, development, and brain mechanisms* (4th ed., Vol. 1., pp. 121–147). Hoboken, NJ, Wiley.

Chawarska, K., Shic, F., Macari, S., Campbell, D. J., Brian, J., Landa, R., . . . Bryson, S. (2014bs). 18-month predictors of later outcomes in younger siblings of children with autism spectrum disorder: A Baby Siblings Research Consortium study. *Journal of the American Academy of Child and Adolescent Psychiatry, 53*(12), 1317–1327.

Cheak-Zamora, N. C., & Farmer, J. E. (2015). The impact of the medical home on access to care for children with autism spectrum disorders. *Journal of Autism and Developmental Disorders, 45*(3), 636–644.

Cicchetti, D. V., Volkmar, F., Klin, A., & Showalter, D. (1995). Diagnosing autism using ICD-10 criteria: A comparison of neural networks and standard multivariate procedures. *Child Neuropsychology, 1*(1), 26–37.

Committee on Practice and Ambulatory Medicine and Bright Futures Periodicity Schedule Workgroup. (2016). 2016 recommendations for preventive pediatric health care. *Pediatrics, 137*, e20153908.

Committee on Practice and Ambulatory Medicine and Bright Futures Steering Committee. (2007). Recommendations for preventive pediatric health care, *Pediatrics, 120*(6), 1376.

Coury, D. (2010). Medical treatment of autism spectrum disorders. *Current Opinion in Neurology, 23*(2), 131–136.

Deonna, T., & Roulet-Perez, E. (2010). Early-onset acquired epileptic aphasia (Landau–Kleffner syndrome, LKS) and regressive autistic disorders with epileptic EEG abnormalities: The continuing debate. *Brain and Development, 32*(9), 746–752.

Durand, V. M. (2008). *When children don't sleep well: Interventions for pediatric sleep disorders, parent workbook.* New York: Oxford University Press.

Farmer, J. E., Clark, M. J., Mayfield, W. A., Cheak-Zamora, N., Marvin, A. R., & Law, P. A. (2014). The relationship between the medical home and unmet needs for children with autism spectrum disorders. *Maternal and Child Health Journal, 18*(3), 672–680.

Fombonne, E., & Chakrabarti, S. (2001). No evidence for a new variant of measles-mumps-rubella-induced autism. *Pediatrics, 108*(4), E58.

Gardener, H., Spiegelman, D., & Buka, S. L. (2009). Prenatal risk factors for autism: Comprehensive meta-analysis. *British Journal of Psychiatry, 195*(1), 7–14.

Gillberg, C., Billstedt, E., Sundh, V., & Gillberg, I. C. (2010). Mortality in autism: A prospective longitudinal community-based study. *Journal of Autism and Developmental Disorders, 40*(3), 352–357.

Goldman, S. E., Richdale, A. L., Clemons, T., & Malow, B. A. (2012). Parental sleep concerns in autism spectrum disorders: Variations from childhood to adolescence. *Journal of Autism and Developmental Disorders, 42*(4), 531–538.

Goldsmith, T. R. (2009). Using virtual reality enhanced behavioral skills training to teach street-crossing skills to children and adolescents with autism spectrum disorders. *Dissertation Abstracts International: Section B: The Sciences and Engineering, 69*(7-B), 4421.

Golnik, A., Scal, P., Wey, A.,& Gaillard, P. (2012). Autism-specific primary care medical home intervention. *Journal of Autism and Developmental Disorders 42*(6), 1087–1093.

Green, D., & Flanagan, D. (2008). Understanding the autistic dental patient. *General Dentistry, 56*(2), 167–171.

Grodberg, D., Siper, P., Jamison, J., Buxbaum, J. D., & Kolevzon, A. (2016). A simplified diagnostic observational assessment of autism spectrum disorder in early childhood. *Autism Research, 9*(4), 443–449.

Howlin, P. (2014). Outcomes in adults with autism spectrum disorders. *Handbook of autism and pervasive developmental disorders, Volume 1: Diagnosis, development, and brain mechanisms* (pp. 97–116). Hoboken, NJ: Wiley.

Hyman, S. L., & Johnson, J. K. (2012). Autism and pediatric practice: Toward a medical home. *Journal of Autism and Developmental Disorders, 42*(6), 1156–1164.

Ibañez, L. V., Stone, W. L., & Coonrod, E. E. (2014). Screening for autism in young children. *Handbook of autism and pervasive developmental disorders: Vol. 2. Assessment, interventions, and policy* (pp. 585–608). Hoboken, NJ: Wiley.

Institute of Medicine. (2004). *Immunization safety review: Vaccines and autism.* Washington DC: National Academies Press.

Isaksen, J., Bryn, V., Diseth, T. H., Heiberg, A., Schjolberg, S., & Skjeldal, O. H. (2013). Children with autism spectrum disorders—the importance of medical investigations. *European Journal of Paediatric Neurology, 17*(1), 68–76.

Johnson, C. P., Myers, S. M., & American Academy of Pediatrics Council on Children with Disabilities. (2007). Identification and evaluation of children with autism spectrum disorders. *Pediatrics, 120*(5), 1183–1215.

Kleinman, J. M., Robins, D. L., Ventola, P. E., Pandey, J., Boorstein, H. C., Esser, E. L., . . . Fein, D. (2008). The Modified Checklist for Autism in Toddlers: A follow-up study investigating the early detection of autism spectrum disorders. *Journal of Autism and Developmental Disorders, 38*(5), 827–839.

Knapp, C., Woodworth, L., Fernandez-Baca, D., Baron-Lee, J., Thompson, L., & Hinojosa, M. (2013). Factors associated with a patient-centered medical home among children with behavioral health conditions. *Maternal and Child Health Journal, 17*(9), 1658–1664.

Kobak, K. A., Stone, W. L., Wallace, E., Warren, Z., Swanson, A., & Robson, K. (2011). A web-based tutorial for parents of young children with autism: Results from a pilot study. *Telemedicine Journal and E-Health, 17*(10), 804–808.

Kuddo, T., & Nelson, K. B. (2003). How common are gastrointestinal disorders in children with autism? *Current Opinion in Pediatrics, 15*(3), 339–343.

Lai, B., Milano, M., Roberts, M. W., & Hooper, S. R. (2012). Unmet dental needs and barriers to dental care among children with autism spectrum disorders. *Journal of Autism and Developmental Disorders, 42*(7), 1294–1303.

Lerner, A. J. (2008). Treatment of pica behavior with olanzapine. *CNS Spectrums, 13*(1), 19.

Levy, S. E., Giarelli, E., Lee, L. C., Schieve, L. A., Kirby, R. S., Cunniff, C., . . . Rice, C. E. (2010). Autism spectrum disorder and co-occurring developmental, psychiatric, and medical conditions among children in multiple populations of the United States. *Journal of Developmental and Behavioral Pediatrics, 31*(4), 267–275.

Levy, S. E., & Hyman, S. L. (2003). Use of complementary and alternative treatments for children with autistic spectrum disorders is increasing. *Pediatric Annals, 32*(10), 685–691.

Lin, S. C., Margolis, B., Yu, S. M., & Adirim, T. A. (2014). The role of medical home in emergency department use for children with developmental disabilities in the United States. *Pediatric Emergency Care, 30*(8), 534–539.

Lord, C., Corsello, C., & Grzadzinski, R. (2014). Diagnostic instruments in autistic spectrum disorders. In F. R. Volkmar, S. J. Rogers, R. Paul, & K. A. Pelphrey (Eds.), *Handbook of autism and pervasive developmental disorders* (4th ed., Vol. 2, pp. 609–660). Hoboken, NJ: Wiley.

Lord, C., & Schopler, E. (1988). Intellectual and developmental assessment of autistic children from preschool to schoolage: Clinical implications of two follow-up studies. In E. Schopler & G. B. Mesibov (Ed.), *Diagnosis and assessment in autism: Current issues in autism* (pp. 167–181). New York: Springer Science+Business Media.

Lyall, K., Schmidt, R. J., & Hertz-Picciotto, I. (2014). Environmental factors in the preconception and prenatal periods in relation to risk for ASD. In F. R. Volkmar, R. Paul, S. J. Rogers, & K. A. Pelphrey (Eds.), *Handbook of autism and pervasive developmental disorders: Vol. 1. Diagnosis, development, and brain mechanisms* (pp. 424–456). Hoboken, NJ: Wiley.

Macari, S. L., Wu, G. C., Powell, K. K., Fontenelle, S., Macris, D. M., & Chawarska, K. (2018). Do parents and clinicians agree on ratings of autism-related behaviors at 12 months of age?: A study of infants at high and low risk for ASD. *Journal of Autism and Developmental Disorders, 48*(4), 1069–1080.

Magnus, P., Birke, C., Vejrup, K., Haugan, A., Alsaker, E., Daltveit, A. K., . . . Stoltenberg, C. (2016). Cohort profile update: The Norwegian Mother and Child Cohort Study (MoBa). *International Journal of Epidemiology, 45*(2), 382–388.

Majnemer, A., & Shevell, M. I. (1995). Diagnostic yield of the neurologic assessment of the developmentally delayed child [see Comments]. *Journal of Pediatrics, 127*(2), 193–199.

Malow, B. A., Adkins, K. W., McGrew, S. G., Wang, L., Goldman, S. E., Fawkes, D., & Burnette, C. (2012). Melatonin for sleep in children with autism: A controlled trial examining dose, tolerability, and outcomes: Erratum. *Journal of Autism and Developmental Disorders, 42*(8), 1738.

Marshall, J., Sheller, B., Williams, B. J., Mancl, L., & Cowan, C. (2007). Cooperation predictors for dental patients with autism. *Pediatric Dentistry, 29*(5), 369–376.

McClure, I. (2014). Developing and implementing practice guidelines. In F. R. Volkmar, R. Paul, S. J. Rogers, & K. A. Pelphrey (Eds.), *Handbook of autism and pervasive developmental disorders: Vol. 2. Assessment, interventions, and policy* (4th ed., pp. 1014–1035). Hoboken, NJ: Wiley.

McPheeters, M. L., Weitlauf, A., Vehorn, A., Taylor, C., Sathe, N. A., Krishnaswami, S., . . . Warren, Z. E. (2016). *Screening for autism spectrum disorder in young children*. Rockville, MD: Agency for Healthcare Research and Quality.

Mrozek-Budzyn, D., Kieltyka, A., & Majewska, R. (2010). Lack of association between measles–mumps–rubella vaccination and autism in children: A case-control study. *Pediatric Infectious Disease Journal, 29*(5), 397–400.

National Research Council. (2001). *Educating young children with autism*. Washington, DC: National Academy Press.

Odom, S. L., Boyd, B. A., Hall, L. J., & Hume, K. A. (2014). Comprehensive treatment models for children and youth with autism spectrum disorders. In F. R. Volkmar, R. Paul, S. J. Rogers, & K. A. Pelphrey (Eds.), *Handbook of autism and pervasive developmental disorders: Vol. 2. Assessment, interventions, and policy* (4th ed., pp. 770–787). Hoboken, NJ: Wiley.

Offit, P. (2008). *Autism's false prophets: Bad science, risky medicine, and the search for a cure*. New York: Columbia University Press.

Øien, R. A., Schjølberg, S., Volkmar, F. R., Shic, F., Cicchetti, D. V., Nordahl-Hansen, A., . . . Chawarska, K. (2018). Clinical features of children with autism who passed 18-month screening. *Pediatrics, 141*(6), e20173596.

Øien, R. A., Siper, P., Kolevzon, A., & Grodberg, D. (2016). Detecting autism spectrum disorder in children with ADHD and social disability. *Journal of Attention Disorders*. [Epub ahead of print]

Ozonoff, S., Iosif, A. M., Baguio, F., Cook, I. C., Hill, M. M., Hutman, T., . . . Young, G. S. (2010). A prospective study of the emergence of early behavioral signs of autism. *Journal of the American Academy of Child and Adolescent Psychiatry, 49*(3), 256–266.

Ozonoff, S., Young, G. S., Carter, A., Messinger, D., Yirmiya, N., Zwaigenbaum, L., . . . Stone, W. L. (2011). Recurrence risk for autism spectrum disorders: A baby siblings research consortium study. *Pediatrics, 128*(3), e488–e495.

Park, S., Cho, S.-C., Cho, I. H., Kim, B.-N., Kim, J.-W., Shin, M.-S., . . . Yoo, H. J. (2012). Sleep problems and their correlates and comorbid psychopathology of children with autism spectrum disorders. *Research in Autism Spectrum Disorders, 6*(3), 1068–1072.

Paul, R., & Fahim, D. (2015). *Let's talk: Navigating communication services and supports for your young child with autism*. Baltimore, MD: Brookes.

Piazza, C. C., Fisher, W. W., Hanley, G. P., LeBlanc, L. A., Worsdell, A. S., Lindauer, S. E., & Keeney, K. M. (1998). Treatment of pica through multiple analyses of its reinforcing functions. *Journal of Applied Behavior Analysis, 31*(2), 165–189.

Reichow, B., & Barton, E. E. (2014). Evidence-based psychosocial interventions for individuals with autism spectrum disorders. In F. R. Volkmar, R. Paul, S. J. Rogers, & K. A. Pelphrey (Eds.), *Handbook of autism and pervasive developmental disorders: Vol. 2. Assessment, interventions, and policy* (4th ed., pp. 969–992). Hoboken, NJ: Wiley.

Reichow, B., Halpern, J. I., Steinhoff, T. B., Letsinger, N., Naples, A., & Volkmar, F. R. (2012a). Characteristics and quality of autism websites. *Journal of Autism and Developmental Disorders, 42*(6), 1263–1274.

Reichow, B., Naples, A., Steinhoff, T., Halpern, J., & Volkmar, F. R. (2012b). Brief report: Consistency of search engine rankings for autism websites. *Journal of Autism and Developmental Disorders, 42*(6), 1275–1279.

Robins, D. L., Casagrande, K., Barton, M., Chen, C.-M.-A., Dumont-Mathieu, T., & Fein, D. (2014). Validation of the Modified Checklist for Autism in Toddlers, revised with follow-up (M-CHAT-R/F). *Pediatrics, 133*(1), 37–45.

Robins, D. L., Fein, D., Barton, M. L., & Green, J. A. (2001). The Modified Checklist for Autism in Toddlers: An initial study investigating the early detection of autism and pervasive developmental disorders. *Journal of Autism and Developmental Disorders, 31*(2), 131–144.

Rutter, M., Bailey, A., & Lord, C. (2003). *The Social Communication Questionnaire: Manual.* Los Angeles: Western Psychological Services.

Rutter, M., & Thapar, A. (2014). Genetics of autism spectrum disorders. In F. R. Volkmar, R. Paul, S. J. Rogers, & K. A. Pelphrey (Eds.), *Handbook of autism and pervasive developmental disorders: Vol. 1. Diagnosis, development, and brain mechanisms* (pp. 411–423). Hoboken, NJ: Wiley.

Schaefer, G. B., Mendelsohn, N. J., & Professional Practice and Guidelines Committee. (2013). Clinical genetics evaluation in identifying the etiology of autism spectrum disorders: 2013 guideline revisions. [Erratum appears in *Genetics in Medicine,* 2013, *15*(8), 669.] *Genetics in Medicine, 15*(5), 399–407.

Schopler, E., Van Bourgondian, M. E., Wellman, G. J., & Love, S. R. (2010). *The Childhood Autism Rating Scale* (2nd ed.) (CARS2). Los Angeles: Western Psychological Services.

Shavelle, R. M., & Strauss, D. (1998). Comparative mortality of persons with autism in California, 1980–1996. *Journal of Insurance Medicine (Seattle), 30*(4), 220–225.

Siu, A. L., U. S. Preventive Services Task Force (USPSTF), Bibbins-Domingo, K., Grossman, D. C., Baumann, L. C., Davidson, K. W., . . . Pignone, M. P. (2016). Screening for autism spectrum disorder in young children: U.S. Preventive Services Task Force recommendation statement. *Journal of the American Medical Association, 315*(7), 691–696.

Siperstein, R., & Volkmar, F. (2004). Brief report: Parental reporting of regression in children with pervasive developmental disorders. *Journal of Autism and Developmental Disorders, 34*(6), 731–734.

Smith, I. C., Reichow, B., & Volkmar, F. R. (2015). The effects of DSM-5 criteria on number of individuals diagnosed with autism spectrum disorder: A systematic review. *Journal of Autism and Developmental Disorders, 45*(8), 2541–2552.

Smith, M. J., Ellenberg, S. S., Bell, L. M., & Rubin, D. M. (2008). Media coverage of the measles-mumps-rubella vaccine and autism controversy and its relationship to MMR immunization rates in the United States. *Pediatrics, 121*(4), e836–e843.

Smith, T., Oakes, L., & Selver, K. (2014). Alternative treatments. In F. R. Volkmar, R. Paul, S. J. Rogers, & K. A. Pelphrey (Eds.), *Handbook of autism and pervasive developmental disorders: Vol. 2. Assessment, interventions, and policy* (4th ed., pp. 1051–1069). Hoboken, NJ: Wiley.

Solomon, O., & Lawlor, M. C. (2013). "And I look down and he is gone": Narrating autism, elopement and wandering in Los Angeles. *Social Science and Medicine, 94*, 106–114.

Stenberg, N. (2015). *Early features and identification of autism spectrum disorder* (C. Stoltenberg, Ed.). Oslo: Faculty of Social Sciences, University of Oslo.

Stenberg, N., Bresnahan, M., Gunnes, N., Hirtz, D., Hornig, M., Lie, K. K., . . . & Schjølberg, S. (2014). Identifying children with autism spectrum disorder at 18 months in a general population sample. *Paediatric and Perinatal Epidemiology, 28*(3), 255–262.

Stone, W. L., Coonrod, E. E., Turner, L. M., & Pozdol, S. L. (2004). Psychometric properties of the STAT for early autism screening. *Journal of Autism and Developmental Disorders, 34*(6), 691–701.

Tammimies, K., Marshall, C. R., Walker, S., Kaur, G., Thiruvahindrapuram, B., Lionel, A. C., . . . Fernandez, B. A. (2015). Molecular diagnostic yield of chromosomal microarray analysis and whole-exome sequencing in children with autism spectrum disorder. *JAMA, 314*(9), 895–903.

U.K. National Screening Committee. (2012, November 13). Screening for autistic spectrum disorders in children under the age of five: Policy position statement and summary. Retrieved July 3, 2017, from *https://legacyscreening.phe.org.uk/autism*.

Volkmar, F. R., Booth, L. L., McPartland, J. C., & Wiesner, L. A. (2014a). Clinical evaluation in multidisciplinary settings. In F. R. Volkmar, R. Paul, S. J. Rogers, & K. A. Pelphrey (Eds.), *Handbook of autism and pervasive developmental disorders: Assessment, interventions, and policy* (4th ed., Vol. 2, pp. 661–672). Hoboken, NJ: Wiley.

Volkmar, F., Siegel, M., Woodbury-Smith, M., King, B., McCracken, J., State, M., & American Academy of Child and Adolescent Psychiatry Committee on Quality Issues. (2014b). Practice parameter for the assessment and treatment of children and adolescents with autism spectrum disorder. *Journal of the American Academy of Child and Adolescent Psychiatry, 53*(2), 237–257.

Volkmar, F. R., & Wiesner, L. (2017). *Essential clincial guide to understanding and treating autism*. Hoboken, NJ, Wiley.

Wakefield, A. J. (1999). MMR vaccination and autism. *The Lancet, 354*(9182), 949–950.

Wang, L. W., Tancredi, D. J., & Thomas, D. W. (2011). The prevalence of gastrointestinal problems in children across the United States with autism spectrum disorders from families with multiple affected members. *Journal of Developmental and Behavioral Pediatrics, 32*(5), 351–360.

Warren, Z., McPheeters, M. L., Sathe, N., Foss-Feig, J. H., Glasser, A., & Veenstra-VanderWeele, J. (2011). A systematic review of early intensive intervention for autism spectrum disorders. *Pediatrics, 127*(5), e1303–e1311.

Warren, Z., Stone, W., & Humberd, Q. (2009). A training model for the diagnosis of autism in community pediatric practice. *Journal of Developmental and Behavioral Pediatrics, 30*(5), 442–446.

Whitehouse, A. J. O., Evans, K., Eapen, V., & Wray, J. (2018). *A national guideline for the assessment and diagnosis of autism spectrum disorders in Australia*. Brisbane, Australia: Cooperative Research Centre for Living with Autism.

Wilson, C., Roberts, G., Gillan, N., Ohlsen, C., Robertson, D., & Zinkstok, J. (2014). The NICE guideline on recognition, referral, diagnosis and management of adults on the autism spectrum. *Advances in Mental Health and Intellectual Disabilities, 8*(1), 3–14.

Yuen, T., Carter, M. T., Szatmari, P., & Ungar, W. J. (2018). Cost-effectiveness of universal or high-risk screening compared to surveillance monitoring in autism spectrum disorder. *Journal of Autism and Developmental Disorders, 48*(9), 2968–2979.

CHAPTER 10

• • • • • • • • •

Advancing Technology to Meet the Needs of Infants and Toddlers at Risk for Autism Spectrum Disorder

Frederick Shic, Kelsey Jackson Dommer, Adham Atyabi,
Marilena Mademtzi, Roald A. Øien, Julie A. Kientz,
and Jessica Bradshaw

Technology permeates our daily lives. Increasing miniaturization, computing power, and connectivity have transformed what once fell under the realm of science fiction into everyday reality. In this chapter, we examine the increasingly diverse roles that technology plays in the lives of infants and toddlers with or at high risk for autism spectrum disorder (ASD). We specifically focus on the novel ways everyday technologies have supported, and will continue to support, positive behavioral change and phenotyping and, ultimately, impact lives.[1]

This chapter is divided into several parts. First, we discuss the physical and cognitive characteristics of early, typical development from 6 to 36 months of age, with an eye toward the constraints these characteristics impose on technology. We contrast these typical developmental trajectories with the atypical trajectories and phenotypic presentations associated with ASD. With an understanding of these capacities and opportunities in mind, we examine the methods by which technological advancements have supported new initiatives into digital phenotyping and how these initiatives, in turn, point toward progress in screening, diagnosis, and capturing individual variation. Next, we examine how technologies have augmented traditional areas of therapy and the unique role this augmentation may play in therapies designed for ASD. Finally, we discuss how a convergence of interdisciplinary advances—across fields of engineering, computer science, developmental science, medicine, and psychology—will pave the way

---

[1] For a broader, in-depth discussion of interactive technologies for individuals with ASD across the lifespan, see Kientz, Goodwin, Hayes, and Abowd (2013).

for the increasing capacity of everyday technologies to advance our understanding of autism and how to define and achieve optimal outcomes.

Physical Attributes: Technology Considerations

Technologies that have seen increasing prominence in recent years for their potential for diagnostic and therapeutic purposes include wearable data collection devices (e.g., activity trackers; Burton et al., 2013; Reinertsen & Clifford, 2018; Tahmasian, Khazaie, Golshani, & Avis, 2013); smart glasses (Firouzian, Asghar, Tervonen, Pulli, & Yamamoto, 2015; Liu, Salisbury, Vahabzadeh, & Sahin, 2017); always-on video and voice-recording systems (Doherty et al., 2013; Dykstra et al., 2013); head-mounted eye trackers (Kim et al., 2014; Vidal, Turner, Bulling, & Gellersen, 2012); augmented and virtual reality systems (Freeman et al., 2017; Turner & Casey, 2014); interactive media (e.g., tablets and smartphones [Bakker, Kazantzis, Rickwood, & Rickard, 2016]); interactive computer games (Horne-Moyer, Moyer, Messer, & Messer, 2014); and passive media (e.g., instructional aids and videos watchable on portable devices such as those described in Golan et al., 2010, and Popple et al., 2016).

Many of these technologies were originally designed with older children or adult users in mind. There has been a recent push to apply these technologies to research on younger populations. However, additional developmental considerations must be made before such technologies can be appropriately used in infant and toddler populations (Lueder & Rice, 2007). These considerations include designing systems that account for the physical size, weight, strength, and motor skills of the child, as well as the unique characteristics of children with ASD in the early developmental period. These attributes change dramatically over the course of early development, with additional individual differences originating from biological (e.g., sex, genetics) and environmental (e.g., nutrition, family dynamics) sources.

Size and Morphology

Body size and shape should be considered during equipment design. Examples include systems that are worn on a child's head, such as head-mounted eye-tracking systems or smart glasses. Among other factors, the physical dimensions of the head will vary in terms of both the age and sex of the child (Table 10.1). The presence of this variability suggests that developers of technological systems worn by infants and toddlers should include, as a key aspect of design, flexibility in accommodating the significant scope of physical form.

For children with or at risk for autism spectrum disorder (ASD), or for children who ultimately develop the disorder, the extent of this variation

TABLE 10.1. Physical Characteristics of Typically Developing Infants and Toddlers

Age	Head circumference (cm)		Weight (kg)		Height (cm)	
	Male	Female	Male	Female	Male	Female
6 months	41.1–46.2	40.1–44.9	6.3–9.9	5.7–9.0	62.2–72.6	60.2–70.4
12 months	44.1–48.6	42.8–47.3	8.5–12.6	7.9–11.6	70.4–81.2	68.4–79.1
24 months	46.3–51.0	45.1–49.8	10.6–15.3	10.1–14.7	81.1–93.5	79.6–92.0
36 months	48.6–52.3	46.0–51.2	12.0–17.5	11.5–17.4	89.3–102.9	88.0–101.7
Adult	54.4–58.4	52.7–56.4	57.4–106.0	47.9–92.3	167.1–186.3	154.7–171.1

Note. Infant and toddler data are 5th–95th percentile range ±2 weeks age in months (adapted from Kuczmarski et al., 2000). Adult ranges are 10th–90th percentiles at 18 years (height and weight: McDowell, Fryar, Ogden, & Flegal, 2008; head circumference: Rollins, Collins, & Holden, 2010).

can be even more extreme. For example, children with both microcephaly and macrocephaly are at increased risk for ASD (Fombonne, Rogé, Claverie, Courty, & Frémolle, 1999), with some children who develop ASD (especially some with known genetic conditions, such as phosphatase and tensin homolog (PTEN) mutations) falling up to 8 standard deviations outside normative head size (Butler et al., 2005). These effects are not only limited to the head; prior work has suggested that children with ASD are, on average, larger in all body dimensions, as compared to control groups (Campbell, Chang, & Chawarska, 2014; Chawarska et al., 2011). As a consequence, technological systems that do not accommodate for extreme variation could risk omitting key groups that are at enhanced risk for ASD—whose physical size may vary into the 99th percentile—from study or application.

Adaptation to the physical form is not limited, however, only to dimensional variance. For example, Miles and colleagues (2005) have examined the increased prevalence of facial dysmorphology in ASD, noting a wide variability that could potentially be considered a natural subgroup within the autism spectrum. The presence of significant dysmorphology in some individuals with ASD emphasizes the need for flexibility in a priori assumptions about the *relationships* between physical features (e.g., distance between the eyes relative to overall size of the head when considering glasses-based technologies), in addition to their range.

Strength and Musculature

Following the question "Does it fit?" one should ask, "Can it be worn?" While also impacted by motor coordination skills, the development of sufficient physical strength is a key aspect of the wearability, manipulability, and usability of technologies for infants and toddlers. Typically, 2-month-old infants will bob their heads when held sitting, but by 4 months they no longer show head lag when pulled to a sitting position (Gerber, Wilks, & Erdie-Lalena, 2010). Moreover, handgrip strength doubles from the first year after birth to the second and triples by the third (Taguchi, Endo, Kurita, & Tamura, 2017), radically changing the ability to both hold and manipulate objects in the environment.

In children with ASD, assumptions regarding sufficiency of strength do not necessarily follow those expected by their typically developing (TD) peers. While studies have been limited, especially in infants, current evidence suggests that older children with ASD show weaker grip strength than TD children (Kern et al., 2013), with the weakness of grip strength associated with increased severity of autism symptoms (Kern et al., 2011). Reduced strength in ASD may limit the usability of some devices.

Diminished physical strength may also play a role in the motor difficulties observed in infant siblings of children with ASD as early as 6 months of age (Iverson et al., 2019). Research has shown that these infant siblings (who are at greater risk for developing ASD themselves) develop postural control in sitting or standing positions later than infants at low risk for developing ASD (Nickel, Thatcher, Keller, Wozniak, & Iverson, 2013). Furthermore, infants who are later diagnosed with ASD show even more impoverished repertoires of motor skills (Nickel et al., 2013). Similarly, high-risk infant siblings and infants later diagnosed with ASD are more likely to show head lag when pulled from a supine to a sitting position (Flanagan, Landa, Bhat, & Bauman, 2012).

Deviation from prototypical expectations of physical strength is yet another consideration in the design of technologies for infants and toddlers with or at risk for ASD. Evidence for diminished muscle strength in this population in early development suggests that lightweight, wieldy designs may be particularly appropriate. Advances in miniaturization, portability, and ability to offload computation via wireless communication make such developments increasingly feasible and may serve to mitigate disparities in application accessibility.

Physical Ability and Motor Skills

In typical development, as children grow physically in size and strength, they also reach major motor milestones, as highlighted in Table 10.2 (American Academy of Pediatrics, 2014, 2017). The specific timing, and even the order, of the attainment of these milestones is highly variable (Vereijken, 2010; Vereijken & Adolph, 1999). Beyond interindividual heterogeneity, acquisition of motor skills during development within an individual is subject to variation in form, function, frequency, and prominence

TABLE 10.2. Physical Ability Milestones in Typical Development

Age	Typical milestones
6 months	• Starts to sit unsupported • Passes objects from one hand to the other
9 months	• Sits unsupported and maneuvers self into seated position • Can pull up to standing and stands with support • Starts to crawl • Can pick up objects with two fingers
12 months	• Pulls up to standing position and walks while holding on to support • Might stand alone or take a few independent steps • Puts items in and takes items out of containers • Points with one finger (and could presumably tap screen with one finger)
18 months	• Walks independently • Needs help in coordinated physical activities (e.g., getting dressed)
24 months	• Is coordinated enough to kick a ball or throw overhand • Can copy or create straight lines and circles with writing tool
36 months	• Is coordinated enough to climb, run, and walk independently up and down stairs • Comfortably holds and uses writing utensil • Works more easily with toys with buttons or moving parts

Note. Adapted from American Academy of Pediatrics (2014, 2017).

as children age. This variation is developmentally meaningful, providing signals regarding neurophysiological and physiological integrity and maturation (Hadders-Algra, 2010; Piek, 2002; Shic & Scassellati, 2007; Thelen, 1995).

In children with ASD, deficits are evident from as early as 6 or 12 months of age in both gross and fine motor skills (as compared to chronological age expectations) and continue to compound as they grow older (Iverson et al., 2019; Lloyd, MacDonald, & Lord, 2013). Although the presence of motor issues in the toddler years is not specific to ASD (Hill, 2001; Shevell, Majnemer, Rosenbaum, & Abrahamowicz, 2001), some evidence suggests that by the second birthday, motor deficits may be especially pronounced, even when compared to toddlers with non-ASD atypical development (Matson, Mahan, Fodstad, Hess, & Neal, 2010). Repertoires of motor skills and movements may be limited and/or less refined or coordinated as compared to chronologically age-matched peers (Esposito, Venuti, Apicella, & Muratori, 2011; Hadders-Algra, 2008). Early motor deficits have been shown to have an impact on later-emerging social and communicative abilities in ASD (Bhat, Galloway, & Landa, 2012; Hellendoorn et al., 2015; Iverson, 2010; LeBarton & Iverson, 2013; Leonard, Bedford, Pickles, Hill, & Team, 2015), potentially due to their seemingly intertwined nature (Bhat, Landa, & Galloway, 2011). While it is important to include accommodations for delayed or deficient motor skills when designing technology, it is equally important to interpret the results of said technology—which will likely demonstrate social, adaptive, or communicative deficits—bearing in mind the reciprocal impact of motor and social communication domains.

Repetitive Behaviors

The occurrence of repetitive motor and self-stimulatory behaviors (e.g., body rocking, arm waving, hand flapping, repetitive object manipulation such as spinning or flipping) is common in typical development and can be considered developmentally appropriate from ages 1 to 4 years (Leekam et al., 2007; Lewis, 2013; Singer, 2009; Subki et al., 2017; Thelen, 1980), resolving as children age (Evans et al., 1997). Research suggests that the presence of greater rhythmical stereotyped movements (stereotypies) is associated with decreased vestibular stimulation (e.g., rocking and bouncing by caregivers) in infants during the first year of life (Thelen, 1980). There appears to be a general relationship between lack of environmental sensory or psychosocial stimulation and stereotypic behaviors, as evidenced by increased rates of stereotypies in blind children (Tröster, Brambring, & Beelmann, 1991) and children with a history of early institutional care (Bos, Zeanah, Smyke, Fox, & Nelson, 2010). Interestingly, stereotypies such as rhythmic body rocking in older deaf children are elevated (Bachara & Phelan, 1980) but seem to be associated with the presence of other comorbid conditions such as vision impairment, learning disability, or autism (Murdoch, 1996).

As compared to typically developing children and children with intellectual disability, children with ASD show increased rates of repetitive sensory motor behaviors in the toddler period between 18 and 24 months of age (Barber, Wetherby, & Chambers, 2012; Lewis & Kim, 2009; Morgan, Wetherby, & Barber, 2008; Watt, Wetherby, Barber, & Morgan, 2008). Specific patterns of repetitive stereotyped behaviors noted by Barber and colleagues (2012) include increased rates in ASD of self-body rubbing, finger stiffening, sensory licking, and object manipulations that include spinning, rolling, moving, clutching, and swiping, as well as decreased rates of banging surfaces with the body. It has been hypothesized that these behaviors serve either to diminish overarousal and maintain sensory homeostatic equilibrium (Hutt, Hutt, Lee, & Ounsted, 1964), or to provide perceptually self-reinforcing sensory stimulation (Lovaas, 1987), among other theories (for a review, see Turner, 1999). Furthermore, elevated rates of repetitive behaviors and atypical object exploration are evident as early as 12 months in infants who have siblings with ASD that eventually develop ASD themselves (Ozonoff et al., 2008; Wolff et al., 2014).

Because restricted, repetitive, and stereotyped behaviors (RRSBs) constitute a core feature of ASD (American Psychiatric Association, 2013), their targeted measurement and quantification through technological systems (e.g., video cameras and computer vision, wearable actigraphy [motion tracking]) are of interest in their own right (discussed in subsequent sections). However, the elevated presence of these behaviors in ASD, and their primary expression in typical development, are points of concern for the design and interpretation of interactive and passive monitoring technologies. First, body movements are known to interfere with multiple technological measurement modalities, particularly (but not limited to) those of an electrical or magnetic form (e.g., electrodermal activity, electroencephalography, magnetic resonance imaging; Brunner et al., 1996; Friston, Williams, Howard, Frackowiak, & Turner, 1996; Gwin, Gramann, Makeig, & Ferris, 2010; Power, Barnes, Snyder, Schlaggar, & Petersen, 2012). For potentially affected measurement modalities, the identification, categorization, and classification of repetitive actions as a separate state for either artifact detection or algorithmic compensation could help prevent inflation of group differences between ASD and control groups (due to the differential expression of RRSBs as they wax and wane through development). Second, the commonality of RRSBs during early development suggests that technological systems designed to operate interactively with infants and toddlers should be designed for robustness against rough and unexpected manipulation and handling. Third, scenarios designed to test or use technologies should consider the potential presence and disruption to the scenario that could be caused by RRSBs. That is, just as the devices should be physically robust to handling, so protocols meant to utilize technologies should be robust to protocol deviations that relate to RRSBs' heterogeneity across development, groups, and individuals. For example, a task that measures cognitive performance in a building task by the number of discrete physical actions taken to achieve a goal may not want to overly penalize RRSBs in the same manner as they would penalize erroneous object placements; a study examining control of virtual objects through hand movements may consider temporal smoothing of object trajectories to mitigate jerky responses caused by repetitive motor behaviors; and protocols with fixed time limits on experimental phases may consider providing greater flexibility for participants with significant RRSBs.

Together with variations in form, strength, and coordination, this section reaffirms our overarching theme that the design of technology for infants and toddlers needs to account for extremely wide ranges of ability, sizes, and child characteristics. Appropriate consideration of this variability will help ensure that individuals at the extreme ends of the bell curve are not left out of the research and development of technologies for infants and toddlers with ASD.

Cognitive/Perceptual Attributes

Development of Sensory Systems

The development of sensory systems, as compared to the development of sensory sensitivity profiles (next section), is another domain of infant and toddler development that demands consideration when developing technological equipment and designing technology-related research studies.

Primary sensory systems, including sight, hearing, and touch, mature rapidly in the first few years after birth in TD infants. For example, visual contrast grating acuity increases 4- to 10-fold during the first year of life, likely supported by foveal maturation, cone migration, and cortically driven spatiotemporal tuning (Wilson, 1988; Yuodelis & Hendrickson, 1986). Contrast grating acuity and high-frequency temporal flicker sensitivity continue to increase up to adult levels by 6–7 years of age (Ellemberg, Lewis, Hong Liu, & Maurer, 1999). Similarly, chromatic detection sensitivity increases by a factor of 30 between 3 months of age, when most TD infants show some color vision (Brown, 1990), and adolescence, with detection thresholds decreasing by a factor of 2 with each doubling of age (Knoblauch, Vital-Durand, & Barbur, 2001).

Compared to visual systems, basic auditory sensory systems are already well developed at birth, with evidence for prenatal programming of auditory processing systems, including newborn sensitivity to maternal voice (Hepper, Scott, & Shahidullah, 1993; Spence & DeCasper, 1987) and native language (Mehler et al., 1988; Moon, Cooper, & Fifer, 1993). As outlined by Werner (2007), early human auditory development can be divided into three stages: (1) maturation of neural encoding of sound postnatally until 6 months of age, during which detection thresholds for especially high-pitch sounds decrease rapidly (e.g., see Tharpe & Ashmead, 2001), reaching adult-like competencies for some tasks (Olsho, Koch, & Halpin, 1987); (2) increasing ability to isolate acoustic cues (e.g., the ability to detect tones in noise, see Leibold & Werner, 2006) and to identify and leverage new cues in decision making (e.g., as evidenced by training for low-frequency tone discrimination in children; Soderquist & Moore, 1970; Zaltz, Ari-Even Roth, Karni, & Kishon-Rabin, 2018), beginning at around 6 months postnatally and extending into the early school years; and (3) increasing flexibility in use of acoustic information extending from early school age through adolescence (e.g., the selective use of multiple auditory cues; see Hazan & Barrett, 2000).

Touch, however, is considered to be the earliest developing sensory system, with reports of embryonic responses to light stroking of the face from as early as 6 weeks gestational age (Montagu, 1986). The cutaneous sensory system, which encompasses tactile, heat, pain, itch, and possibly affiliative or affective sensation, develops rapidly prenatally and during the early postnatal period (McGlone & Reilly, 2010), with multisensory spatial and temporal discrimination capacity available at birth (Filippetti, Johnson, Lloyd-Fox, Dragovic, & Farroni, 2013; Filippetti, Orioli, Johnson, & Farroni, 2015); posture-invariant tactile response developing between 6.5 and 10 months (Bremner, Mareschal, Lloyd-Fox, & Spence, 2008); and body self-awareness maturing through the toddler years (Brownell, Zerwas, & Ramani, 2007).

Across the lifespan, studies have indicated a higher prevalence of atypicalities in sensory system performance in ASD. For instance, recent reviews have indicated higher rates of ophthalmologic and visual impairment (e.g., strabismus) in individuals with ASD relative to the general population (Butchart et al., 2017; Ikeda, Davitt, Ultmann, Maxim, & Cruz, 2013). Interestingly, in terms of psychophysical assessment, several studies have also reported on greater visual discrimination ability in certain task and population contexts in ASD (Bertone, Mottron, Jelenic, & Faubert, 2003, 2005; see Mottron, Dawson, Soulieres, Hubert, & Burack, 2006, for perspectives; see Simmons et al., 2009, for a review). Likewise, auditory impairments, including hearing loss, are also common in ASD (Hitoglou, Ververi, Antoniadis, & Zafeiriou, 2010; O'Connor, 2012; Rosenhall, Nordin, Sandström, Ahlsén, & Gillberg, 1999; Rydzewska et al., 2018). As with vision, islets of increased performance have been reported in auditory tasks in some individuals with ASD (Bonnel et al., 2003). As compared to visual or auditory impairment, examination of impairments associated with touch is less well studied in ASD. Initial reports, primarily based on anecdotal clinical or parent observation, suggested patterns of hyposensitivity to pain in ASD, but definitive evidence of this and of associated opioid enhancement models in ASD are limited (Allely, 2013; Moore, 2015; Whiteley & Shattock, 2002). Recent research and perspectives suggest that observations of pain hyposensitivity may be conflated with atypical expression of pain in ASD (Allely, 2013; Nader, Oberlander, Chambers, & Craig, 2004). In parallel, however, multiple studies have highlighted atypical tactile or somatosensory neurophysiological profiles in ASD and individuals exhibiting traits associated with ASD, consistent both neurophysiologically and psychophysically with deficit models, especially in areas related to affective touch (Cascio et al., 2008, 2012; Kaiser et al., 2016; Puts, Wodka, Tommerdahl, Mostofsky, & Edden, 2014; Voos, Pelphrey, & Kaiser, 2013).

These results have implications for technology development. Even in typical development, the rapid maturation of sensation-related capability, both within specific sensory modalities and cooperatively across modalities, impacts the perception and presumed salience of delivered cues, especially at younger ages. These maturational processes are context specific, with physical maturation of sensing capacities (e.g., visual acuity) acting as a base on which higher-order, more cognitively advanced skills (e.g., object recognition) are built. For infants and toddlers with increased risk for ASD, the increased prevalence of fundamental sensory system deficits is an additional consideration: presumption regarding the accessibility of technological affordances to these children is a concern above and beyond typical concerns of developmental-level appropriateness.

Sensory–Behavioral Profiles

Sensory profiles (which can include hyporesponsiveness, hyperresponsiveness, sensitivity, and sensory-seeking in Dunn's [2014] model) have long been considered a facet of a child's temperamental characteristics (Carey, 1970; Colombo & Fagen, 2014; Fullard, McDevitt, & Carey, 1984; Thomas & Chess, 1968; Thomas, Chess, Birch, Hertzig, & Korn, 1963). Systematic relationships among sensory profiles, developmental outcomes, and clinically relevant phenotypes have made the study of sensory sensitivities and responses an area of continued and active research in infancy and the toddler years (Carey, 1972; Dunn & Daniels, 2002; Nakagawa, Sukigara, Miyachi, & Nakai, 2016; O'boyle & Rothbart, 1996). As expected of features associated with child temperament, significant variations in sensory profiles are evident even in typical populations. However, the uncommon nature of some specific forms of sensitivities increases the utility of sensory profiling for understanding or predicting clinical conditions such as anxiety, depression, ADHD, and ASD (Dunn & Bennett, 2002; Engel-Yeger et al., 2016; Ermer & Dunn, 1998; Green & Ben-Sasson, 2010; Robertson & Baron-Cohen, 2017). In ASD, sensory profiles can be quite heterogeneous, with recent studies highlighting the possible existence of sensory-based subtypes within the spectrum (see DeBoth & Reynolds, 2017, for a review; cf. Little, Dean, Tomchek, & Dunn, 2017, in typical development). These efforts note a range of impacted sensory systems (e.g., touch, taste, sounds) as well as extended variability both in the clinical significance of impairment (from severe to minor to not present) and the sensory profile presentation (e.g., higher prevalence of both hyporesponsivity as well as overresponsivity; for recent perspectives on unified nomenclature and profiling, see Schaaf & Lane, 2015).

Sensory issues are more prevalent in toddlers with ASD than in toddlers with other developmental disabilities as well with typical development (Rogers, Hepburn, & Wehner, 2003). Recent work has shown that toddlers with ASD, compared to both their chronologically-age-matched and mental-age-matched typical peers, show lower awareness and more avoidance, but also higher sensitivity to sensations, suggesting an extreme sensory modulation profile for toddlers with ASD (Ben-Sasson et al., 2007). Subgroup cluster analysis in 170 toddlers with ASD revealed several clusters of sensory behaviors, with approximately half of the toddlers belonging to a cluster with higher frequencies of both under- and overresponsivity together with lower sensory seeking, and two groups of approximately equal proportion, one demonstrating low levels of sensory symptoms and the other demonstrating high levels (Ben-Sasson et al., 2008). In 2-year-old toddlers with ASD, sensory overresponsivity is predictive of comorbid anxiety symptoms 1 year later (Green, Ben-Sasson, Soto, & Carter, 2012). In even younger infants, prospective studies have highlighted atypical visual behaviors toward objects (e.g. peering) between 12 and 18 months of age in infants later diagnosed with ASD (Ozonoff et al., 2008; Zwaigenbaum et al., 2005, 2009) as well as potentially inhibited development of more efficient and flexible visual-orienting behaviors (Elsabbagh et al., 2013).

These results highlight the high prevalence of sensory issues in infants and toddlers with ASD as well as its heterogeneity across the spectrum. For this reason, it is important to consider the temperamental characteristics of the individual infant or toddler, and, more specifically, their sensory sensitivities, lack of sensitivities, and response behaviors, in the design and deployment of technology-based systems. This could include incorporation of longer periods of acclimation or protracted desensitization as well as other behavioral techniques as commonly applied in varied fields from dentistry (Hernandez & Ikkanda, 2011; Luscre & Center, 1996) to MRI (Nordahl et al., 2016), including positive praise, visual schedules, presentation of choices, and use of preferred reinforcers. These technological systems could also include increased flexibility with regard to specific sensory qualities of interactive technologies, so as to best adapt to the needs of an individual child (e.g., outer layers of physical devices that could be swapped for different tactile properties; adjustment of the brightness, refresh rates, or visual qualities of video monitors; customizable filters; or selections for sounds and noises). In addition, the high frequency of sensory-related issues experienced by children with ASD highlights the utility of sensory profiling prior to technology use, as well as the design of deployment protocols that flexibly accommodate for a wide range of sensory-related responses (including aversion). Finally, it is important to note that sensory underresponsivity also frequently occurs in toddlers with ASD. While underresponsivity to sensory cues of a social or communicative origin overlap with the fundamental social interaction deficits in ASD, underresponsivity to other environmental sensations, such as loud sounds and bright or flashing lights, can also occur. For this reason, cues for guiding attention toward specific attributes of a technological system (e.g., buttons meant to be pressed) may benefit from multimodal designs (e.g., including synchronized flashing of lights with sounds), and the interpretation of technology usage should consider hyper- and hyposensory perspectives in addition to core social autism symptoms.

Cognitive Development[2]

Cognitive development, encompassing attention, memory, and language processes, drives the way in which infants and toddlers construct, organize, and interact with their environment. Many cognitive skills, particularly language, are learned via repeated, affectively laden social interactions with caregivers. It may not be surprising, then, that normative acquisition of cognitive milestones is delayed in many children with ASD. For some, these delays appear as early as 6 months of age (Estes et al., 2015). Research suggests that neurodevelopmental systems supporting cognitive development, including sustained attention, cognitive flexibility, executive functioning, and social reward systems, are atypical for children with ASD (O'Hearn, Asato, Ordaz, & Luna, 2008). Delayed achievement of cognitive milestones (see Table 10.3) is a common first concern for parents, and cognitive deficits are among the most comorbid features of ASD (Barbaro & Dissanayake, 2012; Zwaigenbaum, Bryson, & Garon, 2013). Language delays occur in about 60% of children with ASD (May et al., 2018), and about 44% of children with ASD are also diagnosed with intellectual disability (Baio, 2012). Attention-deficit/hyperactivity disorder (ADHD) is also highly comorbid, with rates of dual ADHD and ASD diagnoses ranging from 50 to 83% (May et al., 2018).

Although many children with ASD exhibit atypical cognitive functioning, there remains a substantial proportion of the ASD population for whom these abilities are relatively preserved (for perspectives, see Happé, 1999; Mottron et al., 2006). Underlying this phenotypic heterogeneity may be even more variable biological and neural pathways leading to ability and disability (Happé, Ronald, & Plomin, 2006). Technology can not only help to capture key elements of highly variable cognitive profiles in infants and toddlers with ASD, but can also link the behavioral phenotype with specific neural underpinnings. Moreover, cognitive differences create unique challenges for traditional assessment and treatment methods, which technology may be able to overcome. For example, classic theory of mind tasks require robust receptive language skills, but creative use of technology can

---

[2]The cognitive and psychological development of infants and toddlers with or at high risk for autism is more extensively discussed by Emily Campi, Catherine Lord, and Rebecca Grzadzinski (Chapter 2, this volume) and Jonathan Green (Chapter 8, this volume).

TABLE 10.3. Cognitive Ability Milestones Applicable to Technology Assessment and Intervention

Age	Typical milestones
6 months	• Knows familiar faces compared to a stranger • Babbles • Responds to name • Demonstrates sustained attention
9 months	• Understands "no" • Imitates sounds and gestures • Watches path of moving objects • Searches for hidden objects
12 months	• Asks for help by giving objects or pointing • Repeats sounds/actions to get attention • Responds to simple directions/requests • Understands and uses basic communicative gestures (waving, shaking head, etc.) • Tries to repeat words • Looks at pictures of named objects
18 months	• Hands objects to others to initiate play (joint attention/prompt to engage) • Has several-word expressive vocabulary • Scribbles for fun • Follows one-step directions without any informative gestures
24 months	• Imitates complex actions • Includes other children in play • Points to object being named • Sorts by shape/color • Engages in pretend play • Follows a two-step instruction
36 months	• Takes turns • Understands concept of "mine" versus "yours" • Follows instruction with two to three steps • Completes three- to four-piece puzzles

Note. Adapted from American Academy of Pediatrics (2014, 2017).

evaluate the same construct in the absence of language (Senju, Southgate, White, & Frith, 2009). Still, it is imperative to consider how these cognitive differences may constrain the application of technology and interpretation of findings.

The use of technology with children with ASD without consideration for cognitive differences can lead to inherent, unintended bias. Consider the use of eye tracking in children with ASD. Verbal and nonverbal cues to "look at the screen" or "stay still" may be less effective for children with communicative issues. Visual and auditory aspects of experimental and calibration stimuli may be more or less distracting to infants with varying attention regulation and impulse control abilities. Other technologies may rely on imitation (e.g., "push this button like me") and social reward strategies, both of which may be less effective for children with ASD. Because many of these skills are naturally robust in TD children, researchers may not even realize the extent to which their procedures rely on these abilities and therefore confound task performance with task comprehension.

Furthermore, children with ASD and cognitive deficits are all too frequently excluded from participation in technology-based studies. The equipment and procedures are usually novel for children with ASD, which can be challenging for those with cognitive inflexibility and impaired language skills. Many technology-based operations are lengthy, and participants are subject to significant wait time for setup and calibration procedures. Intellectual, language, and attention deficits make this process extremely challenging and sometimes impossible.

On the other hand, technology may provide a new way for children with ASD to organize and construct their world in a way that better matches their cognitive style. As such, technological advances hold an enormous opportunity for treatment of specific deficits.

Technological Methods Augmenting Screening and Phenotyping[3]

The development of systems for augmenting early identification of autism symptoms and for tracking the presentation of children with ASD has been and continues to be a prominent and concerted area of clinical and research activity. Digital or technology-based platforms offer multiple avenues for examining early indicators of autism and for tracking the progression of the condition across development. Broadly, digital systems used in phenotyping

---

[3] More details on early screening and diagnosis are presented by Fred R. Volkmar and Roald Øien (Chapter 1, this volume).

infants and toddlers can be broken into two categories: those that obtain information through a secondary source (e.g., parent-based questionnaires) and those that take their measurements directly from children (e.g., video-based annotation of behaviors).

Advantages of Translating Traditional Screening Systems to a Digital Format

Screening measures used to detect the earliest signs of developmental risk (in infancy and toddlerhood) rely predominantly on parent-report measures. One of the most straightforward applications of technology to early screening is the translation of traditionally pen-and-paper surveys and interviews into a digital format. Despite its straightforwardness, the use of a digital format offers several advantages, as highlighted by Harrington, Bai, and Perkins (2013) in a paper describing a deployment of an electronic version of the widely used Modified Checklist for Autism in Toddlers (M-CHAT; Robins, Fein, Barton, & Green, 2001). First, scoring can be automated rather than calculated by hand. In Harrington's study, 17% of paper M-CHATs were scored incorrectly, and one-third of those mistakes led to an erroneous assessment of autism risk.

Second, a digital format offers the possibility of streamlining questions through serial presentation of choice-and-branching logic. For example, in the more recent M-CHAT-R/F (Revised with Follow-Up), an initial battery of 20 questions administered to parents classifies toddlers into three risk groups: low, medium, and high. Toddlers in the low-risk group are considered likely negatives for ASD, and those in the high-risk category are immediately recommended for referral for formal diagnosis and early intervention services. The medium-risk category, however, warrants greater scrutiny. Traditionally, an interview is conducted with caregivers to further clarify the child's risk. This interview involves a prescribed set of questions, with subsequent questions dependent on prior answers. Although such a process is highly effective when administered by a trained administrator, it relies on additional personnel to conduct the interview. This inserts a lag, which can be considerable given that parents may have left the screening site by the time the instrument is scored and can result in data loss if caregivers are unable to be contacted for follow-up. The use of digital branching logic atop automated scoring can efficiently deliver follow-up questions as needed, resulting in less use of human resources (especially in follow-up), a more streamlined experience for caregivers, and more timely and efficient receipt of screening concerns for clinicians.

Third, digital systems can allow faster incorporation of data into electronic health records, with suggestions and recommendations for pathways to service, when necessary, automated and optimized. Campbell and colleagues (2017) showed that use of digital administration of the

M-CHAT-R/F increased accurate electronic health record documentation from 54 to 92% and the administration of appropriate follow-up actions based on screening results from 25 to 85%. Similarly, Bauer, Sturm, Carroll, and Downs (2013) report on the addition of an autism module to a computer decision support system in community pediatric clinics and found that 70% of staff users reported that the automation aided in adherence to recommended guidelines for screening and care.

Finally, digital systems have the ability to incorporate other methods for encouraging engagement in the screening process and motivating its use. For example, the Baby Steps system (Kientz, Arriaga, & Abowd, 2009) used a digital baby book metaphor and allowed for sentimental recordkeeping alongside developmental screening using the Ages and Stages Questionnaire (Squires et al., 2009) to motivate parent engagement and decrease parent anxiety. Technology-based systems may also provide reminders and flexible formats to allow for a wider reach of these parent-completed screeners.

Increased Accessibility through Mobile Technologies

In addition, the increasing penetration of mobile technologies globally, especially mobile phones, affords increasing accessibility of developmental screening directly to caregivers. Estimates of population accessibility to cell phones, for example, range from 44 to 91% in sub-Saharan Africa, for example (GSM Association, 2018; Pew Research Center, 2018). This may have advantages for accessibility to developmental screening questionnaires and surveys, even where clinical and developmental expertise or access to validated screening instruments is difficult to access locally (Durkin et al., 2015). For example, Brooks, Haynes, Smith, McFadden, and Robins (2016) demonstrated that web-based autism screening increased participation and follow-up rates in an underresourced urban clinic setting serving a primarily minority population.

Multiple strategies exist for using mobile technologies to access hard-to-reach populations, including interactive voice response (e.g., prescripted audio surveys with information gathered through dial pad responses), voice calling, text messaging, and customized mobile applications (Firchow & Mac Ginty, 2017). The increased accessibility afforded by mobile technologies can be deep as well as broad, expanding not only the size of the community that can gain access to screening technologies, but also the richness of information gained. For example, Suh, Porter, Racadio, Sung, and Kientz (2017) used a text-messaging-based approach to longitudinally assess developmental risk over extended periods of time. Dense, longitudinal tracking of behaviors could help to achieve goals of developmental monitoring while increasing the objectivity and stability of derived measures.

Leveraging Multimedia Presentation and Capture Capabilities of Mobile Technologies

Newer mobile technologies, especially smartphones and tablets, are becoming increasingly prevalent globally (Pew Research Center Global Attitudes and Trends, 2016) and offer a range of capabilities that will potentially increase the power and utility of early developmental screening systems. For example, screening using video examples and animations to clarify questions to caregivers have been highlighted in several reports (Macari et al., 2018; Mamun et al., 2016; Marrus et al., 2015, 2018; Shic et al., 2018; Wilkinson et al., 2018). Janvier and colleagues (2016) developed the Developmental Check-In, a screening system that uses pictures of behaviors to clarify developmental questions. This measure does not require an electronic implementation but, like traditional text-based screening, could be digitally adapted for greater flexibility. In similar vein, Bardhan and colleagues (2016) described a smartphone system that augmented M-CHAT questions with pictorial representation in a digital framework for data collection and referral to services.

In addition, multimedia capabilities of modern mobile technologies extend not only to the presentation of multimedia content but also to its capture. In the most straightforward form, smartphone systems with video-capture capabilities provide an easily accessible means for recording the early developmental behaviors of children, an approach successfully used in multiple retrospective studies of infant and toddler behavior to understand the earliest manifestations of autism (Baranek, 1999; Osterling & Dawson, 1994; Roche et al., 2018; Werner, Dawson, Osterling, & Dinno, 2000; Wilson et al., 2017; for discussions, see Baranek et al., 2005; Costanzo et al., 2015; Zwaigenbaum et al., 2007). Telemedicine approaches are also viable and offer a way for developmental specialists to observe, comment on, and interactively guide the probing of key behaviors relevant to identification of early autism symptoms (Buttross, Curtis, Lucas, & Annett, 2018). Modern implementations take such capabilities one step further, wedding video capture with automatically guided behavioral probes administered by parents, so as to enable more structured rating of child behaviors (Kanne, Carpenter, & Warren, 2018; Sarkar et al., 2018).

Machine Learning and Computer Vision

Developmental screening and phenotypic profiling also benefit from advances in computational analytics that have already impacted multiple facets of society and the economy. Notable among these advances is the adoption of machine learning techniques that employ datacentric approaches to improve the efficiency, automation, and performance of digital tools (Abbas, Garberson, Glover, & Wall, 2018; Ben-Sasson, Robins, & Yom-Tov, 2018; Thabtah, 2018, 2019; Thabtah, Kamalov, & Rajab, 2018).

In addition, data-mining techniques have been used to provide additional clarity regarding the nature of early autism symptom profiles, as exemplified by clustering techniques applied to behavioral and survey data in high-risk infant siblings of children with ASD (Bussu et al., 2018; Chawarska et al., 2014; Rowberry et al., 2015).

Data-mining and machine learning advances in phenotyping applications for infants and toddlers with or at high risk for ASD generally follow similar investigations into the characterization of autism symptoms in older children (Abbas et al., 2018; Bone et al., 2016; Wall, 2013; Wall, Kosmicki, DeLuca, Harstad, & Fusaro, 2012). Similarly, they come with analogous and important considerations and caveats regarding their deployment and use, notably the care in which datasets need to be assembled, analyzed, and interpreted (Bone et al., 2015).

Beyond investigating behavioral and survey data, machine learning methods have also been used (1) to study abnormalities and differences in neuro-responses (EEG, MEG, MRI) and bio-responses (eye tracking, heart rate, motor, etc.) in infants at high risk for autism from TD infants by modeling and stratifying early brain and biological development (Crippa et al., 2015; Emerson et al., 2017; Hazlett et al., 2017) and (2) to study abnormal usage patterns of mobile, video, and gaming platforms as a means of stratifying children with or at high risk of autism from their peers (Anzulewicz, Sobota, & Delafield-Butt, 2016; Atyabi et al., 2017; Li et al., 2018).

Computer vision techniques, combined with machine learning approaches, enabled by digital platforms, are also becoming increasingly prominent in the phenotyping of children with ASD in the early developmental period. They offer the promise of circumventing the laborious process of training raters to hand-code behaviors observed through multimedia data streams (e.g., children's voices and behavioral reactions to a task), as well as increasing objectivity through the extraction of quantitative metrics of performance. These methods have been highlighted by a number of studies (Campbell et al., 2018; Fusaro et al., 2014; Hashemi et al., 2012, 2015, 2018; Tariq et al., 2018), including studies where presentation of stimuli via tablets is combined with digital recording and coding of affective facial response by infants with ASD (Campbell et al., 2018) and automatic detection of eye contact in children with ASD in live behavioral interactions (Chong et al., 2017; Edmunds et al., 2017; Rehg, Rozga, Abowd, & Goodwin, 2014; Rehg, 2011; Ye et al., 2012, 2015).

Other Sensing Technologies

While a large proportion of technology development associated with digital phenotyping of behaviors in ASD is focused on smartphones and mobile technologies such as tablets, progress using other sensing and interactive technologies is also rapidly advancing. These technologies include eye-tracking systems, wearables (movement trackers, electrodermal activity monitors, sleep monitors), voice analysis systems, and touch systems (for detailed discussion across the lifespan in ASD, see Cabibihan et al., 2017). This section briefly summarizes major themes relating to each of these technologies.

Eye Tracking

Eye tracking has become a prominent tool in the investigation of early signatures of atypical visual social cognition and attention in individuals with ASD (for reviews, see Chita-Tegmark, 2016; Frazier et al., 2017). A minority of eye-tracking research in ASD focuses on infants and toddlers, but this work has already generated a large number of insights. For example, we know that toddlers with ASD focus less on the faces of simulated interactive partners than TD toddlers (Chawarska, Macari, & Shic, 2012; Chawarska & Shic, 2009; Shic, Bradshaw, Klin, Scassellati, & Chawarska, 2011). They also demonstrate visual scanning patterns that differ from TD toddlers during initiation of joint attention tasks, but they do not significantly differ in their response to joint attention tasks (Billeci et al., 2016). More broadly, infants and toddlers with ASD show decreased visual preference for social information compared to nonsocial information (Klin, Lin, Gorrindo, Ramsay, & Jones, 2009; Pierce et al., 2015). Recent work using gaze-contingent eye tracking (i.e., using eye tracking to automatically and adaptively modify visual inputs per participant) has also shown atypicalities in learning about and responding to the value of social information (Vernetti, Senju, Charman, Johnson, & Gliga, 2018; Wang, DiNicola, Heymann, Hampson, & Chawarska, 2017). Applications of computational and statistical methods have further revealed the fine-grained structure of atypical attention in ASD (Campbell, Shic, Macari, & Chawarska, 2014; Chawarska, Ye, Shic, & Chen, 2015; Wang, Campbell, Macari, Chawarska, & Shic, 2018), with implications supporting the development of more optimized systems for early detection of ASD and for the prediction of treatment outcomes (Murias et al., 2018).

Results from studies of infant siblings of children with ASD who are at high risk for developing ASD themselves have shown similarly promising results. Near 6 months of age, infant siblings with a later diagnosis of ASD show decreased looking at faces (Chawarska, Macari, & Shic, 2013), erratic scanning patterns while looking at speaking faces (Shic, Macari, & Chawarska, 2014), and atypical attentional disengagement profiles (Elison et al., 2013). These high-risk infants that develop ASD also show atypical developmental trajectories of face scanning through early infancy and the toddler years (Jones & Klin, 2013), nuanced joint attention difficulties at 13 months of age (Bedford et al., 2012), and, surprisingly, increased efficiency at visual search at 9 months of age (Gliga et al., 2015).

Although research is still ongoing (for commentary on future directions and field recommendations, see Shic, 2016), these results highlight the
promise of eye tracking for identifying and understanding the earliest manifestations of atypical social attention in infants and toddlers who will later
receive a clinical diagnosis of ASD. Eye tracking is an enormously flexible
technology that is noninvasive and highly tolerated by very young children
(for discussions, see Karatekin, 2007; Shic, 2013a). While gaze-contingent
eye tracking is still a nascent technology, it also holds the potential for
developing systems that help to train social attention as well as monitor it
(Powell, Wass, Erichsen, & Leekam, 2016; Vernetti et al., 2018; Wang et
al., 2015, 2017; Wass, Porayska-Pomsta, & Johnson, 2011).

Wearables

For infants and toddlers who later receive a diagnosis of ASD, the use of
wearable technologies can be difficult owing to challenges with sensory
input, unique sensory needs, and language impairments, all of which may
affect compliance. However, several recent studies have highlighted their
potential. For example, electrodermal activity monitors (also known as
skin-conductance detectors or galvanic skin response detectors) have been
used in toddlers with ASD to highlight relationships between increases in
electrodermal response to mechanical toys and increased presence of repetitive behaviors (Prince et al., 2017). Actigraphy has been used to illuminate
atypical sleep patterns in older children with ASD (Wiggs & Stores, 2004),
but little information is available regarding its application in toddlers and
infants with or at risk for ASD. Similar systems have been reported for
tracking repetitive behaviors in toddlers and infants, as well as in older children (Min, Tewfik, Kim, & Menard, 2009; Tapia, Intille, Lopez, & Larson, 2006). As improvements in miniaturization and advances in hardware
platforms and software algorithms continue, however, we should see an
increased prevalence of wearable technologies in applications for the early
developmental periods of ASD. Ideally, many of the technological systems
and applications described in this chapter will benefit from these advances
as well as from a wearable form-factor that can increase the pervasiveness of
their operation and their ability to generate large, dense, continuous datasets
describing patterns relevant to, and possibly redefining, clinical phenotype.

Voice Analysis Systems

The relatively recent development of practicable voice analysis systems,
consisting of compact digital recorders and automated analysis software,
has significantly advanced research on speech development (Oller et al.,
2010). This technology allows thousands of hours of audio data, including child-produced vocalizations and the child's acoustic environment,

to be collected in natural settings (e.g., the home or school). Interest in speech development and language acquisition has prompted many infant and toddler researchers to adopt systems such as the Language ENvironment Analysis (LENA) hardware and software system. LENA recorders are small and wireless and can be affixed directly to the child's clothing for day-long acoustic recordings in the home and other natural environments. LENA software processes continuous audio stream and segment vocalizations, which can be classified by speaker (e.g., female adult, child) and used to determine frequency counts of adult words, child vocalizations, and conversational turns (Xu, Yapanel, & Gray, 2009). Additionally, measures such as the Automatic Vocalization Assessment (AVA) have been developed to analyze child vocalizations and to determine expressive language level, represented by a standard score, which correlates with clinical assessments of language (Richards et al., 2017).

LENA technology has shown great potential for clinical practice related to early screening, detection of language disorders, and treatment response. It has high reliability and validity (Woynaroski et al., 2017; Xu et al., 2009; Yoder, Oller, Richards, Gray, & Gilkerson, 2013) and can collect and analyze massive amounts of acoustic data present in the child's language-learning environment. These features may allow for more efficient and nuanced measurement of child speech than some standardized clinical assessments, which are most commonly used in practice. Using LENA, researchers have found that children with ASD differ from typically developing children in their acoustic environments and language use. Conversational turns tend to be lower in frequency and shorter in duration for children with ASD than for TD children (Warren et al., 2009). In addition, children with ASD make fewer and less contingent vocalizations and produce fewer canonical syllables (Oller et al., 2010; Warlaumont, Richards, Gilkerson, & Oller, 2014; Warren et al., 2009). Advancing this work, Harbison et al. (2018) recently proposed a measure of child vocal reciprocity to be used as a predictor of response to treatment in clinical practice for children with ASD. In a novel application of LENA technology, Pawar et al. (2017) developed a laughter detector, which allows for estimation of affect in older children with ASD. These systems can also be used to identify impoverished language environments, which may have a particularly significant impact on the language development of infants and toddlers with or at risk for ASD, and which may prove invaluable for guiding language interventions (Gilkerson et al., 2017).

Pitfalls and Potential Drawbacks to Digital Phenotyping Implementations

It is important to note the potential disadvantages associated with digital phenotyping implementations. As an example, we consider the case of early ASD screening, which is among the most mature digital phenotyping approaches used in infants and toddlers who receive a diagnosis of ASD.

First, the digital systems used in screening (typically, mobile phones or tablets) themselves are an added expense (as compared to pen and paper). Care must be taken to ensure that the systems are not lost either intentionally or unintentionally. They are also susceptible to breakage and malfunction in ways paper is not.

Second, while the delivery of questions themselves can be quite efficient, surrounding infrastructure must be developed in order to maintain the operation of electronic survey systems, including (1) secure communication channels for data transfer; (2) secure locking of data contained in the system (in case of system loss); (3) daily maintenance of systems, including ensuring that systems are charged and are functioning correctly; (4) backend data services for collecting and organizing data as well as for disseminating information along relevant communication lines (e.g., reporting results to clinicians); (5) creation of tracking systems to guard against data loss and to match survey answers to the identity of child records; and (6) consideration of multiple points of failure and adequate solutions to address those vulnerabilities (e.g., wireless communication infrastructure breakdown; caregivers not fully filling out systems or letting the system time-out due to excessive delay; parents entering wrong or mismatched identifying information to child records). Many of these difficulties can also have analogues in traditional pen-and-paper-based methodologies, but they can be compounded by perceptions of infallibility by the users and staff deploying electronic screening systems.

Third, it is not clear that electronic and pen-and-paper-based methodologies used in screening generate the same results. While it seems, as in Harrington et al.'s study (2013), that digital systems are highly accepted and sometimes even preferred as compared to traditional pen-and-paper, there is currently a lack of information regarding discrepancies in psychometric properties between the two implementations, just as there is little research describing the effects of different techniques for administering questions (e.g., one question at a time versus questions in a list; use of scroll bars and navigation buttons; usability issues related to sizes of check boxes; selection sensitivities; or other user interface options) and their impact on the psychometric or usability properties of digital screening systems.

Finally, it is clear that, while an interview process and the ability to accommodate "free-form answers" (e.g., marking when a question does not make sense to you) can allow for respondent variability that can be challenging to analyze in a structured fashion, it also allows for the prompting of bidirectional discussion, which can enrich the screening or diagnostic process in a way that fully automated systems cannot.

These difficulties are shared by other digital phenotyping solutions, which, to achieve practical utility, will need to address many of the same infrastructural, cost, and psychometric evaluative investigations to which traditional assessment is subject. Areas of potential vulnerability will require more research to fully disassemble and understand and should be weighed against the potential advantages that digital format phenotyping systems allow.

Technological Methods Augmenting Treatment and Monitoring[4]

There is significant evidence suggesting that early intervention improves developmental outcomes for individuals with ASD (Zwaigenbaum et al., 2015), and there is an ongoing effort to lower the age of reliable diagnosis to improve early access to intervention services (Koegel, Koegel, Ashbaugh, & Bradshaw, 2014). Thanks to the advancements made over the last decade, ASD can be reliably diagnosed in infants as young as 24 months (Guthrie, Swineford, Nottke, & Wetherby, 2013; Ozonoff et al., 2015), especially in clinic-referred populations (Chawarska, Klin, Paul, & Volkmar, 2007). Still, by this age, many children with ASD have missed out on countless learning opportunities, and many are already significantly behind their TD peers in key social and language milestones. Many of these early foundational milestones, such as joint attention, imitation, gesture use, and language acquisition, serve to scaffold the development of later, more sophisticated skills. Infants and toddlers who do not receive early intervention may miss critical windows of opportunity to hone these foundational skills, which may interfere with timely development of advanced adaptive abilities, such as executive functioning, emotion regulation, social skills, and academic achievement. The most empirically validated treatment strategies for infants and toddlers with or at risk for ASD fall under the umbrella of naturalistic developmental behavioral interventions (NDBIs; Bradshaw, Steiner, Gengoux, & Koegel, 2015; Schreibman et al., 2015). Research on technological approaches to early intervention in the infant and toddler years is still emerging, but this area holds promise for creatively addressing early deficits.

Technology can provide a means of augmenting treatment delivery or making it more accessible. For example, bug-in-ear coaching (Ottley & Hanline, 2014; Ottley, 2016) has been used to provide real-time feedback for optimizing treatment delivery and education for both parents and professionals. Telehealth technology has been used to train parents of infants and toddlers with ASD in intervention strategies (Vismara et al., 2018).

---

[4]For more detailed discussion on evidence-based practices for early intervention, see the discussion by Katarzyna Chawarska, Suzanne L. Macari, Angelina Vernetti, and Ludivine Brunissen (Chapter 5, this volume).

Web-based teaching materials have been used to supplement knowledge or instruction for parents and providers (Hamad, Serna, Morrison, & Fleming, 2010; Jang et al., 2012; Kobak, Stone, Wallace, et al., 2011) using techniques that have also been applied to early identification (Kobak, Stone, Ousley, & Swanson, 2011; Koegel et al., 2005). However, most technology-based intervention research, including interactive computer games, computer-aided instruction, and social robots, are designed primarily for use with school-age children, adolescents, and adults (Bölte, Golan, Goodwin, & Zwaigenbaum, 2010). Outside of telehealth approaches designed to augment or increase the accessibility of behavioral interventions, there is a dearth of research focused on using technology-based interventions for infants and toddlers. The following sections focus on technologies developed primarily for older children with ASD, with a focus on how some of these technologies can be or are currently being extended downward to younger ages.

Interactive Games and Computer-Assisted Instruction

Educational games and serious gaming have a long history in special education. Research has focused primarily on skill remediation and augmentation of traditional intervention in older children (Horne-Moyer et al., 2014; Noor, Shahbodin, & Pee, 2012; Rego, Moreira, & Reis, 2010; Ritterfeld, Cody, & Vorderer, 2009; Whyte, Smyth, & Scherf, 2014). These domains often use internal measures of game performance to track the trajectory of skill development within the specific context of each game (Shute, Ventura, Bauer, & Zapata-Rivera, 2009). Less explored, but highly valuable, is the use of gaming platforms to extract measures associated with clinical phenotype. Several studies have shown relationships between patterns of play and autism-related profiles in older children and adults (Anzulewicz et al., 2016; Li et al., 2018; Tanaka et al., 2010; Weng et al., 2015; Wolf et al., 2008). However, due to infants' and toddlers' (with or without ASD) relatively immature perceptual-cognitive-motor capabilities, the use of interactive digital gaming systems to effect or monitor meaningful relationships with clinically relevant profiles remains a relatively unexplored area of research. Anzulewicz and colleagues (2016) showed that gesture and play patterns during a digital "sharing" activity (where the child user had to split a fruit into pieces and then give the pieces to digital characters) and a digital tracing/coloring activity could be combined with machine learning techniques to differentially classify children with ASD from TD children as young as 3 years of age with 93% accuracy.

Recent large-scale work (involving $n = 366$ TD infants and toddlers) has shown that a toddler's use of touchscreen interfaces (especially scrolling) is associated with fine motor milestones (Bedford, Saez de Urabain,

Cheung, Karmiloff-Smith, & Smith, 2016). Given the demonstrated relationships between fine motor performance in infancy and later autism severity in infants at high risk for developing ASD (Iverson et al., 2019), studies of typical development, such as Bedford and colleagues' work (2016), highlights potential applications in examining developmental profiles in children with ASD.

Similarly, there is a dearth of knowledge regarding the use of video game approaches for either remediation or behavioral intervention in toddlers or infants who ultimately receive a diagnosis of ASD. However, research has evaluated these systems for preschoolers (e.g., see Fletcher-Watson, Pain, Hammond, Humphry, & McConachie, 2016, for an example and discussion regarding game designs for very young children with ASD) and there is extensive information regarding the use of games across the lifespan in ASD (Boyd et al., 2017; Mehl-Schneider & Steinmetz, 2014; Ploog, Scharf, Nelson, & Brooks, 2013; Shic, 2013b; Whyte et al., 2014). Even outside of ASD, there is little work in this early age range (Jurdi, Montaner, Garcia-Sanjuan, Jaen, & Nacher, 2018), though some preliminary guidelines for designing health care games for toddlers have been described (Høiseth, Giannakos, Alsos, Jaccheri, & Asheim, 2013). At the same time, development and research evaluation for games and computer-assisted instruction systems for the early developmental periods of ASD have increased in recent years. For example, one recent study describes a multimonitor system designed to teach social attention skills to toddlers with ASD (specifically, response to name; Zheng et al., 2015). Several studies have shown positive results using computer-assisted teaching methods. For example, Moore and Calvert (2000) described increased attention and vocabulary retention in children with ASD as young as 3 years of age using computer instruction relative to teacher instruction. Other platforms provide opportunities for learning, augmenting educational delivery by a therapist or educator in a computer-assisted format. For example, Herrera et al. (2012) describe a Kinect-based body-tracking video game that allows for the teaching of collaborative and turn-taking skills, while Simmons, Paul, and Shic (2016) describe a visualization system for teaching prosodic aspects of speech to children with ASD. An even larger body of research has begun considering how more traditional behavior modeling techniques such as video modeling (Bellini & Akullian, 2007; Charlop-Christy, Le, & Freeman, 2000; Ganz, Earles-Vollrath, & Cook, 2011) can be enhanced by the multimedia and portability capabilities afforded by mobile devices (Cihak, Fahrenkrog, Ayres, & Smith, 2010; Popple et al., 2016). Finally, promising results show the feasibility and potential advantages in typically developing infants and toddlers in learning from teleconference instruction (Myers, LeWitt, Gallo, & Maselli, 2017), especially in co-viewing situations where the parent models responses desired from the child (Strouse, Troseth, O'Doherty, & Saylor, 2018).

Robots and Smart Toys

With the rapid growth in technology and artificial intelligence in recent years, researchers have also begun to explore the possible therapeutic benefits of robots for ASD. There is a growing body of research in socially assistive robotics (SAR), which aims to assist special populations via robots designed specifically for social interactions. Potential interventions for individuals with ASD have been highlighted as a promising application for SAR (Scassellati, Admoni, & Matarić, 2012) for several reasons (Cabibihan, Javed, Ang, & Aljunied, 2013; Scassellati, 2005). First, socially assistive robots can be designed to facilitate social interactions—an area of particular challenge for children with ASD. Second, the features of social robots are well suited to the strengths and preferences of children with ASD: these children tend to show preferences for (and strengths in comprehending) physical and systematic phenomena (Auyeung et al., 2009; Dawson, Soulieres, Gernsbacher, & Mottron, 2007; Turner-Brown, Lam, Holtzclaw, Dichter, & Bodfish, 2011), but they can show discomfort with the complexity and unpredictability of the social world (Bellini, 2006). Robots offer a unique combination of object-like simplicity and predictable behavior, together with human-like social behaviors (Thill, Pop, Belpaeme, Ziemke, & Vanderborght, 2012). As a result, children with ASD might feel more comfortable interacting with them (Kim et al., 2015), which can serve to diminish initial or continuing barriers toward reception of interventional content.

Socially interactive robots can be designed to communicate, express, and perceive emotions, contribute to social interactions, interpret natural cues, and help children develop social competencies (Fong, Nourbakhsh, & Dautenhahn, 2003). Today, social robots are being used as tools to teach skills to children with autism, emphasize social affordances (for a discussion of social affordances and their role in ASD, see Valenti & Gold, 1991; Loveland, 1991), promote play, and elicit desired behaviors. Robots can be used to create interesting, appealing, and meaningful social scenarios to facilitate interactions with other children. The role of a robot in an interactive context can take on many forms, including (1) diagnostic agent, (2) friendly playmate, (3) behavior-eliciting agent, (4) social mediator, (5) social actor, and (6) personal therapist (Cabibihan et al., 2013). These roles can be grouped into two main applications of social robotics for autism: diagnostic tool and therapy agent.

Robots as a Diagnostic Tool

While much of the work examining the utility of SAR in autism research has focused on efforts toward intervention systems, there have also been considerable advances in the design and implementation of phenotyping and diagnostic evaluation systems embedded atop robotic platforms (for relevant methods, see the section "Technological Methods Augmenting Screening and Phenotyping" earlier in this chapter). In robotics, sensing and action work hand in hand: without appropriate systems to evaluate child performance, robots seeking an ultimately social therapeutic or educational goal cannot be truly automated. Wizard of Oz (WoZ) approaches (Riek, 2012), in which a human observer remote-controls a robot's response, avoid the burden of having to design and deploy appropriate detection and sensing systems but fall short of the potential of robotics for achieving practical, augmentative solutions for therapy because a human remains "in the loop." If a human is required to directly intervene in the robot's responses in real time, there is no net savings of therapist effort. Still, it is important to note that even without automated sensing and evaluation methods, there may be advantages to using robots as a tool for augmenting the diagnostic process. For example, complex actions can be preprogrammed to be triggered by a remote human observer, combining the advantages of telehealth with standardization offered by scripted, preprogrammed robotic behavioral probes. The elimination or reduction of a human intermediary's presence in the diagnostic process can also provide a window into developmental skills in the absence of confounding factors related to disparities in social proclivities or understanding. This latter facet of robotic presentation and interaction may lead to advantages similar to those observed in IQ tests, where individuals with ASD were found to perform at a higher level in nonverbal tests of fluid intelligence as compared to standard IQ tests mediated through language (Dawson et al., 2007). These aspects work in concert with the advantages highlighted in the previous section regarding comfort and motivation for children with ASD, potentially leading to highly effective methods to isolate and quantify child behavioral profiles. It should be noted, however, that responses by children with ASD may not be representative of what might be expected in comparable human interaction scenarios.

Scassellati (2005) identified multiple quantitative metrics of social response, including measures of attention, position tracking, auditory preferences, and prosodic qualities of speech, that, when built into robotic platforms, could help augment the diagnostic process for individuals with ASD. While most systems employing such metrics work in synergy with an associated therapeutic goal, some efforts have been made to use these measures directly to reveal clinically relevant child aspects. In toddlers and preschool-age children with (Boccanfuso et al., 2016) and without (Boccanfuso et al., 2015) ASD, patterns of interaction with a low-cost, commercially available robotic ball, programmed to emulate stylized emotional behaviors, were shown to be associated with developmental ability. Zheng and colleagues (2015) described an automated robot system, appropriate for use with toddlers, that could automatically evaluate and respond to toddler joint attention probe responses using a graded prompt hierarchy. Similar work by the same group later showed that head positions under human–robot inter-action conditions could predict behaviorally assessed response-to-joint-attention skills in 2 1/2-year-old children (Nie et al., 2018). Kumazaki and colleagues (2019) described enactment of gold-standard autism behavioral assessment probes (Autism Diagnostic Observation Schedule: Lord et al., 2012) using a robot in 5- to 6-year-old children, noting that younger par-ticipants were often fearful of the robots. With careful and selective rede-sign of robot components, such work could herald next-generation robotic phenotyping tools for use with much younger populations.

Robots as a Therapy Agent

There has been considerable discussion regarding the role of robots in therapies for children with developmental conditions such as ASD (Begum, Serna, & Yanco, 2016; Diehl et al., 2014; Diehl, Schmitt, Villano, & Crow-ell, 2012; Pennisi et al., 2016; Rabbitt, Kazdin, & Scassellati, 2015; Scas-sellati et al., 2012). As with research in detection and phenotyping, most robotic work in autism research has been conducted with children who are school-age or older. As expected, much of this work focuses on strategies for ameliorating deficits in skills known to be developmentally or behav-iorally linked with social ability. For example, several studies have exam-ined robot systems designed to promote imitation (Duquette, Michaud, & Mercier, 2008; Fujimoto, Matsumoto, De Silva, Kobayashi, & Higashi, 2011; Zheng et al., 2014) or joint attention skills (Boccanfuso et al., 2017; Kozima, Nakagawa, & Yasuda, 2007; Nagai, Asada, & Hosoda, 2002; Scassellati, 1999; Scassellati et al., 2018; Warren et al., 2013; Zheng et al., 2015). Recently, progress has shifted away from WoZ systems toward sys-tems that are more fully autonomous. In toddlers and young children with ASD, recent work has shown that repeated joint-attention probes admin-istered autonomously by a robot four times over a period of a month led to improvements in joint attention skills, with no evidence of diminished attention to the robot over repeated sessions (Zheng et al., 2018). Scassellati and colleagues (2018) demonstrated improvements in social skills in older children with ASD after a one month in-home intervention in which social skills games were conducted or facilitated daily by an autonomous, socially assistive robot. Results showed improvements in children's joint-attention skills in probes administered by a human examiner, suggesting general-ization of learning. This study is notable as it at least partially achieves what has long been considered a necessary step toward using robots as a practical tool for augmenting therapy: longer-term, sustained, remote, and autonomous engagement with children with ASD, which achieved general-izable improvements.

In addition to social skills, several studies have also shown robot sys-tems or protocols that impact other domains known often to be affected in individuals with ASD. For instance, Pennisi and colleagues (2016), in their review of robots in autism research, found positive support for the notion that robots might provide therapists and teachers with new means to connect with individuals with ASD during support sessions. They reported that participants with ASD showed, in addition to social behavior toward robots, reduced repetitive and stereotyped behaviors (e.g., Michaud et al., 2007) and increased spontaneous use of language in sessions with a robot, compared to sessions with an experimenter (e.g., Kim et al., 2013). Srinivasan and colleagues (2015a) showed that the longitudinal use of a robot in motor-play-based activities was associated with body coordination improvements in children with ASD. However, other reports based on overlapping data from this study reported reductions in positive affect over time with the robot (Srinivasan, Park, Neely, & Bhat, 2015b). Also noted was diminished social looking relative to a rhythm-based intervention (Srinivasan, Eigsti, Neely, & Bhat, 2016). The latter studies emphasize the importance of context in the simultaneous design of robot platforms and treatment protocols. As with treatment in general, careful monitoring and attention to the metrics of appropriate functional gains are essential to the appropriate deployment and goal of improvement for the individual.

While robotics work in autism research has been proceeding rapidly toward achieving the goal of complementing and augmenting diagnostic or therapeutic clinical practice, current evidence in the field does not yet support widespread deployment. Most ASD–robot studies involve a small number of participants ($n < 10$) and focus on the engineering or theoretical aspects of human–robot interactions. However, surveys of accumulated knowledge regarding robot applications for individuals with ASD highlight the potential. With the increasing success of small-scale studies, more rigorous evidence as to the effectiveness of robot-assisted interventions for individuals with autism will likely follow in subsequent years. However, results presented by Srinivasan and colleagues (2015b, 2016), who compared a robot-based intervention against other novel interventions as well as a control condition, provide caution that results with robots are not uniformly positive. These findings highlight the idea that the context of the robot protocol may be as important, and potentially more important, than the robot platform itself. Future work will need to bridge knowledge gaps regarding the utility of robot-assisted diagnostics and therapies, addressing questions about *for whom* these (sometimes costly) technologies will be of value and *what form* this value will take.

Smart Toys, Challenges in Privacy, and Knowledge Gaps

To an extent, robots could be seen as a specific instantiation of the broader class of smart toys. Smart toys are objects, designed typically for children, that utilize computing power to gather data, process information, and/or modify inherent capabilities and affordances available to users (Cagiltay, Kara, & Aydin, 2014; D'Hooge, Dalton, Shwe, Lieberman, & O'Malley, 2000; Goldstein, Buckingham, & Brougere, 2004). Smart toys enable bi-directional interactions between the child and the smart toy, a process that can increase engagement and enhance learning (Cagiltay et al., 2014). Smart toy designs have been created with the goals of early detection and phenotyping of developmental disorders and/or motor difficulties (Campolo et al., 2006; Escobedo, Ibarra, Hernandez, Alvelais, & Tentori, 2014; García, Ruiz, Rivera, Vadillo, & Duboy, 2017; Westeyn et al., 2012). Recent explorations have further examined their utility in an interventional context (Ekin, Cagiltay, & Karasu, 2018; Escobedo et al., 2014).

Yet, these new capabilities come with the need for new considerations. Digital systems that collect or aggregate data pose unique and fundamental questions regarding the privacy of children and families (Hung, Iqbal, Huang, Melaisi, & Pang, 2016; Rafferty et al., 2017; Taylor & Michael, 2016). As an example, Ramalho (2017), in a perspective article, uses events surrounding a once popular children's toy, the Furby, to illustrate privacy concerns regarding smart toys in our daily lives and as an extended metaphor for societal complicity in eroding barriers between public and private spaces in the digital age. Sensitive branches of the U.S. government once banned the Furby in offices for fear that it would record audio (in reality, the Furby had no recording capability). Yet there remains some suspicion that some Furbies were modified with eavesdropping capabilities. Further, more modern iterations of the Furby (e.g., Furby Connect) as well as other popular Internet-connected toys may also pose security issues in allowing malicious control (Frenkel, 2018). In some cases, parent agreements for use of these toys make it too easy for parents to ignore "the fine print" regarding information sharing, allowing child–toy interactions that the child believes to be private to become public (Jones & Meurer, 2016). For children with ASD, the risks include exposing sensitive medical information as well as leading to "social network mishaps," which can compound difficulties in social peer networks.

The unrealistic expectation that caregivers fully understand the potentially complex nature of smart toys and other adaptive tools for their children poses yet another challenge. Whereas a standard toy has affordances, hazards, and play life cycles that are often comprehendible at a glance, the capabilities, functions, and responses that a smart toy can take on can be as complex as their programming. Further, overlooked engineering aspects, such as performance in low-battery states, wire shorts, and other technical mishaps, add more uncertainties to predictions of performance over the lifespan of use. For tools designed for infants and toddlers, especially for those with developmental issues such as ASD, appropriate monitoring systems should be in place to ensure that the quality of smart toy functionality and its use fall in line with caregiver expectations. This issue is especially important when therapeutic outcome is dependent on smart toy use, as a malfunctioning system risks sending a child down a less optimal developmental, educational, or therapeutic trajectory.

Finally, because smart toys and digital interactive systems are relatively recent, less is known about the optimal strategies for providing developmental gains for either typical or atypical populations. Arnott, Palaiologou, and Gray (2018), in a preface to a special issue on the new ecology of digital devices, toys, and games, note that research should move beyond the question of whether digital systems should be included in children's lives (as they already are and will continue to be) and toward a more comprehensive perspective of the quality of technological experiences in digital play. Fleer (2016) examines epistemological questions regarding the nature and essence of digital play and concludes that digital play exists as something more than what the traditional definition indicates. Expanding on Lev Vygostky's conception of play, Fleer states that digital play is characterized by four aspects: (1) imaginary digital situations, (2) digital talk in those situations, (3) transformation of digital elements to create new digital situations, giving digital play a new sense, and (4) "porous boundaries between digital play and social pretend play situations" (p. 79). This fourth element describes mutual interactions and enmeshment between virtual and physical "real-world" imaginary play situations. As we continue to consider the challenges involved in creating technologies to support the lives of children with ASD in their earliest developmental periods, it will be necessary to reconcile—and perhaps expand upon—emerging philosophical frameworks, with classical perspectives on deficits in social imagination in ASD (Wing, Gould, & Gillberg, 2011). These efforts may yield more powerful models that can be used to conceptualize the optimal allocation of technological tools to enrich long-term trajectories of quality of life for individuals with ASD, grounded in the most critical periods of early development.

Alternative and Augmentative Communication and Speech-Generating Devices

A substantial 25% of children who receive a diagnosis of ASD never develop functional verbal communication (Eigsti, de Marchena, Schuh, & Kelley, 2011; Rose, Trembath, Keen, & Paynter, 2016). These children are often referred to as minimally verbal or nonverbal. Minimally verbal children fail to use language in a functional way across settings and have little spoken language or display echolalia (Tager-Flusberg & Kasari, 2013). Alternative and augmentative communication (AAC) systems are often utilized in early intervention to address these language deficits. The primary function of AAC systems is to serve as a supplement or a replacement for verbal language (Beukelman & Mirenda, 2013; Schlosser & Sigafoos, 2006). While there exist an enormous number of potential AAC modalities (e.g., forms by which AAC can mediate communication, such as nonverbal gestures and expressions, symbol cards representing concepts, and digital systems translating touch patterns to speech), here we consider two primary AAC system types: unaided and aided. Unaided AAC systems rely on the user physically communicating—for example, using sign language or other manual gestures. Alternatively, aided AAC systems use symbolic representations such as pictures or symbols as the primary communication medium and rely on external equipment. Aided AAC systems include the Picture Exchange Communication System (PECS) or speech-generating devices (SGDs; e.g., GoTalk). SGDs have been in use for decades. The initial technology used symbols that produced digitized speech. Though effective, early systems were often cumbersome, expensive, and not easily accessible. Recently, the integration of SGD systems into smartphones and tablets has vastly increased the accessibility and convenience of SGD AAC systems. Advances in developing variants that use eye tracking rather than physical touch have opened doors even further for those with motor impairments (Sharma & Abrol, 2013). Even more cutting-edge research has explored the direct mapping of brain activity for communication (Lazarou, Nikolopoulos, Petrantonakis, Kompatsiaris, & Tsolaki, 2018).

However, the continual digitalization and miniaturization of such assistive tools also present unique challenges for certain populations. For those with motor impairment or atypicalities, the use of smartphones and tablets can be more challenging than dedicated buttons with concrete, physical form and demand-specific considerations in design (Chen, Savage, Chourasia, Wiegmann, & Sesto, 2013). Additionally, digital apps and more physical, manual systems may not be as interchangeable as is often assumed. For example, an individual switching from a manual AAC system to an app-based system, or vice versa, may produce significant transition challenges. In addition, there are disadvantages in relying solely on a digital device for communication, as they might not be appropriate or functional in a wide range of settings (e.g., outdoor activities where the system is exposed to the elements, in very cold climates where the user must wear gloves or mittens, or during a gym class or swimming lessons at a pool where the expensive device may get damaged). When possible, it is advisable that users be taught how to use multiple communication systems so that communication will still be possible even in situations in which the use of a specific device is not practical or is unavailable.

This said, a growing body of research shows strong effects and emerging support for aided AAC systems (Ganz et al., 2011; Logan, Iacono, & Trembath, 2017). Learning to comfortably use AAC and SGD systems often requires discrete trial training. This involves teaching minimally verbal individuals to request objects, typically by offering the individuals desirable rewards (e.g., preferred foods, snacks, or toys; Lancioni et al., 2007; Schlosser & Sigafoos, 2006). However, an increasing amount of research now supports using more naturalistic models. Research has demonstrated that when a child displays a preference for a given modality (e.g., SGD or PECS), applying that modality significantly improves the results of the AAC intervention (van der Meer, Sigafoos, O'Reilly, & Lancioni, 2011). Historically, one limitation of the research studying the effects of AAC systems was that most studies were conducted as single-case experimental designs, making it difficult to draw statistical inferences regarding the effects of AAC interventions (Ganz et al., 2011; Logan et al., 2017). A more recent and comprehensive study was conducted by Kasari and colleagues (2014). In this study, 61 minimally verbal children with autism, 5 to 8 years of age, received 6 months of an NDBI (joint attention symbolic play engagement and regulation [JASPER]). Participants were randomly assigned to either augment their treatment with the addition of an AAC with SGD or to receive only the traditional intervention. The study team found that the addition of an AAC improved the effectiveness of the intervention. However, this is one of very few studies employing a more empirical, statistical model on a larger sample to study the additional benefits of aided AAC systems. More well-designed research is necessary to further explore the efficacy of different modalities. Recent recommendations suggest that research examining interventions utilizing aided AAC systems should consider incidental communications and the use of these systems in situations that promote spontaneous social communication and interaction, with particular focus on naturalistic reinforcement to enable social communication across activities (Logan et al., 2017).

As with other classes of technology-based interventions, less is known about the efficacy of SGDs and other digital AACs for toddlers and infants at risk for autism. However, a review by Branson and Demchak (2009) on 12 studies involving 190 participants 16 to 36 months of age noted that there was little evidence for a minimum age for use of an AAC, though age did appear to influence the selection of AAC type (aided or unaided). This review found that symbol-based PECS was slightly more effective than sign language, but highlighted the greater importance of consistent and appropriate use of AAC by families. In addition, the review cautioned that a variety of AAC modalities should be considered to ensure that a child does not miss opportunities for communicative learning. While many of the conclusions of this review are as true today as they were a decade ago when the review was written, it preceded the explosion of mobile technologies supporting AAC applications and could therefore benefit from being revisited.

The added usability and convenience of AAC apps with SGD and PECS support on smartphones and tablets are making these systems increasingly popular. Additionally, the cost of such systems has decreased dramatically since the introduction of tablet-based mobile devices such as the iPad. A plethora of communication and AAC apps are available for download. Some of the most popular apps are *Proloquo2go, TouchChat HD, iPrompts,* and *I Can Speak* ("App Annie," 2017). However, the magnitude and variation of options to choose from poses a larger problem: the lack of empirical research into the effectiveness of each app leaves users vulnerable to being misled by unfounded promises or frustrated by lack of results. In Apple's AppStore, these apps are typically found in the "Education" section, which does not require FDA approval for listing. However, AAC systems are often placed in the same category as medical devices (Centers for Medicare and Medicaid Services, 2015). This may drive users to both inherently trust the available systems and feel a (potentially unnecessary) need to access these systems in order to provide the best and most recent advances for their children. The accessibility of these apps is pivotal to maintain, as they represent an affordable option for both schools and caregivers. Nevertheless, more generalizable research on their effectiveness should be a focus for developers and researchers to ensure that stakeholders are not misled in their search for more effective communication modalities. Further, Davidoff (2017) offers a cautionary note regarding the use of screens and technology in supporting communicative intervention: "The danger of communication and play apps is focusing on the technology more than on the child and communicative interaction" (p. 51). It is still largely unknown how technology-based applications would fare in effectiveness compared to other, more traditional AAC modalities, especially if those traditional methods were met by the same level of effort, innovation, enthusiasm, and dedicated resources in development.

Considering the Negative Impacts of Technology on Children

While the development of technological tools for aiding the lives of the youngest children affected by ASD is both exciting and highly promising, it is important to realize there are trade-offs and potential drawbacks to their use. As a case in point, the controversies (and pediatric recommendations) surrounding the use of electronic screens by infants and toddlers illustrates why, despite their many advantages and high potential for improving lives, one should use caution in incorporating technologies into the daily routine of infants and toddlers with or at risk for ASD.

In 2016, the American Academy of Pediatrics released a series of recommendations for infant and toddler screen media use (Council on Communications and Media, 2016). Included was the recommendation that infants under 18 months of age have limited to no exposure to traditional screen-based media outside of video chat calls. This recommendation was based on the concern that screen time can replace valuable face-to-face learning as well as physical activity and exploration. No physical health concerns were cited in making these recommendations beyond impact of time lost, which might otherwise be spent in activities that would strengthen child musculature.

Media consumption is becoming an unavoidable fact of life; even the American Academy of Pediatrics (AAP) recognizes its occasional necessity. The AAP advises preparing a "media plan" for children over 18 months of age to set ground rules for media use, and research has provided additional guidelines to be incorporated into that plan to allow for the best possible outcome of media exposure. The effects of media use and concerns about the amount of media consumption in children have been the focus of much study (for a review in infancy, see Christakis, 2009; for a large meta-analysis in adolescents, see Orben & Przybylski, 2019). On one side of the argument, researchers have found that screen-based, passive media is not a more effective teaching instrument than in-person interaction before the age of 3 (Anderson & Pempek, 2005; Barr & Hayne, 1999; Troseth & DeLoache, 1998). However, there are characteristics that allow for media use leading to better imitation, learning, and preservation of skills (Kirkorian, Wartella, & Anderson, 2008). These factors include repetition: allowing children to watch the same content multiple times promotes greater learning and better retention (Anderson et al., 2000; Barr, Muentener, Garcia, Fujimoto, & Chávez, 2007; Lauricella, Pempek, Barr, & Calvert, 2010; Skouteris & Kelly, 2006). Interactivity, which includes speaking with a child about the content, plot, and characters, and reflecting back characters' feelings and overall themes, is recommended during media use (Guernsey, 2012; Lauricella et al., 2010). In part, this allows for greater face-to-face interaction so that media use does not replace valuable learning opportunities. It also allows for greater vocabulary input and modeling of reflection, empathy, and logical thinking. It is important to remember, however, that interactivity has still been shown in some studies to be significantly less effective than nonmedia-based, human-only demonstrations and interactions (e.g., Moser et al., 2015). The final factor in improved outcome from media use is, perhaps, the most obvious one: to allow a child to engage only with media that shows age-appropriate content (Zimmerman & Christakis, 2005).

Currently, no research suggests that the AAP recommendations and other general guidelines regarding screen use in infants and toddlers with ASD should be more relaxed than those for their typically developing peers. Indeed, there are some indications that children with ASD struggle with excessive use of screen media throughout their lives (Mazurek, Shattuck, Wagner, & Cooper, 2012; Mazurek & Wenstrup, 2012; See & Navarro, 2018; Shane & Albert, 2008). For this reason, additional caution may in fact be warranted for infants at risk for ASD and toddlers with ASD (e.g., for a perspective on children with ASD, see Westby, 2018). However, it is important to note that descriptions regarding excessive use of screen media in ASD do not refer to technology-based systems designed to provide therapeutic benefit (either directly or through monitoring of behaviors). Nor do they necessarily refer to digital systems specifically designed to preserve the advantages of traditional toys (Hiniker, Lee, Kientz, & Radesky, 2018). Furthermore, it is not clear whether excessive screen use reflects a causal relationship with the inherent social challenges associated with the condition. This means that due to a more limited engagement in activities involving direct interactions with peers (Ratcliff, Hong, & Hilton, 2018), screen media use arises to fill the void. Yet to be clarified, especially for the youngest individuals affected by ASD, is the role excessive screen media use has in increasing sustained social difficulties for individuals with ASD, as well as its potential positive aspects (e.g., social interactions via multiplayer gaming, topics of discussion with real-world peers, management of stress; Anderson, 2016; Bishop-Fitzpatrick, DaWalt, Greenberg, & Mailick, 2017; Ng, 2017; Ringland, Wolf, Faucett, Dombrowski, & Hayes, 2016; Stone, Mills, & Saggers, 2019; for additional perspectives, see Ferguson, 2018).

In summary, careful monitoring and control of media consumption (interactive or not) is recommended for infants and toddlers with or without ASD. The same caveats apply to any technology, including monitoring, educational, or interventional tools. As with medicine, the dose is important. Care should be taken to ensure that the use of technologies does not pass the point of efficacy and enter into the area of abuse. Guidelines for such recommendations remain to be established, but given the heterogeneity of the autism spectrum, they are likely to be highly personalized.

Summary and Discussion

This chapter provides a brief overview on the rapidly evolving landscape of technological tools designed for infants and toddlers with or at risk for ASD. There are many challenges in designing these tools for this age range, the most significant being the nature of development itself: infants and toddlers experience rapid and expansive physical and cognitive changes in the early months and years of life. Physical changes include morphological, musculoskeletal, and neural development. These advances occur concurrently with motor skill acquisition and sensory system improvements and refinements, which influence how technologies can be applied and manipulated. Cognitive changes are also profound as children learn to understand cause and effect, develop self-awareness and understand their physical existence, create a language schema with continuous environmental enrichment, engage in joint attention and learn selectively from others via observational learning, and begin to conceptualize that others have a viewpoint and understanding that is different from their own—all within the first 3 years of life. This prolific accumulation of skills and knowledge intrinsically creates highly varied profiles for individual children as they progress through their own developmental trajectory.

Yet, despite this variability in development, reliable milestones are commonly met by specific ages in typical development. For children with ASD, achieving these milestones at expected points in chronological development is not guaranteed. Developmental profiles are more varied, with delays occurring in a heterogeneous manner across time and across skills. Simultaneously, in the second year of life, for many individuals with ASD, the first positive behavioral indicators of ASD begin to manifest overtly. These signals include increased prominence of atypical behaviors, including pronounced repetitive behaviors, hypo- or hypersensory sensitivities, and regression or plateauing of motoric, social-cognitive, or communicative skills. Development of one-size-fits-all technologies that can meet the needs of all individuals on the spectrum is a practical impossibility. As such, the first step in technological development is to consider for which children and for what purpose a technology is meant to serve.

Recent advances in miniaturization and decreasing hardware and software development costs have made possible the accelerating progress in technology development for the youngest individuals affected by ASD. In part, these efforts include translation of prior physical instantiated systems, such as early screening for ASD, into accessible digital systems. But beyond the straightforward translation of prior methods, technology advancements also offer new forms of presentation, such as multimedia expression, new sensing modalities, computer vision techniques, and the synthesis of data delivery and data collection using machine learning and other advanced analytical techniques. These approaches may provide new ways of generating, validating, and iterating upon the development of novel biomarkers for ASD.

Toward Digital Biomarkers for Infants and Toddlers

Biomarkers for psychiatric conditions reflect quantifiable indices, associated with the biological mechanism underlying pathological processes, that can inform treatment decision making and planning. Mobile health applications have been heralded as a promising platform by which biomarkers of multiple forms (e.g., physiological, cognitive, or behavioral) can be collected and integrated into comprehensive records reflecting an individual's state and projected future, both for children with ASD (Tryfona, Oatley, Calderon, & Thorne, 2016) and for the field of psychiatry in general (Adams et al., 2017). These digital biomarkers could work hand in hand with classical therapies, as well as with more recent software and hardware technology solutions, and are augmented by a host of other potential behavioral, neurobehavioral, and physiological biomarkers such as eye tracking, wearable sensors, and voice analysis systems. A key question is what a biomarker represents, and to what purpose a specific biomarker effectively can be deployed. Equally important are consideration of the need (i.e., the specific problem a biomarker is meant to address) and, working backward, the question of how we can align the state of the art in our knowledge of different kinds of technological solutions to optimize or create new paradigms and new modalities that can serve as biomarkers for that specific need.

Biomarker technologies can help to fill the monitoring component of flexible, adaptable, and personalizable therapeutics. One of the greatest advantages of technology-enhanced therapies is the ability to adapt quickly to the learning of participants, and this adaptation necessitates appropriate sensing and quantifiable measures upon which to base decisions. Our discussion of technology-enhanced therapies therefore interleaved discussion relating to monitoring and diagnostics within the different classes of considered technological systems. This approach highlights just how intertwined monitoring and treatment can be when considering technology supports for individuals with ASD. At the same time, it is important to note that the relationships are not symmetric: while every adaptive treatment needs an object to adapt to (i.e., some measure it uses to make a decision), biomarkers and related measures and metrics do not presuppose specific interventions. Rather, marker tasks and technologies can be broader windows into developmental or clinical questions regarding the individual. As such, they can be used for stratification of samples into more homogeneous subgroups as well as for intervention selection and decision making. Still, we would argue that a tighter wedding of monitoring systems to therapies may provide more optimal predictions for those therapies, just as the development of biomarkers for specific purposes provides additional opportunities for optimization of those purposes. As the field progresses, it is hoped that a deeper, conceptual understanding of relevant ASD-related clinical axes and how they relate to specific biomarker modalities is achieved, informing the development and adaption of specific technology tools in specific circumstances.

Appraising the Risks and Drawbacks of Technology

While powerful, we have also used this discussion to highlight some of the potential drawbacks of technology-enhanced systems for phenotyping or treatment. In our discussion of digital phenotyping, we noted that digital infrastructure can be expensive. In our experiences, a digital solution is not always the simplest, most cost-effective, or the most elegant. Creation of practical, usable technological tools to support individuals with ASD requires commitment to open communication and to potentially conflicting incentives and goals among multiple stakeholders, including engineers, clinicians, entrepreneurs, and the larger ASD community (Brosnan, Parsons, Good, & Yuill, 2016; Kim, Paul, Shic, & Scassellati, 2012; Shic et al., 2015). Yet, the design of prototype systems is a necessity for creation of more optimal, fine-tuned, subsequent iterations. Deciding to embark on the development of a digital platform should thus constitute careful consideration of the long-term vision of technology-as-an-outcome and the advantages such a digital or technology-based format will provide above and beyond simpler, manual approaches. In our discussion of smart toys, we raised concerns that digital implementations suffer from some unique issues, such as concerns regarding security and privacy, that manual alternatives do not face or face differently (e.g., the possibility of losing a laptop containing a database of clinical phenotypes of patients vs. the comparable misplacement of an entire cabinet of files). We also discussed how the complexity of smart systems (including smart toys, robots, and other adaptive technologies) can confound appraisal and adoption decisions by caregivers, and we highlighted the need for more powerful analytical and conceptual frameworks to give this process some clarity. Similarly, throughout this chapter, especially in our section on AAC and SGDs, we highlighted gaps in research knowledge, uncertainties regarding optimal form and function, and the relative dearth of information on infants and toddlers who receive a diagnosis of ASD. Finally, we discussed the potential negative impacts of technology on children and, based on the propensity for excessive use of screen media by older children with ASD, urged caution and careful monitoring of technology systems for use with infants and toddlers.

Concluding Remarks

Despite these limitations, the broad field of technology use in phenotyping and novel therapies is still extraordinarily promising. Advances are occurring rapidly—perhaps so rapidly that they are outstripping our capacity to analyze them rigorously in a traditional fashion. As we move into the next generation of technological innovations, it may become necessary to adopt hybrid approaches in evaluation, blending new analytical and data collection tools with large samples and traditional statistical approaches. Such approaches (e.g., Atyabi et al., 2017) can combine multiple perspectives from data science, engineering, psychology, psychiatry, speech pathology, developmental medicine, and special education in order to create new methods for not only practical goals (such as treatment optimization), but also for understanding—and redefining—our fundamental conceptualization of the nature of ASD.

ACKNOWLEDGMENTS

We thank Jay Martini, Tawny Tsang, Minhang Xie, and Katherine Riley for their helpful review and editing of this chapter. This work was made possible through funding, resources, and experiences provided by National Institutes of Health Grants K01 MH104739, R21 MH102572, and R21 MH103550; National Science Foundation Expedition in Computing No. 1139078 (Socially Assistive Robotics and Cyber-enabled Discovery and Innovation No. 0835767); and the Associates of the Yale Child Study Center. Views in this chapter are those of the authors and do not reflect the opinions of any funding agency.

REFERENCES

Abbas, H., Garberson, F., Glover, E., & Wall, D. P. (2018). Machine learning approach for early detection of autism by combining questionnaire and home video screening. *Journal of the American Medical Informatics Association, 25*(8), 1000–1007.

Adams, Z., McClure, E. A., Gray, K. M., Danielson, C. K., Treiber, F. A., & Ruggiero, K. J. (2017). Mobile devices for the remote acquisition of physiological and behavioral biomarkers in psychiatric clinical research. *Journal of Psychiatric Research, 85*, 1–14.

Allely, C. S. (2013). Pain sensitivity and observer perception of pain in individuals with autistic spectrum disorder. *Scientific World Journal, 2013*, Article ID 916178.

American Academy of Pediatrics. (2014). *Caring for your baby and young child: Birth to age 5* (6th ed., rev.). New York: Bantam.

American Academy of Pediatrics. (2017). *Bright futures: Guidelines for health supervision of infants, children, and adolescents* (4th ed.). Elk Grove Village, IL: Author.

American Psychiatric Association. (2013). *Diagnostic and statistical manual of mental disorders* (5th ed.). Arlington, VA: Author.

Anderson, D. R., Bryant, J., Wilder, A., Santomero, A., Williams, M., & Crawley, A. M. (2000). Researching Blue's Clues: Viewing behavior and impact. *Media Psychology, 2*(2), 179–194.

Anderson, D. R., & Pempek, T. A. (2005). Television and very young children. *American Behavioral Scientist, 48*(5), 505–522.

Anderson, K. (2016). The Board Game Club; The ASHA leader. Retrieved from *https://leader.pubs.asha.org/doi/abs/10.1044/leader.HYTT.21092016.40*.

Anzulewicz, A., Sobota, K., & Delafield-Butt, J. T. (2016). Toward the autism motor signature: Gesture patterns during smart tablet gameplay identify children with autism. *Scientific Reports, 6*, 31107.

App Annie. (2017). Retrieved January 23, 2019, from *www.appannie.com/en*.

Arnott, L., Palaiologou, I., & Gray, C. (2018). Digital devices, Internet-enabled toys and digital games: The changing nature of young children's learning ecologies, experiences and pedagogies. *British Journal of Educational Technology, 49*(5), 803–806.

Atyabi, A., Li, B., Ahn, Y. A., Kim, M., Barney, E., & Shic, F. (2017). An exploratory analysis targeting diagnostic classification of AAC app usage patterns. In *2017 International Joint Conference on Neural Networks* (pp. 1633–1640). Hoffman Estates, IL: International Neural Networks Society.

Auyeung, B., Wheelwright, S., Allison, C., Atkinson, M., Samarawickrema, N., &

Baron-Cohen, S. (2009). The Children's Empathy Quotient and Systemizing Quotient: Sex differences in typical development and in autism spectrum conditions. *Journal of Autism and Developmental Disorders, 39*(11), 1509–1521.

Bachara, G. H., & Phelan, W. J. (1980). Rhythmic movement in deaf children. *Perceptual and Motor Skills, 50*(3, Pt. 1), 933–934.

Baio, J. (2012). Prevalence of autism spectrum disorders: Autism and Developmental Disabilities Monitoring Network, 14 sites, United States, 2008. *Morbidity and Mortality Weekly Report, 61*(SS03), 1–19.

Bakker, D., Kazantzis, N., Rickwood, D., & Rickard, N. (2016). Mental health smartphone apps: Review and evidence-blased recommendations for future developments. *JMIR Mental Health, 3*(1), e7.

Baranek, G. T. (1999). Autism during infancy: A retrospective video analysis of sensory-motor and social behaviors at 9–12 months of age. *Journal of Autism and Developmental Disorders, 29*(3), 213–224.

Baranek, G. T, Barnett, C. R., Adams, E. M., Wolcott, N. A., Watson, L. R., & Crais, E. R. (2005). Object play in infants with autism: Methodological issues in retrospective video analysis. *American Journal of Occupational Therapy, 59*(1), 20–30.

Barbaro, J., & Dissanayake, C. (2012). Early markers of autism spectrum disorders in infants and toddlers prospectively identified in the Social Attention and Communication Study. *Autism, 17*(1), 64–86.

Barber, A. B., Wetherby, A. M., & Chambers, N. W. (2012). Brief report: Repetitive behaviors in young children with autism spectrum disorder and developmentally similar peers: A follow up to Watt et al. (2008). *Journal of Autism and Developmental Disorders, 42*(9), 2006–2012.

Bardhan, S., Mridha, G. M. M. M., Ahmed, E., Ullah, M. A., Ahmed, H. U., Akhter, S., . . . Mamun, K. A. A. (2016). Autism Barta—A smart device based automated autism screening tool for Bangladesh. In *5th International Conference on Informatics, Electronics and Vision* (ICIEV) (pp. 602–607).

Barr, R., & Hayne, H. (1999). Developmental changes in imitation from television during Infancy. *Child Development, 70*(5), 1067–1081.

Barr, R., Muentener, P., Garcia, A., Fujimoto, M., & Chávez, V. (2007). The effect of repetition on imitation from television during infancy. *Developmental Psychobiology, 49*(2), 196–207.

Bauer, N. S., Sturm, L. A., Carroll, A. E., & Downs, S. M. (2013). Computer decision support to improve autism screening and care in community pediatric clinics. *Infants and Young Children, 26*(4), 306.

Bedford, R., Elsabbagh, M., Gliga, T., Pickles, A., Senju, A., Charman, T., & Johnson, M. H. (2012). Precursors to social and communication difficulties in infants at-risk for autism: Gaze following and attentional engagement. *Journal of Autism and Developmental Disorders, 42*(10), 2208–2218.

Bedford, R., Saez de Urabain, I. R., Cheung, C. H. M., Karmiloff-Smith, A., & Smith, T. J. (2016). Toddlers' fine motor milestone achievement is associated with early touchscreen scrolling. *Frontiers in Psychology, 7*, 1108.

Begum, M., Serna, R. W., & Yanco, H. A. (2016). Are robots ready to deliver autism interventions?: A comprehensive review. *International Journal of Social Robotics, 8*(2), 157–181.

Bellini, S. (2006). The development of social anxiety in adolescents with autism spectrum disorders. *Focus on Autism and Other Developmental Disabilities, 21*(3), 138–145.

Bellini, S., & Akullian, J. (2007). A meta-analysis of video modeling and video self-modeling interventions for children and adolescents with autism spectrum disorders. *Exceptional Children, 73*(3), 264–287.

Ben-Sasson, A., Cermak, S. A., Orsmond, G. I., Tager-Flusberg, H., Carter, A. S., Kadlec, M. B., & Dunn, W. (2007). Extreme sensory modulation behaviors in toddlers with autism spectrum disorders. *American Journal of Occupational Therapy, 61*(5), 584–592.

Ben-Sasson, A., Cermak, S. A., Orsmond, G. I., Tager-Flusberg, H., Kadlec, M. B., & Carter, A. S. (2008). Sensory clusters of toddlers with autism spectrum disorders: Differences in affective symptoms. *Journal of Child Psychology and Psychiatry, 49*(8), 817–825.

Ben-Sasson, A., Robins, D. L., & Yom-Tov, E. (2018). Risk assessment for parents who suspect their child has autism spectrum disorder: Machine learning approach. *Journal of Medical Internet Research, 20*(4), e134.

Bertone, A., Mottron, L., Jelenic, P., & Faubert, J. (2003). Motion perception in autism: A "complex" issue. *Journal of Cognitive Neuroscience, 15*(2), 218–225.

Bertone, A., Mottron, L., Jelenic, P., & Faubert, J. (2005). Enhanced and diminished visuo-spatial information processing in autism depends on stimulus complexity. *Brain, 128*(10), 2430–2441.

Beukelman, D. R., & Mirenda, P. (2013). *Augmentative and alternative communication: Supporting children and adults with complex communication needs.* Baltimore: Brookes.

Bhat, A. N., Galloway, J. C., & Landa, R. J. (2012). Relation between early motor delay and later communication delay in infants at risk for autism. *Infant Behavior and Development, 35*(4), 838–846.

Bhat, A. N., Landa, R. J., & Galloway, J. C. (2011). Current perspectives on motor functioning in infants, children, and adults with autism spectrum disorders. *Physical Therapy, 91*(7), 1116–1129.

Billeci, L., Narzisi, A., Campatelli, G., Crifaci, G., Calderoni, S., Gagliano, A., . . . Comminiello, V. (2016). Disentangling the initiation from the response in joint attention: An eye-tracking study in toddlers with autism spectrum disorders. *Translational Psychiatry, 6*(5), e808.

Bishop-Fitzpatrick, L., DaWalt, L. S., Greenberg, J. S., & Mailick, M. R. (2017). Participation in recreational activities buffers the impact of perceived stress on quality of life in adults with autism spectrum disorder. *Autism Research, 10*(5), 973–982.

Boccanfuso, L., Barney, E., Foster, C., Ahn, Y. A., Chawarska, K., Scassellati, B., & Shic, F. (2016). Emotional robot to examine differences in play patterns and affective response of children with and without ASD. In the *Eleventh ACM/IEEE International Conference on Human Robot Interaction* (pp. 19–26). Piscataway, NJ: IEEE Press.

Boccanfuso, L., Kim, E. S., Snider, J. C., Wang, Q., Wall, C. A., DiNicola, L., . . . Shic, F. (2015). Autonomously detecting interaction with an affective robot to explore connection to developmental ability. In 2015 International Conference on Affective Computing and Intelligent Interaction (ACII) (pp. 1–7).

Boccanfuso, L., Scarborough, S., Abramson, R. K., Hall, A. V., Wright, H. H., & O'Kane, J. M. (2017). A low-cost socially assistive robot and robot-assisted intervention for children with autism spectrum disorder: Field trials and lessons learned. *Autonomous Robots, 41*(3), 637–655.

Bölte, S., Golan, O., Goodwin, M. S., & Zwaigenbaum, L. (2010). What can innovative technologies do for autism spectrum disorders? *Autism, 14*(3), 155–159.

Bone, D., Bishop, S. L., Black, M. P., Goodwin, M. S., Lord, C., & Narayanan, S.

S. (2016). Use of machine learning to improve autism screening and diagnostic instruments: Effectiveness, efficiency, and multi-instrument fusion. *Journal of Child Psychology and Psychiatry, 57*(8), 927–937.

Bone, D., Goodwin, M. S., Black, M. P., Lee, C.-C., Audhkhasi, K., & Narayanan, S. (2015). Applying machine learning to facilitate autism diagnostics: Pitfalls and promises. *Journal of Autism and Developmental Disorders, 45*(5), 1121–1136.

Bonnel, A., Mottron, L., Peretz, I., Trudel, M., Gallun, E., & Bonnel, A.-M. (2003). Enhanced pitch sensitivity in individuals with autism: A signal detection analysis. *Journal of Cognitive Neuroscience, 15*(2), 226–235.

Bos, K. J., Zeanah, C. H., Smyke, A. T., Fox, N. A., & Nelson, C. A. (2010). Stereotypies in children with a history of early institutional care. *Archives of Pediatrics and Adolescent Medicine, 164*(5), 406–411.

Boyd, L. E., Ringland, K. E., Faucett, H., Hiniker, A., Klein, K., Patel, K., & Hayes, G. R. (2017). Evaluating an iPad game to address overselectivity in preliterate AAC users with minimal verbal behavior. In *Proceedings of the 19th International ACM SIGACCESS Conference on Computers and Accessibility* (pp. 240–249). New York: ACM.

Bradshaw, J., Steiner, A. M., Gengoux, G., & Koegel, L. K. (2015). Feasibility and effectiveness of very early intervention for infants at-risk for autism spectrum disorder: A systematic review. *Journal of Autism and Developmental Disorders, 45*(3), 778–794.

Branson, D., & Demchak, M. (2009). The use of augmentative and alternative communication methods with infants and toddlers with disabilities: A research review. *Augmentative and Alternative Communication, 25*(4), 274–286.

Bremner, A. J., Mareschal, D., Lloyd-Fox, S., & Spence, C. (2008). Spatial localization of touch in the first year of life: Early influence of a visual spatial code and the development of remapping across changes in limb position. *Journal of Experimental Psychology: General, 137*(1), 149–162.

Brooks, B. A., Haynes, K., Smith, J., McFadden, T., & Robins, D. L. (2016). Implementation of web-based autism screening in an urban clinic. *Clinical Pediatrics, 55*(10), 927–934.

Brosnan, M., Parsons, S., Good, J., & Yuill, N. (2016). How can participatory design inform the design and development of innovative technologies for autistic communities? *Journal of Assistive Technologies, 10*(2), 115–120.

Brown, A. M. (1990). Development of visual sensitivity to light and color vision in human infants: A critical review. *Vision Research, 30*(8), 1159–1188.

Brownell, C. A., Zerwas, S., & Ramani, G. B. (2007). "So big": The development of body self-awareness in toddlers. *Child Development, 78*(5), 1426–1440.

Brunner, D., Vasko, R., Detka, C., Monahan, J., Reynolds, C. R., & Kupfer, D. (1996). Muscle artifacts in the sleep EEG: Automated detection and effect on all-night EEG power spectra. *Journal of Sleep Research, 5*(3), 155–164.

Burton, C., McKinstry, B., Szentagotai Tătar, A., Serrano-Blanco, A., Pagliari, C., & Wolters, M. (2013). Activity monitoring in patients with depression: A systematic review. *Journal of Affective Disorders, 145*(1), 21–28.

Bussu, G., Jones, E. J. H., Charman, T., Johnson, M. H., Buitelaar, J. K., Baron-Cohen, S., . . . BASIS Team. (2018). Prediction of autism at 3 years from behavioural and developmental measures in high-risk infants: A longitudinal cross-domain classifier analysis. *Journal of Autism and Developmental Disorders, 48*(7), 2418–2433.

Butchart, M., Long, J. J., Brown, M., McMillan, A., Bain, J., & Karatzias, T. (2017).

Autism and visual impairment: A review of the literature. *Review Journal of Autism and Developmental Disorders, 4*(2), 118–131.

Butler, M. G., Dasouki, M. J., Zhou, X.-P., Talebizadeh, Z., Brown, M., Takahashi, T. N., ... Eng, C. (2005). Subset of individuals with autism spectrum disorders and extreme macrocephaly associated with germline PTEN tumour suppressor gene mutations. *Journal of Medical Genetics, 42*(4), 318–321.

Buttross, S., Curtis, J., Lucas, A., & Annett, R. (2018). Forging a new path to early discovery: Parterning childcare centers with telemedicine for developmental screening: *Pediatrics, 141*(1 Meeting Abstract), 50.

Cabibihan, J.-J., Javed, H., Aldosari, M., Frazier, T. W., & Elbashir, H. (2017). Sensing technologies for autism spectrum disorder screening and intervention. *Sensors (Basel), 17*(1), 46.

Cabibihan, J.-J., Javed, H., Ang, M., & Aljunied, S. M. (2013). Why robots?: A survey on the roles and benefits of social robots in the therapy of children with autism. *International Journal of Social Robotics, 5*(4), 593–618.

Cagiltay, K., Kara, N., & Aydin, C. C. (2014). Smart toy based learning. In J. M. Spector, M. D. Merrill, J. Elen, & M. J. Bishop (Eds.), *Handbook of research on educational communications and technology* (pp. 703–711). New York: Springer.

Campbell, D. J., Chang, J., & Chawarska, K. (2014). Early generalized overgrowth in autism spectrum disorder: Prevalence rates, gender effects, and clinical outcomes. *Journal of the American Academy of Child and Adolescent Psychiatry, 53*(10), 1063–1073.

Campbell, D. J., Shic, F., Macari, S., & Chawarska, K. (2014). Gaze response to dyadic bids at 2 years related to outcomes at 3 years in autism spectrum disorders: A subtyping analysis. *Journal of Autism and Developmental Disorders, 44*(2), 431–442.

Campbell, K., Carpenter, K. L. H., Espinosa, S., Hashemi, J., Qiu, Q., Tepper, M., ... Dawson, G. (2017). Use of a digital modified checklist for autism in toddlers—Revised with follow-up to improve quality of screening for autism. *Journal of Pediatrics, 183*, 133–139.

Campbell, K., Carpenter, K. L., Hashemi, J., Espinosa, S., Marsan, S., Borg, J. S., ... Dawson, G. (2018). Computer vision analysis captures atypical attention in toddlers with autism. *Autism, 23*(3), 619–628.

Campolo, D., Molteni, M., Guglielmelli, E., Keller, F., Laschi, C., & Dario, P. (2006). Towards development of biomechatronic tools for early diagnosis of neurodevelopmental disorders. In *2006 International Conference of the IEEE Engineering in Medicine and Biology Society* (pp. 3242–3245).

Carey, W. B. (1970). A simplified method for measuring infant temperament. *Journal of Pediatrics, 77*(2), 188–194.

Carey, W. B. (1972). Clinical applications of infant temperament measurements. *Journal of Pediatrics, 81*(4), 823–828.

Cascio, C., McGlone, F., Folger, S., Tannan, V., Baranek, G., Pelphrey, K. A., & Essick, G. (2008). Tactile perception in adults with autism: A multidimensional psychophysical study. *Journal of Autism and Developmental Disorders, 38*(1), 127–137.

Cascio, C. J., Moana-Filho, E. J., Guest, S., Nebel, M. B., Weisner, J., Baranek, G. T., & Essick, G. K. (2012). Perceptual and neural response to affective tactile texture stimulation in adults with autism spectrum disorders. *Autism Research, 5*(4), 231–244.

Centers for Medicare and Medicaid Services. (2015). National Coverage Determination

(NCD) for speech generating devices (50.1). Retrieved January 14, 2019, from *www.cms.gov/medicare-coverage-database.*

Charlop-Christy, M. H., Le, L., & Freeman, K. A. (2000). A comparison of video modeling with in vivo modeling for teaching children with autism. *Journal of Autism and Developmental Disorders, 30*(6), 537–552.

Chawarska, K., Campbell, D., Chen, L., Shic, F., Klin, A., & Chang, J. (2011). Early generalized overgrowth in boys with autism. *Archives of General Psychiatry, 68*(10), 1021–1031.

Chawarska, K., Klin, A., Paul, R., & Volkmar, F. (2007). Autism spectrum disorder in the second year: Stability and change in syndrome expression. *Journal of Child Psychology and Psychiatry, 48*(2), 128–138.

Chawarska, K., Macari, S., & Shic, F. (2012). Context modulates attention to social scenes in toddlers with autism. *Journal of Child Psychology and Psychiatry, and Allied Disciplines, 53*(8), 903–913.

Chawarska, K., Macari, S., & Shic, F. (2013). Decreased spontaneous attention to social scenes in 6-month-old infants later diagnosed with autism spectrum disorders. *Biological Psychiatry, 74*(3), 195–203.

Chawarska, K., & Shic, F. (2009). Looking but not seeing: Atypical visual scanning and recognition of faces in 2- and 4-year-old children with autism spectrum disorder. *Journal of Autism and Developmental Disorders, 39*(12), 1663–1672.

Chawarska, K., Shic, F., Macari, S., Campbell, D. J., Brian, J., Landa, R., . . . Bryson, S. (2014). 18-month predictors of later outcomes in younger siblings of children with autism spectrum disorder: A Baby Siblings Research Consortium study. *Journal of the American Academy of Child and Adolescent Psychiatry, 53*(12), 1317–1327.

Chawarska, K., Ye, S., Shic, F., & Chen, L. (2015). Multilevel differences in spontaneous social attention in toddlers with autism spectrum disorder. *Child Development, 87*(2), 543–557.

Chen, K. B., Savage, A. B., Chourasia, A. O., Wiegmann, D. A., & Sesto, M. E. (2013). Touch screen performance by individuals with and without motor control disabilities. *Applied Ergonomics, 44*(2), 297–302.

Chita-Tegmark, M. (2016). Social attention in ASD: A review and meta-analysis of eye-tracking studies. *Research in Developmental Disabilities, 48*, 79–93.

Chong, E., Chanda, K., Ye, Z., Southerland, A., Ruiz, N., Jones, R. M., . . . Rehg, J. M. (2017). Detecting gaze towards eyes in natural social interactions and its use in child assessment. *Proceedings of the ACM on Interactive, Mobile, Wearable Ubiquitous Technology, 1*(3), 43:1–43:20.

Christakis, D. A. (2009). The effects of infant media usage: What do we know and what should we learn? *Acta Paediatrica, 98*(1), 8–16.

Cihak, D., Fahrenkrog, C., Ayres, K. M., & Smith, C. (2010). The use of video modeling via a video iPod and a system of least prompts to improve transitional behaviors for students with autism spectrum disorders in the general education classroom. *Journal of Positive Behavior Interventions, 12*(2), 103–115.

Colombo, J., & Fagen, J. (2014). *Individual differences in infancy: Reliability, stability, and prediction.* New York: Psychology Press.

Costanzo, V., Chericoni, N., Amendola, F. A., Casula, L., Muratori, F., Scattoni, M. L., & Apicella, F. (2015). Early detection of autism spectrum disorders: From retrospective home video studies to prospective "high risk" sibling studies. *Neuroscience and Biobehavioral Reviews, 55*, 627–635.

Council on Communications and Media. (2016). Media and young minds. *Pediatrics, 138*(5), e20162591.

Crippa, A., Salvatore, C., Perego, P., Forti, S., Nobile, M., Molteni, M., & Castiglioni, I. (2015). Use of machine learning to identify children with autism and their motor abnormalities. *Journal of Autism and Developmental Disorders, 45*(7), 2146–2156.

Davidoff, B. E. (2017). AAC with energy—Earlier. *The ASHA Leader.* Retrieved from *https://leader.pubs.asha.org/doi/abs/10.1044/leader.FTR2.22012017.48.*

Dawson, M., Soulieres, I., Gernsbacher, M. A., & Mottron, L. (2007). The level and nature of autistic intelligence. *Psychological Science, 18*(8), 657–662.

DeBoth, K. K., & Reynolds, S. (2017). A systematic review of sensory-based autism subtypes. *Research in Autism Spectrum Disorders, 36,* 44–56.

D'Hooge, H., Dalton, L., Shwe, H., Lieberman, D., & O'Malley, C. (2000). Smart toys: Brave new world? In *CHI '00 Extended Abstracts on Human Factors in Computing Systems* (pp. 247–248). New York: ACM.

Diehl, J. J., Crowell, C. R., Villano, M., Wier, K., Tang, K., & Riek, L. D. (2014). Clinical applications of robots in autism spectrum disorder diagnosis and treatment. In V. B. Patel, V. R. Preedy, & C. R. Martin (Eds.), *Comprehensive guide to autism* (pp. 411–422). New York: Springer.

Diehl, J. J., Schmitt, L. M., Villano, M., & Crowell, C. R. (2012). The clinical use of robots for individuals with autism spectrum disorders: A critical review. *Research in Autism Spectrum Disorders, 6*(1), 249–262.

Doherty, A. R., Hodges, S. E., King, A. C., Smeaton, A. F., Berry, E., Moulin, C. J. A., . . . Foster, C. (2013). Wearable cameras in health: The state of the art and future possibilities. *American Journal of Preventive Medicine, 44*(3), 320–323.

Dunn, W. (2014). *Child Sensory Profile—2: User's manual.* Bloomington, MN: Pearson.

Dunn, W., & Bennett, D. (2002). Patterns of sensory processing in children with attention deficit hyperactivity disorder. *OTJR: Occupation, Participation and Health, 22*(1), 4–15.

Dunn, W., & Daniels, D. B. (2002). Initial development of the infant/toddler sensory profile. *Journal of Early Intervention, 25*(1), 27–41.

Duquette, A., Michaud, F., & Mercier, H. (2008). Exploring the use of a mobile robot as an imitation agent with children with low-functioning autism. *Autonomous Robots, 24*(2), 147–157.

Durkin, M. S., Elsabbagh, M., Barbaro, J., Gladstone, M., Happe, F., Hoekstra, R. A., . . . Shih, A. (2015). Autism screening and diagnosis in low resource settings: Challenges and opportunities to enhance research and services worldwide. *Autism Research, 8*(5), 473–476.

Dykstra, J. R., Sabatos-DeVito, M. G., Irvin, D. W., Boyd, B. A., Hume, K. A., & Odom, S. L. (2013). Using the Language ENvironment Analysis (LENA) system in preschool classrooms with children with autism spectrum disorders. *Autism, 17*(5), 582–594.

Edmunds, S. R., Rozga, A., Li, Y., Karp, E. A., Ibañez, L. V., Rehg, J. M., & Stone, W. L. (2017). Brief report: Using a point-of-view camera to measure eye gaze in young children with autism spectrum disorder during naturalistic social interactions: A pilot study. *Journal of Autism and Developmental Disorders, 47*(3), 898–904.

Eigsti, I.-M., de Marchena, A. B., Schuh, J. M., & Kelley, E. (2011). Language acquisition in autism spectrum disorders: A developmental review. *Research in Autism Spectrum Disorders, 5*(2), 681–691.

Ekin, C. C., Cagiltay, K., & Karasu, N. (2018). Effectiveness of smart toy applications in teaching children with intellectual disability. *Journal of Systems Architecture,* *89,* 41–48.

Elison, J. T., Paterson, S. J., Wolff, J. J., Reznick, J. S., Sasson, N. J., Gu, H., . . . Piven, J. (2013). White matter microstructure and atypical visual orienting in 7-month-olds at risk for autism. *American Journal of Psychiatry, 170*(8), 899–908.

Ellemberg, D., Lewis, T. L., Hong Liu, C., & Maurer, D. (1999). Development of spatial and temporal vision during childhood. *Vision Research, 39*(14), 2325–2333.

Elsabbagh, M., Fernandes, J., Jane Webb, S., Dawson, G., Charman, T., & Johnson, M. H. (2013). Disengagement of visual attention in infancy is associated with emerging autism in toddlerhood. *Biological Psychiatry, 74*(3), 189–194.

Emerson, R. W., Adams, C., Nishino, T., Hazlett, H. C., Wolff, J. J., Zwaigenbaum, L., . . . Piven, J. (2017). Functional neuroimaging of high-risk 6-month-old infants predicts a diagnosis of autism at 24 months of age. *Science Translational Medicine, 9*(393), eaag2882.

Engel-Yeger, B., Muzio, C., Rinosi, G., Solano, P., Geoffroy, P. A., Pompili, M., . . . Serafini, G. (2016). Extreme sensory processing patterns and their relation with clinical conditions among individuals with major affective disorders. *Psychiatry Research, 236,* 112–118.

Ermer, J., & Dunn, W. (1998). The sensory profile: A discriminant analysis of children with and without disabilities. *American Journal of Occupational Therapy, 52*(4), 283–290.

Escobedo, L., Ibarra, C., Hernandez, J., Alvelais, M., & Tentori, M. (2014). Smart objects to support the discrimination training of children with autism. *Personal Ubiquitous Computing, 18*(6), 1485–1497.

Esposito, G., Venuti, P., Apicella, F., & Muratori, F. (2011). Analysis of unsupported gait in toddlers with autism. *Brain and Development, 33*(5), 367–373.

Estes, A., Munson, J., Rogers, S. J., Greenson, J., Winter, J., & Dawson, G. (2015). Long-term outcomes of early intervention in 6-year-old children with autism spectrum disorder. *Journal of the American Academy of Child and Adolescent Psychiatry, 54*(7), 580–587.

Evans, D. W., Leckman, J. F., Carter, A., Reznick, J. S., Henshaw, D., King, R. A., & Pauls, D. (1997). Ritual, habit, and perfectionism: The prevalence and development of compulsive-like behavior in normal young children. *Child Development, 68*(1), 58–68.

Ferguson, C. J. (2018). Children should not be protected from using interactive screens. In C. J. Ferguson (Ed.), *Video game influences on aggression, cognition, and attention* (pp. 83–91). Cham, Switzerland: Springer International.

Filippetti, M. L., Johnson, M. H., Lloyd-Fox, S., Dragovic, D., & Farroni, T. (2013). Body perception in newborns. *Current Biology, 23*(23), 2413–2416.

Filippetti, M. L., Orioli, G., Johnson, M. H., & Farroni, T. (2015). Newborn body perception: Sensitivity to spatial congruency. *Infancy, 20*(4), 455–465.

Firchow, P., & Mac Ginty, R. (2017). Including hard-to-access populations using mobile phone surveys and participatory indicators. *Sociological Methods and Research, 49*(1), 133–160.

Firouzian, A., Asghar, Z., Tervonen, J., Pulli, P., & Yamamoto, G. (2015). Conceptual design and implementation of indicator-based smart glasses: A navigational device for remote assistance of senior citizens suffering from memory loss. In *2015 9th International Symposium on Medical Information and Communication Technology (ISMICT)* (pp. 153–156).

Flanagan, J. E., Landa, R., Bhat, A., & Bauman, M. (2012). Head lag in infants at risk for autism: A preliminary study. *American Journal of Occupational Therapy, 66*(5), 577–585.

Fleer, M. (2016). Theorising digital play: A cultural-historical conceptualisation of children's engagement in imaginary digital situations. *International Research in Early Childhood Education, 7*(2), 75–90.

Fletcher-Watson, S., Pain, H., Hammond, S., Humphry, A., & McConachie, H. (2016). Designing for young children with autism spectrum disorder: A case study of an iPad app. *International Journal of Child-Computer Interaction, 7*, 1–14.

Fombonne, E., Rogé, B., Claverie, J., Courty, S., & Frémolle, J. (1999). Microcephaly and macrocephaly in autism. *Journal of Autism and Developmental Disorders, 29*(2), 113–119.

Fong, T., Nourbakhsh, I., & Dautenhahn, K. (2003). A survey of socially interactive robots. *Robotics and Autonomous Systems, 42*(3–4), 143–166.

Frazier, T. W., Strauss, M., Klingemier, E. W., Zetzer, E. E., Hardan, A. Y., Eng, C., & Youngstrom, E. A. (2017). A meta-analysis of gaze differences to social and non-social information between individuals with and without autism. *Journal of the American Academy of Child and Adolescent Psychiatry, 56*(7), 546–555.

Freeman, D., Reeve, S., Robinson, A., Ehlers, A., Clark, D., Spanlang, B., & Slater, M. (2017). Virtual reality in the assessment, understanding, and treatment of mental health disorders. *Psychological Medicine, 47*(14), 2393–2400.

Frenkel, S. (2018, January 2). A cute toy just brought a hacker into your home. *The New York Times.* Retrieved from *www.nytimes.com/2017/12/21/technology/connected-toys-hacking.html.*

Friston, K. J., Williams, S., Howard, R., Frackowiak, R. S. J., & Turner, R. (1996). Movement-related effects in fMRI time-series. *Magnetic Resonance in Medicine, 35*(3), 346–355.

Fujimoto, I., Matsumoto, T., De Silva, P. R. S., Kobayashi, M., & Higashi, M. (2011). Mimicking and evaluating human motion to improve the imitation skill of children with autism through a robot. *International Journal of Social Robotics, 3*(4), 349–357.

Fullard, W., McDevitt, S. C., & Carey, W. B. (1984). Assessing temperament in one- to three-year-old children. *Journal of Pediatric Psychology, 9*(2), 205–217.

Fusaro, V. A., Daniels, J., Duda, M., DeLuca, T. F., D'Angelo, O., Tamburello, J., . . . Wall, D. P. (2014). The potential of accelerating early detection of autism through content analysis of youtube videos. *PLOS ONE, 9*(4), e93533.

Ganz, J. B., Earles-Vollrath, T. L., & Cook, K. E. (2011). Video modeling. *Teaching Exceptional Children, 43*(6), 8–19.

García, M. A. G., Ruiz, M. L. M., Rivera, D., Vadillo, L., & Duboy, M. A. V. (2017). A smart toy to enhance the decision-making process at children's psychomotor delay screenings: A pilot study. *Journal of Medical Internet Research, 19*(5), e171.

Gerber, R. J., Wilks, T., & Erdie-Lalena, C. (2010). Developmental milestones: Motor development. *Pediatrics in Review, 31*(7), 267–277.

Gilkerson, J., Richards, J. A., Warren, S. F., Montgomery, J. K., Greenwood, C. R., Oller, D. K., . . . Paul, T. D. (2017). Mapping the early language environment using all-day recordings and automated analysis. *American Journal of Speech-Language Pathology, 26*(2), 248–265.

Gliga, T., Bedford, R., Charman, T., Johnson, M. H., Baron-Cohen, S., Bolton, P., . . . Tucker, L. (2015). Enhanced visual search in infancy predicts emerging autism symptoms. *Current Biology, 25*(13), 1727–1730.

Golan, O., Ashwin, E., Granader, Y., McClintock, S., Day, K., Leggett, V., & Baron-

Cohen, S. (2010). Enhancing emotion recognition in children with autism spectrum conditions: An intervention using animated vehicles with real emotional faces. *Journal of Autism and Developmental Disorders, 40*(3), 269–279.

Goldstein, J., Buckingham, D., & Brougere, G. (2004). *Toys, games, and media.* New York: Routledge.

Green, S. A., & Ben-Sasson, A. (2010). Anxiety disorders and sensory over-responsivity in children with autism spectrum disorders: Is there a causal relationship? *Journal of Autism and Developmental Disorders, 40*(12), 1495–1504.

Green, S. A., Ben-Sasson, A., Soto, T. W., & Carter, A. S. (2012). Anxiety and sensory over-responsivity in toddlers with autism spectrum disorders: Bidirectional effects across time. *Journal of Autism and Developmental Disorders, 42*(6), 1112–1119.

GSM Association. (2018). The mobile economy—Sub-Saharan Africa 2018. Retrieved from *www.gsma.com/mobileeconomy/sub-saharan-africa*.

Guernsey, L. (2012). *Screen time: How electronic media—from baby videos to educational software—affects your young child.* New York: Basic Books.

Guthrie, W., Swineford, L. B., Nottke, C., & Wetherby, A. M. (2013). Early diagnosis of autism spectrum disorder: Stability and change in clinical diagnosis and symptom presentation. *Journal of Child Psychology and Psychiatry, 54*(5), 582–590.

Gwin, J. T., Gramann, K., Makeig, S., & Ferris, D. P. (2010). Removal of movement artifact from high-density EEG recorded during walking and running. *Journal of Neurophysiology, 103*(6), 3526–3534.

Hadders-Algra, M. (2008). Reduced variability in motor behaviour: An indicator of impaired cerebral connectivity? *Early Human Development, 84*(12), 787–789.

Hadders-Algra, M. (2010). Variation and cariability: Key words in human motor development. *Physical Therapy, 90*(12), 1823–1837.

Hamad, C. D., Serna, R. W., Morrison, L., & Fleming, R. (2010). Extending the reach of early intervention training for practitioners: A preliminary investigation of an online curriculum for teaching behavioral intervention knowledge in autism to families and service providers. *Infants and Young Children, 23*(3), 195–208.

Happé, F. (1999). Autism: Cognitive deficit or cognitive style? *Trends in Cognitive Sciences, 3*(6), 216–222.

Happé, F., Ronald, A., & Plomin, R. (2006). Time to give up on a single explanation for autism. *Nature Neuroscience, 9*(10), 1218.

Harbison, A. L., Woynaroski, T. G., Tapp, J., Wade, J. W., Warlaumont, A. S., & Yoder, P. J. (2018). A new measure of child vocal reciprocity in children with autism spectrum disorder. *Autism Research, 11*(6), 903–915.

Harrington, J. W., Bai, R., & Perkins, A. M. (2013). Screening children for autism in an urban clinic using an electronic M-CHAT. *Clinical Pediatrics, 52*(1), 35–41.

Hashemi, J., Campbell, K., Carpenter, K., Harris, A., Qiu, Q., Tepper, M., . . . Sapiro, G. (2015). A scalable app for measuring autism risk behaviors in young children: A technical validity and feasibility study. In *Proceedings of the 5th EAI International Conference on Wireless Mobile Communication and Healthcare* (pp. 23–27). Brussels, Belgium: Institute for Computer Sciences, Social-Informatics and Telecommunications Engineering.

Hashemi, J., Dawson, G., Carpenter, K. L. H., Campbell, K., Qiu, Q., Espinosa, S., . . . Sapiro, G. (2018). Computer vision analysis for quantification of autism risk behaviors. *IEEE Transactions on Affective Computing,* pp. 1–12.

Hashemi, J., Spina, T. V., Tepper, M., Esler, A., Morellas, V., Papanikolopoulos, N., & Sapiro, G. (2012). Computer vision tools for the non-invasive assessment of autism-related behavioral markers. *ArXiv:1210.7014 [Cs.CV]*. Retrieved from *http://arxiv.org/abs/1210.7014*.

Hazan, V., & Barrett, S. (2000). The development of phonemic categorization in children aged 6–12. *Journal of Phonetics, 28*(4), 377–396.

Hazlett, H. C., Gu, H., Munsell, B. C., Kim, S. H., Styner, M., Wolff, J. J., . . . the IBIS Network. (2017). Early brain development in infants at high risk for autism spectrum disorder. *Nature, 542*(7641), 348–351.

Hellendoorn, A., Wijnroks, L., van Daalen, E., Dietz, C., Buitelaar, J. K., & Leseman, P. (2015). Motor functioning, exploration, visuospatial cognition and language development in preschool children with autism. *Research in Developmental Disabilities, 39*, 32–42.

Hepper, P. G., Scott, D., & Shahidullah, S. (1993). Newborn and fetal response to maternal voice. *Journal of Reproductive and Infant Psychology, 11*(3), 147–153.

Hernandez, P., & Ikkanda, Z. (2011). Applied behavior analysis: Behavior management of children with autism spectrum disorders in dental environments. *Journal of the American Dental Association, 142*(3), 281–287.

Herrera, G., Casas, X., Sevilla, J., Rosa, L., Pardo, C., Plaza, J., . . . Le Groux, S. (2012). Pictogram room: Natural interaction technologies to aid in the development of children with autism. *Annuary of Clinical and Health Psychology, 8*, 39–44.

Hill, E. L. (2001). Non-specific nature of specific language impairment: A review of the literature with regard to concomitant motor impairments. *International Journal of Language and Communication Disorders, 36*(2), 149–171.

Hiniker, A., Lee, B., Kientz, J. A., & Radesky, J. S. (2018). Let's play!: Digital and analog play between preschoolers and parents. In *Proceedings of the 2018 CHI Conference on Human Factors in Computing Systems* (pp. 1–659). New York: ACM.

Hitoglou, M., Ververi, A., Antoniadis, A., & Zafeiriou, D. I. (2010). Childhood autism and auditory system abnormalities. *Pediatric Neurology, 42*(5), 309–314.

Høiseth, M., Giannakos, M. N., Alsos, O. A., Jaccheri, L., & Asheim, J. (2013). Designing healthcare games and applications for toddlers. In *Proceedings of the 12th International Conference on Interaction Design and Children* (pp. 137–146). New York: ACM.

Horne-Moyer, H. L., Moyer, B. H., Messer, D. C., & Messer, E. S. (2014). The use of electronic games in therapy: A review with clinical implications. *Current Psychiatry Reports, 16*(12), 520.

Hung, P. C. K., Iqbal, F., Huang, S.-C., Melaisi, M., & Pang, K. (2016). A glance of child's play privacy in smart toys. In X. Sun, A. Liu, H.-C. Chao, & E. Bertino (Eds.), *Cloud Computing and Security* (pp. 217–231). Cham, Switzerland: Springer International.

Hutt, C., Hutt, S. J., Lee, D., & Ounsted, C. (1964). Arousal and childhood autism. *Nature, 204*(4961), 908–909.

Ikeda, J., Davitt, B. V., Ultmann, M., Maxim, R., & Cruz, O. A. (2013). Brief report: Incidence of ophthalmologic disorders in children with autism. *Journal of Autism and Developmental Disorders, 43*(6), 1447–1451.

Iverson, J. M. (2010). Developing language in a developing body: The relationship between motor development and language development. *Journal of Child Language, 37*(2), 229–261.

Iverson, J., Shic, F., Wall, C. A., Chawarska, K., Curtin, S., Estes, A., . . . Young, G. (2019). Early motor abilities in infants at heightened vs. low risk for ASD: A Baby Siblings Research Consortium (BSRC) study. *Journal of Abnormal Psychology, 128*(1), 69–80.

Jang, J., Dixon, D. R., Tarbox, J., Granpeesheh, D., Kornack, J., & de Nocker, Y. (2012). Randomized trial of an eLearning program for training family members of children with autism in the principles and procedures of applied behavior analysis. *Research in Autism Spectrum Disorders, 6*(2), 852–856.

Janvier, Y. M., Harris, J. F., Coffield, C. N., Louis, B., Xie, M., Cidav, Z., & Mandell, D. S. (2016). Screening for autism spectrum disorder in underserved communities: Early childcare providers as reporters. *Autism, 20*(3), 364–373.

Jones, M. L., & Meurer, K. (2016). Can (and should) Hello Barbie keep a secret? In *2016 IEEE International Symposium on Ethics in Engineering, Science and Technology (ETHICS)* (pp. 1–6).

Jones, W., & Klin, A. (2013). Attention to eyes is present but in decline in 2–6-month-old infants later diagnosed with autism. *Nature, 504*(7480), 427–431.

Jurdi, S., Montaner, J., Garcia-Sanjuan, F., Jaen, J., & Nacher, V. (2018). A systematic review of game technologies for pediatric patients. *Computers in Biology and Medicine, 97,* 89–112.

Kaiser, M. D., Yang, D. Y.-J., Voos, A. C., Bennett, R. H., Gordon, I., Pretzsch, C., . . . Pelphrey, K. A. (2016). Brain mechanisms for processing affective (and nonaffective) touch are atypical in autism. *Cerebral Cortex, 26*(6), 2705–2714.

Kanne, S. M., Carpenter, L. A., & Warren, Z. (2018). Screening in toddlers and preschoolers at risk for autism spectrum disorder: Evaluating a novel mobile-health screening tool. *Autism Research, 11*(7), 1038–1049.

Karatekin, C. (2007). Eye tracking studies of normative and atypical development. *Developmental Review, 27*(3), 283–348.

Kasari, C., Kaiser, A., Goods, K., Nietfeld, J., Mathy, P., Landa, R., . . . Almirall, D. (2014). Communication interventions for minimally verbal children with autism: A sequential multiple assignment randomized trial. *Journal of the American Academy of Child and Adolescent Psychiatry, 53*(6), 635–646.

Kern, J. K., Geier, D. A., Adams, J. B., Troutman, M. R., Davis, G., King, P. G., & Geier, M. R. (2011). Autism severity and muscle strength: A correlation analysis. *Research in Autism Spectrum Disorders, 5*(3), 1011–1015.

Kern, J. K., Geier, D. A., Adams, J. B., Troutman, M. R., Davis, G. A., King, P. G., & Geier, M. R. (2013). Handgrip strength in autism spectrum disorder compared with controls. *Journal of Strength and Conditioning Research, 27*(8), 2277–2281.

Kientz, J. A., Arriaga, R. I., & Abowd, G. D. (2009). Baby Steps: Evaluation of a system to support record-keeping for parents of young children. In *Proceedings of the SIGCHI Conference on Human Factors in Computing Systems* (pp. 1713–1722). New York: ACM.

Kientz, J. A., Goodwin, M. S., Hayes, G. R., & Abowd, G. D. (2013). Interactive technologies for autism. *Synthesis Lectures on Assistive, Rehabilitative, and Health-Preserving Technologies, 2*(2), 1–177.

Kim, E. S., Berkovits, L. D., Bernier, E. P., Leyzberg, D., Shic, F., Paul, R., & Scassellati, B. (2013). Social robots as embedded reinforcers of social behavior in children with autism. *Journal of Autism and Developmental Disorders, 43*(5), 1038–1049.

Kim, E. S., Daniell, C. M., Makar, C., Elia, J., Scassellati, B., & Shic, F. (2015). Potential clinical impact of positive affect in robot interactions for autism intervention. In *2015 International Conference on Affective Computing and Intelligent Interaction (ACII)* (pp. 8–13).

Kim, E. S., Naples, A., Gearty, G. V., Wang, Q., Wallace, S., Wall, C., . . . Shic, F. (2014). Development of an untethered, mobile, low-cost head-mounted eye tracker. In

Proceedings of the Symposium on Eye Tracking Research and Applications (pp. 247–250). New York: ACM.

Kim, E. S., Paul, R., Shic, F., & Scassellati, B. (2012). Bridging the research gap: Making HRI useful to individuals with autism. *Journal of Human-Robot Interaction, 1*(1), 26–54.

Kirkorian, H. L., Wartella, E. A., & Anderson, D. R. (2008). Media and young children's learning. *The Future of Children, 18*(1), 39–61.

Klin, A., Lin, D., Gorrindo, P., Ramsay, G., & Jones, W. (2009). Two-year-olds with autism orient to non-social contingencies rather than biological motion. *Nature, 459*(7244), 257–261.

Knoblauch, K., Vital-Durand, F., & Barbur, J. L. (2001). Variation of chromatic sensitivity across the life span. *Vision Research, 41*(1), 23–36.

Kobak, K. A., Stone, W. L., Ousley, O. Y., & Swanson, A. (2011). Web-based training in early autism screening: Results from a pilot study. *Telemedicine and E-Health, 17*(8), 640–644.

Kobak, K. A., Stone, W. L., Wallace, E., Warren, Z., Swanson, A., & Robson, K. (2011). A web-based tutorial for parents of young children with autism: Results from a pilot study. *Telemedicine and E-Health, 17*(10), 804–808.

Koegel, L. K., Koegel, R. L., Ashbaugh, K., & Bradshaw, J. (2014). The importance of early identification and intervention for children with or at risk for autism spectrum disorders. *International Journal of Speech-Language Pathology, 16*(1), 50–56.

Koegel, L. K., Koegel, R. L., Nefdt, N., Fredeen, R., Klein, E. F., & Bruinsma, Y. E. M. (2005). First S.T.E.P: A model for the early identification of children with autism spectrum disorders. *Journal of Positive Behavior Interventions, 7*(4), 247–252.

Kozima, H., Nakagawa, C., & Yasuda, Y. (2007). Children–robot interaction: A pilot study in autism therapy. *Progress in Brain Research, 164,* 385–400.

Kuczmarski, R. J., Ogden, C. L., Grummer-Strawn, L. M., Flegal, K. M., Guo, S. S., Wei, R., . . . Johnson, C. L. (2000). *CDC growth charts: United States* (No. 314; Advance Data from Vital and Health Statistics, pp. 1–27). Washington, DC: National Center for Health Statistics.

Kumazaki, H., Muramatsu, T., Yoshikawa, Y., Yoshimura, Y., Ikeda, T., Hasegawa, C., . . . Kikuchi, M. (2019). Brief report: A novel system to evaluate autism spectrum disorders using two humanoid robots. *Journal of Autism and Developmental Disorders, 49*(4), 1709–1716.

Lancioni, G. E., O'Reilly, M. F., Cuvo, A. J., Singh, N. N., Sigafoos, J., & Didden, R. (2007). PECS and VOCAs to enable students with developmental disabilities to make requests: An overview of the literature. *Research in Developmental Disabilities, 28*(5), 468–488.

Lauricella, A. R., Pempek, T. A., Barr, R., & Calvert, S. L. (2010). Contingent computer interactions for young children's object retrieval success. *Journal of Applied Developmental Psychology, 31*(5), 362–369.

Lazarou, I., Nikolopoulos, S., Petrantonakis, P. C., Kompatsiaris, I., & Tsolaki, M. (2018). EEG-based brain–computer interfaces for communication and rehabilitation of people with motor impairment: A novel approach of the 21st century. *Frontiers in Human Neuroscience, 12,* 14.

LeBarton, E. S., & Iverson, J. M. (2013). Fine motor skill predicts expressive language in infant siblings of children with autism. *Developmental Science, 16*(6), 815–827.

Leekam, S., Tandos, J., McConachie, H., Meins, E., Parkinson, K., Wright, C., . . . Couteur, A. L. (2007). Repetitive behaviours in typically developing 2-year-olds. *Journal of Child Psychology and Psychiatry, 48*(11), 1131–1138.

Leibold, L. J., & Werner, L. A. (2006). Effect of masker-frequency variability on the detection performance of infants and adults. *Journal of the Acoustical Society of America, 119*(6), 3960–3970.

Leonard, H. C., Bedford, R., Pickles, A., Hill, E. L., & Team, B. (2015). Predicting the rate of language development from early motor skills in at-risk infants who develop autism spectrum disorder. *Research in Autism Spectrum Disorders, 13,* 15–24.

Lewis, M. (2013). Stereotyped movement disorder. In F. R. Volkmar (Ed.), *Encyclopedia of autism spectrum disorders* (pp. 2997–3003). New York: Springer.

Lewis, M., & Kim, S.-J. (2009). The pathophysiology of restricted repetitive behavior. *Journal of Neurodevelopmental Disorders, 1*(2), 114.

Li, B., Atyabi, A., Kim, M., Barney, E., Ahn, A. Y., Luo, Y., . . . Shic, F. (2018). Social influences on executive functioning in autism: Design of a mobile gaming platform. In *Proceedings of the 2018 CHI Conference on Human Factors in Computing Systems* (pp. 1–443:13). New York: ACM.

Little, L. M., Dean, E., Tomchek, S. D., & Dunn, W. (2017). Classifying sensory profiles of children in the general population. *Child Care, Health and Development, 43*(1), 81–88.

Liu, R., Salisbury, J. P., Vahabzadeh, A., & Sahin, N. T. (2017). Feasibility of an autism-focused augmented reality smartglasses system for social communication and behavioral coaching. *Frontiers in Pediatrics, 5,* 145.

Lloyd, M., MacDonald, M., & Lord, C. (2013). Motor skills of toddlers with autism spectrum disorders. *Autism, 17*(2), 133–146.

Logan, K., Iacono, T., & Trembath, D. (2017). A systematic review of research into aided AAC to increase social-communication functions in children with autism spectrum disorder. *Augmentative and Alternative Communication, 33*(1), 51–64.

Lord, C., Rutter, M., DiLavore, P. C., Risi, S., Gotham, K., & Bishop, S. L. (2012). *Autism Diagnostic Observation Schedule, 2nd ed. (ADOS-2) Manual (Part 1): Modules 1–4.* Torrance, CA: Western Psychological Services.

Lovaas, O. I. (1987). Behavioral treatment and normal educational and intellectual functioning in young autistic children. *Journal of Consulting and Clinical Psychology, 55*(1), 3–9.

Loveland, K. A. (1991). Social affordances and interaction: II. Autism and the affordances of the human environment. *Ecological Psychology, 3*(2), 99–119.

Lueder, R., & Rice, V. J. B. (2007). *Ergonomics for children: Designing products and places for toddler to teens.* Boca Raton: CRC Press.

Luscre, D. M., & Center, D. B. (1996). Procedures for reducing dental fear in children with autism. *Journal of Autism and Developmental Disorders, 26*(5), 547–556.

Macari, S., Chawarska, K., Kim, E. S., Wall, C., Wilkinson, M., Barney, E., . . . Shic, F. (2018, May). *A multimedia screening system to predict ASD symptoms in diverse community settings: Preliminary convergent and concurrent validity.* Abstract presented at the 2018 International Society for Autism Research (INSAR 2018), Rotterdam, the Netherlands.

Mamun, K. A. A., Bardhan, S., Ullah, M. A., Anagnostou, E., Brian, J., Akhter, S., & Rabbani, M. G. (2016). Smart autism—A mobile, interactive and integrated framework for screening and confirmation of autism. In *2016 38th Annual International Conference of the IEEE Engineering in Medicine and Biology Society (EMBC)* (pp. 5989–5992).

Marrus, N., Glowinski, A. L., Jacob, T., Klin, A., Jones, W., Drain, C. E., . . . Constantino, J. N. (2015). Rapid video-referenced ratings of reciprocal social behavior in toddlers: A twin study. *Journal of Child Psychology and Psychiatry, 56*(12), 1338–1346.

Marrus, N., Kennon-McGill, S., Harris, B., Zhang, Y., Glowinski, A. L., & Constantino, J. N. (2018). Use of a video scoring anchor for rapid serial assessment of social communication in toddlers. *Journal of Visualized Experiments, 133,* 57041.

Matson, J. L., Mahan, S., Fodstad, J. C., Hess, J. A., & Neal, D. (2010). Motor skill abilities in toddlers with autistic disorder, pervasive developmental disorder-not otherwise specified, and atypical development. *Research in Autism Spectrum Disorders, 4*(3), 444–449.

May, T., Brignell, A., Hawi, Z., Brereton, A., Tonge, B., Bellgrove, M. A., & Rinehart, N. J. (2018). Trends in the overlap of autism spectrum disorder and attention deficit hyperactivity disorder: Prevalence, clinical management, language and genetics. *Current Developmental Disorders Reports, 5*(1), 49–57.

Mazurek, M. O., Shattuck, P. T., Wagner, M., & Cooper, B. P. (2012). Prevalence and correlates of screen-based media use among youths with autism spectrum disorders. *Journal of Autism and Developmental Disorders, 42*(8), 1757–1767.

Mazurek, M. O., & Wenstrup, C. (2012). Television, video game and social media use among children with ASD and typically developing siblings. *Journal of Autism and Developmental Disorders, 43*(6), 1258–1271.

McDowell, M. A., Fryar, C. D., Ogden, C. L., & Flegal, K. M. (2008). Anthropometric reference data for children and adults: United States, 2003–2006. *National Health Statistics Reports, 10,* 5.

McGlone, F., & Reilly, D. (2010). The cutaneous sensory system. *Neuroscience and Biobehavioral Reviews, 34*(2), 148–159.

Mehl-Schneider, T., & Steinmetz, S. (2014). Video games as a form of therapeutic intervention for children with autism spectrum disorders. In N. R. Silton (Ed.), *Video games as a form of therapeutic intervention for children with autism spectrum disorders.* IGI Global. Retrieved from *www.igi-global.com/chapter/video-games-as-a-form-of-therapeutic-intervention-for-children-with-autism-spectrum-disorders/99569.*

Mehler, J., Jusczyk, P., Lambertz, G., Halsted, N., Bertoncini, J., & Amiel-Tison, C. (1988). A precursor of language acquisition in young infants. *Cognition, 29*(2), 143–178.

Michaud, F., Salter, T., Duquette, A., Mercier, H., Lauria, M., Larouche, H., & Larose, F. (2007). Assistive technologies and child-robot interaction. *2007 AAAI Spring Symposium Series Papers: Multidisciplinary Collaboration for Socially Assistive Robotics* (pp. 1–5).

Miles, J. H., Takahashi, T. N., Bagby, S., Sahota, P. K., Vaslow, D. F., Wang, C. H., . . . Farmer, J. E. (2005). Essential versus complex autism: Definition of fundamental prognostic subtypes. *American Journal of Medical Genetics Part A, 135A*(2), 171–180.

Min, C. H., Tewfik, A. H., Kim, Y., & Menard, R. (2009). Optimal sensor location for body sensor network to detect self-stimulatory behaviors of children with autism spectrum disorder. *Conference Proceedings at the IEEE Engineering in Medicine and Biology Society, 2009,* 3489–3492.

Montagu, A. (1986). *Touching: The human significance of the skin* (3rd ed.). New York: William Morrow Paperbacks.

Moon, C., Cooper, R. P., & Fifer, W. P. (1993). Two-day-olds prefer their native language. *Infant Behavior and Development, 16*(4), 495–500.

Moore, D. J. (2015). Acute pain experience in individuals with autism spectrum disorders: A review. *Autism, 19*(4), 387–399.

Moore, M., & Calvert, S. (2000). Brief report: Vocabulary acquisition for children with autism: Teacher or computer instruction. *Journal of Autism and Developmental Disorders, 30*(4), 359–362.

Morgan, L., Wetherby, A. M., & Barber, A. (2008). Repetitive and stereotyped movements in children with autism spectrum disorders late in the second year of life. *Journal of Child Psychology and Psychiatry, and Allied Disciplines, 49*(8), 826–837.

Moser, A., Zimmermann, L., Dickerson, K., Grenell, A., Barr, R., & Gerhardstein, P. (2015). They can interact, but can they learn?: Toddlers' transfer learning from touchscreens and television. *Journal of Experimental Child Psychology, 137,* 137–155.

Mottron, L., Dawson, M., Soulieres, I., Hubert, B., & Burack, J. (2006). Enhanced perceptual functioning in autism: An update, and eight principles of autistic perception. *Journal of Autism and Developmental Disorders, 36*(1), 27–43.

Murdoch, H. (1996). Stereotyped behaviors in deaf and hard of hearing children. *American Annals of the Deaf, 141*(5), 379–386.

Murias, M., Major, S., Davlantis, K., Franz, L., Harris, A., Rardin, B., . . . Dawson, G. (2018). Validation of eye-tracking measures of social attention as a potential biomarker for autism clinical trials. *Autism Research, 11*(1), 166–174.

Myers, L. J., LeWitt, R. B., Gallo, R. E., & Maselli, N. M. (2017). Baby FaceTime: Can toddlers learn from online video chat? *Developmental Science, 20*(4), e12430.

Nader, R., Oberlander, T. F., Chambers, C. T., & Craig, K. D. (2004). Expression of pain in children with autism. *Clinical Journal of Pain, 20*(2), 88.

Nagai, Y., Asada, M., & Hosoda, K. (2002). Developmental learning model for joint attention. *Proceedings of the IEEE/RSJ International Conference on Intelligent Robots and Systems, 1,* 932–937.

Nakagawa, A., Sukigara, M., Miyachi, T., & Nakai, A. (2016). Relations between temperament, sensory processing, and motor coordination in 3-year-old children. *Frontiers in Psychology, 7,* 623.

Ng, L. E. (2017). Technology as an extension of the self: Socialising through technology for young people with autism. In A. Marcus & W. Wang (Eds.), *Design, user experience, and usability: Understanding users and contexts* (pp. 393–402). Cham, Switzerland: Springer International.

Nickel, L. R., Thatcher, A. R., Keller, F., Wozniak, R. H., & Iverson, J. M. (2013). Posture development in infants at heightened versus low risk for autism spectrum disorders. *Infancy, 18*(5), 639–661.

Nie, G., Zheng, Z., Johnson, J., Swanson, A. R., Weitlauf, A. S., Warren, Z. E., & Sarkar, N. (2018). Predicting response to joint attention performance in human–human interaction based on human-robot interaction for young children with autism spectrum disorder. In *2018 27th IEEE International Symposium on Robot and Human Interactive Communication (RO-MAN)* (pp. 1–4).

Noor, H. A. M., Shahbodin, F., & Pee, N. C. (2012). Serious game for autism children: Review of literature. *World Academy of Science, Engineering and Technology: International Journal of Social, Behavioral, Educational, Economic, Business and Industrial Engineering, 6*(4), 554–559.

Nordahl, C. W., Mello, M., Shen, A. M., Shen, M. D., Vismara, L. A., Li, D., . . . Amaral, D. G. (2016). Methods for acquiring MRI data in children with autism spectrum disorder and intellectual impairment without the use of sedation. *Journal of Neurodevelopmental Disorders, 8*(1), 20.

O'boyle, C. G., & Rothbart, M. K. (1996). Assessment of distress to sensory stimulation in early infancy through parent report. *Journal of Reproductive and Infant Psychology, 14*(2), 121–132.

O'Connor, K. (2012). Auditory processing in autism spectrum disorder: A review. *Neuroscience and Biobehavioral Reviews, 36*(2), 836–854.

O'Hearn, K., Asato, M., Ordaz, S., & Luna, B. (2008). Neurodevelopment and executive function in autism. *Development and Psychopathology, 20*(4), 1103–1132.

Oller, D. K., Niyogi, P., Gray, S., Richards, J. A., Gilkerson, J., Xu, D., . . . Warren, S. F. (2010). Automated vocal analysis of naturalistic recordings from children with autism, language delay, and typical development. *Proceedings of the National Academy of Sciences, 107*(30), 13354–13359.

Olsho, L. W., Koch, E. G., & Halpin, C. F. (1987). Level and age effects in infant frequency discrimination. *Journal of the Acoustical Society of America, 82*(2), 454–464.

Orben, A., & Przybylski, A. K. (2019). The association between adolescent well-being and digital technology use. *Nature Human Behaviour, 3,* 173–182.

Osterling, J., & Dawson, G. (1994). Early recognition of children with autism: A study of first birthday home videotapes. *Journal of Autism and Developmental Disorders, 24*(3), 247–257.

Ottley, J. R. (2016). Real-time coaching with bug-in-ear technology: A practical approach to support families in their child's development. *Young Exceptional Children, 19*(3), 32–46.

Ottley, J. R., & Hanline, M. F. (2014). Bug-in-ear coaching: Impacts on early childhood educators' practices and associations with toddlers' expressive communication. *Journal of Early Intervention, 36*(2), 90–110.

Ozonoff, S., Macari, S., Young, G. S., Goldring, S., Thompson, M., & Rogers, S. J. (2008). Atypical object exploration at 12 months of age is associated with autism in a prospective sample. *Autism, 12*(5), 457–471.

Ozonoff, S., Young, G. S., Landa, R. J., Brian, J., Bryson, S., Charman, T., . . . Iosif, A.-M. (2015). Diagnostic stability in young children at risk for autism spectrum disorder: A Baby Siblings Research Consortium study. *Journal of Child Psychology and Psychiatry, 56*(9), 988–998.

Pawar, R., Albin, A., Gupta, U., Rao, H., Carberry, C., Hamo, A., . . . Clements, M. A. (2017). Automatic analysis of LENA recordings for language assessment in children aged five to fourteen years with application to individuals with autism. In *2017 IEEE EMBS International Conference on Biomedical Health Informatics (BHI)* (pp. 245–248).

Pennisi, P., Tonacci, A., Tartarisco, G., Billeci, L., Ruta, L., Gangemi, S., & Pioggia, G. (2016). Autism and social robotics: A systematic review. *Autism Research, 9*(2), 165–183.

Pew Research Center. (2018). Basic mobile phones more common than smartphones in sub-Saharan Africa. Retrieved from *www.pewglobal.org/2018/10/09/majorities-in-sub-saharan-africa-own-mobile-phones-but-smartphone-adoption-is-modest.*

Pew Research Center Global Attitudes and Trends. (2016). Smartphone ownership and internet usage continues to climb in emerging economies. Retrieved from *www.pewglobal.org/2016/02/22/smartphone-ownership-and-internet-usage-continues-to-climb-in-emerging-economies.*

Piek, J. P. (2002). The role of variability in early motor development. *Infant Behavior and Development, 25*(4), 452–465.

Pierce, K., Marinero, S., Hazin, R., McKenna, B., Barnes, C. C., & Malige, A. (2015). Eye tracking reveals abnormal visual preference for geometric images as an early biomarker of an autism spectrum disorder subtype associated with increased symptom severity. *Biological Psychiatry, 79*(8), 657–666.

Ploog, B. O., Scharf, A., Nelson, D., & Brooks, P. J. (2013). Use of computer-assisted technologies (CAT) to enhance social, communicative, and language development in children with autism spectrum disorders. *Journal of Autism and Developmental Disorders, 43*(2), 301–322.

Popple, B., Wall, C., Flink, L., Powell, K., Discepolo, K., Keck, D., . . . Shic, F. (2016). Brief report: Remotely delivered video modeling for improving oral hygiene in children with ASD: A pilot study. *Journal of Autism and Developmental Disorders, 46*(8), 2791–2796.

Powell, G., Wass, S. V., Erichsen, J. T., & Leekam, S. R. (2016). First evidence of the feasibility of gaze-contingent attention training for school children with autism. *Autism, 20*(8), 927–937.

Power, J. D., Barnes, K. A., Snyder, A. Z., Schlaggar, B. L., & Petersen, S. E. (2012). Spurious but systematic correlations in functional connectivity MRI networks arise from subject motion. *NeuroImage, 59*(3), 2142–2154.

Prince, E. B., Kim, E. S., Wall, C. A., Gisin, E., Goodwin, M. S., Simmons, E. S., . . . Shic, F. (2017). The relationship between autism symptoms and arousal level in toddlers with autism spectrum disorder, as measured by electrodermal activity. *Autism: International Journal of Research and Practice, 21*(4), 504–508.

Puts, N. A. J., Wodka, E. L., Tommerdahl, M., Mostofsky, S. H., & Edden, R. A. E. (2014). Impaired tactile processing in children with autism spectrum disorder. *Journal of Neurophysiology, 111*(9), 1803–1811.

Rabbitt, S. M., Kazdin, A. E., & Scassellati, B. (2015). Integrating socially assistive robotics into mental healthcare interventions: Applications and recommendations for expanded use. *Clinical Psychology Review, 35*, 35–46.

Rafferty, L., Hung, P. C. K., Fantinato, M., Peres, S. M., Iqbal, F., Kuo, S.-Y., & Huang, S.-C. (2017). Towards a privacy rule conceptual model for smart toys. In J. K. T. Tang & P. C. K. Hung (Eds.), *Computing in smart toys* (pp. 85–102). Cham, Switzerland: Springer International.

Ramalho, M. I. (2017). The private is public or Furbies are us. *E-Cadernos Ces* (27).

Ratcliff, K., Hong, I., & Hilton, C. (2018). Leisure participation patterns for school age youth with autism spectrum disorders: Findings from the 2016 National Survey of Children's Health. *Journal of Autism and Developmental Disorders, 48*(11), 3783–3793.

Rego, P., Moreira, P. M., & Reis, L. P. (2010). *Serious games for rehabilitation: A survey and a classification towards a taxonomy.* Paper presented at 5th Iberian Conference on Information Systems and Technologies (CISTI), Santiago de Compostela, Spain.

Rehg, J. M. (2011). Behavior imaging: Using computer vision to study autism. *Twelfth IAPR Conference on Machine Vision Applications (MVA2011), 11*, 14–21.

Rehg, J. M., Rozga, A., Abowd, G. D., & Goodwin, M. S. (2014). Behavioral imaging and autism. *IEEE Pervasive Computing, 13*(2), 84–87.

Reinertsen, E., & Clifford, G. D. (2018). A review of physiological and behavioral monitoring with digital sensors for neuropsychiatric illnesses. *Physiological Measurement, 39*(5), 05TR01.

Richards, J. A., Xu, D., Gilkerson, J., Yapanel, U., Gray, S., & Paul, T. (2017). Automated assessment of child vocalization development using LENA. *Journal of Speech, Language, and Hearing Research, 60*(7), 2047–2063.

Riek, L. D. (2012). Wizard of Oz studies in HRI: A systematic review and new reporting guidelines. *Journal of Human-Robot Interaction, 1*(1), 119–136.

Ringland, K. E., Wolf, C. T., Faucett, H., Dombrowski, L., & Hayes, G. R. (2016). "Will I always be not social?": Re-conceptualizing sociality in the context of a minecraft community for autism. In *Proceedings of the 2016 CHI Conference on Human Factors in Computing Systems* (pp. 1256–1269). New York: ACM.

Ritterfeld, U., Cody, M., & Vorderer, P. (2009). *Serious games: Mechanisms and effects.* New York: Routledge.

Robertson, C. E., & Baron-Cohen, S. (2017). Sensory perception in autism. *Nature Reviews Neuroscience, 18*(11), 671–684.

Robins, D. L., Fein, D., Barton, M. L., & Green, J. A. (2001). The Modified Checklist for Autism in Toddlers: An initial study investigating the early detection of autism and pervasive developmental disorders. *Journal of Autism and Developmental Disorders, 31*(2), 131–144.

Roche, L., Zhang, D., Bartl-Pokorny, K. D., Pokorny, F. B., Schuller, B. W., Esposito, G., . . . Marschik, P. B. (2018). Early vocal development in autism spectrum disorder, Rett syndrome, and fragile x syndrome: Insights from studies using retrospective video analysis. *Advances in Neurodevelopmental Disorders, 2*(1), 49–61.

Rogers, S. J., Hepburn, S., & Wehner, E. (2003). Parent reports of sensory symptoms in toddlers with autism and those with other developmental disorders. *Journal of Autism and Developmental Disorders, 33*(6), 631–642.

Rollins, J. D., Collins, J. S., & Holden, K. R. (2010). United States head circumference growth reference charts: Birth to 21 years. *Journal of Pediatrics, 156*(6), 907–913.

Rose, V., Trembath, D., Keen, D., & Paynter, J. (2016). The proportion of minimally verbal children with autism spectrum disorder in a community-based early intervention programme. *Journal of Intellectual Disability Research, 60*(5), 464–477.

Rosenhall, U., Nordin, V., Sandström, M., Ahlsén, G., & Gillberg, C. (1999). Autism and hearing loss. *Journal of Autism and Developmental Disorders, 29*(5), 349–357.

Rowberry, J., Macari, S., Chen, G., Campbell, D., Leventhal, J. M., Weitzman, C., & Chawarska, K. (2015). Screening for autism spectrum disorders in 12-month-old high-risk siblings by parental report. *Journal of Autism and Developmental Disorders, 45*(1), 221–229.

Rydzewska, E., Hughes-McCormack, L. A., Gillberg, C., Henderson, A., MacIntyre, C., Rintoul, J., & Cooper, S.-A. (2018). Prevalence of long-term health conditions in adults with autism: Observational study of a whole country population. *BMJ Open, 8*(8), e023945.

Sarkar, A., Wade, J., Swanson, A., Weitlauf, A., Warren, Z., & Sarkar, N. (2018). A data-driven mobile application for efficient, engaging, and accurate screening of ASD in toddlers. In M. Antona & C. Stephanidis (Eds.), *Universal access in human-computer interaction. methods, technologies, and users* (pp. 560–570). Cham, Switzerland: Springer International.

Scassellati, B. (1999). Imitation and mechanisms of joint attention: A developmental structure for building social skills on a humanoid robot. *Computation for Metaphors, Analogy and Agents, 1562,* 176–195.

Scassellati, B. (2005). Quantitative metrics of social response for autism diagnosis. In

IEEE International Workshop on Robot and Human Interactive Communication, 2005 (pp. 585–590).

Scassellati, B., Admoni, H., & Matarić, M. (2012). Robots for use in autism research. *Annual Review of Biomedical Engineering, 14*(1), 276–294.

Scassellati, B., Boccanfuso, L., Huang, C.-M., Mademtzi, M., Qin, M., Salomons, N., . . . Shic, F. (2018). Improving social skills in children with ASD using a long-term, in-home social robot. *Science Robotics, 3*(21), eaat7544.

Schaaf, R. C., & Lane, A. E. (2015). Toward a best-practice protocol for assessment of sensory features in ASD. *Journal of Autism and Developmental Disorders, 45*(5), 1380–1395.

Schlosser, R. W., & Sigafoos, J. (2006). Augmentative and alternative communication interventions for persons with developmental disabilities: Narrative review of comparative single-subject experimental studies. *Research in Developmental Disabilities, 27*(1), 1–29.

Schreibman, L., Dawson, G., Stahmer, A. C., Landa, R., Rogers, S. J., McGee, G. G., . . . Halladay, A. (2015). Naturalistic developmental behavioral interventions: Empirically validated treatments for autism spectrum disorder. *Journal of Autism and Developmental Disorders, 45*(8), 2411–2428.

See, P. C. S., & Navarro, J. O. (2018). Association of media screening time and high-risk developmental disabilities among toddlers and preschoolers seen in a tertiary hospital's center for developmental pediatrics from January 2015–December 2015. *Pediatrics, 142*(1, Meeting Abstract), 781.

Senju, A., Southgate, V., White, S., & Frith, U. (2009). Mindblind eyes: An absence of spontaneous theory of mind in Asperger syndrome. *Science, 325*(5942), 883–885.

Shane, H. C., & Albert, P. D. (2008). Electronic screen media for persons with autism spectrum disorders: Results of a survey. *Journal of Autism and Developmental Disorders, 38*(8), 1499–1508.

Sharma, A., & Abrol, P. (2013). Research issues in designing improved eye gaze based HCI techniques for augmentative and alternative communication. *International Journal of Emerging Technologies in Computational and Applied Sciences, 6*(2), 149–153.

Shevell, M. I., Majnemer, A., Rosenbaum, P., & Abrahamowicz, M. (2001). Etiologic determination of childhood developmental delay. *Brain and Development, 23*(4), 228–235.

Shic, F. (2013a). Eye-tracking. In F. R. Volkmar (Ed.), *Encyclopedia of autism spectrum disorders* (pp. 1208–1213). New York: Springer.

Shic, F. (2013b). Video games, use of. In F. R. Volkmar (Ed.), *Encyclopedia of autism spectrum disorders* (pp. 3255–3265). New York: Springer.

Shic, F. (2016). Eye tracking as a behavioral biomarker for psychiatric conditions: The road ahead. *Journal of the American Academy of Child and Adolescent Psychiatry, 55*(4), 267–268.

Shic, F., Bradshaw, J., Klin, A., Scassellati, B., & Chawarska, K. (2011). Limited activity monitoring in toddlers with autism spectrum disorder. *Brain Research, 1380*, 246–254.

Shic, F., Chawarska, K., Kim, E. S., Wall, C., Wilkinson, M., Barney, E., . . . Macari, S. (2018, May). *A multimedia screening system to predict later ASD symptoms in diverse community settings: A machine-learning design for infants and toddlers.* Abstract presented at the 2018 International Society for Autism Research (INSAR 2018), Rotterdam, the Netherlands.

Shic, F., Macari, S., & Chawarska, K. (2014). Speech disturbs face scanning in 6-month-old infants who develop autism spectrum disorder. *Biological Psychiatry, 75*(3), 231–237.

Shic, F., & Scassellati, B. (2007). Pitfalls in the modeling of developmental systems. *International Journal of Humanoid Robotics, 4*(2), 435–454.

Shic, F., Smith, D., Horsburgh, B., Hollander, E., Rehg, J. M., & Goodwin, M. (2015). Catalysts for change: The role of small business funders in the creation and dissemination of innovation. *Journal of Autism and Developmental Disorders, 45*(12), 3900–3904.

Shute, V. J., Ventura, M., Bauer, M., & Zapata-Rivera, D. (2009). Melding the power of serious games and embedded assessment to monitor and foster learning. *Serious Games: Mechanisms and Effects, 2*, 295–321.

Simmons, D. R., Robertson, A. E., McKay, L. S., Toal, E., McAleer, P., & Pollick, F. E. (2009). Vision in autism spectrum disorders. *Vision Research, 49*(22), 2705–2739.

Simmons, E. S., Paul, R., & Shic, F. (2016). Brief report: A mobile application to treat prosodic deficits in autism spectrum disorder and other communication impairments: A pilot study. *Journal of Autism and Developmental Disorders, 46*(1), 320–327.

Singer, H. S. (2009). Motor stereotypies. *Seminars in Pediatric Neurology, 16*(2), 77–81.

Skouteris, H., & Kelly, L. (2006). Repeated-viewing and co-viewing of an animated video?: An examination of factors that impact on young children's comprehension of video content. *Australian Journal of Early Childhood, 31*(3), 22–30.

Soderquist, D. R., & Moore, M. J. (1970). Effect of training on frequency discrimination in primary school children. *Journal of Auditory Research, 10*(3), 185–192.

Spence, M. J., & DeCasper, A. J. (1987). Prenatal experience with low-frequency maternal-voice sounds influence neonatal perception of maternal voice samples. *Infant Behavior and Development, 10*(2), 133–142.

Squires, J., Bricker, D., Twombly, E., Nickel, R., Clifford, D. J., Murphy, K., . . . Farrell, J. (2009). *Ages and Stages Questionnaires®, Third Edition (ASQ-3™): A parent-completed child monitoring system* (3rd ed.). Baltimore: Brookes.

Srinivasan, S. M., Eigsti, I.-M., Neely, L., & Bhat, A. N. (2016). The effects of embodied rhythm and robotic interventions on the spontaneous and responsive social attention patterns of children with autism spectrum disorder (ASD): A pilot randomized controlled trial. *Research in Autism Spectrum Disorders, 27*, 54–72.

Srinivasan, S. M., Kaur, M., Park, I. K., Gifford, T. D., Marsh, K. L., & Bhat, A. N. (2015a). The effects of rhythm and robotic interventions on the imitation/praxis, interpersonal synchrony, and motor performance of children with autism spectrum disorder (ASD): A pilot randomized controlled trial. *Autism Research and Treatment, 2015*, e736516.

Srinivasan, S. M., Park, I. K., Neely, L. B., & Bhat, A. N. (2015b). A comparison of the effects of rhythm and robotic interventions on repetitive behaviors and affective states of children with autism spectrum disorder (ASD). *Research in Autism Spectrum Disorders, 18*, 51–63.

Stone, B. G., Mills, K. A., & Saggers, B. (2019). Online multiplayer games for the social interactions of children with autism spectrum disorder: A resource for inclusive education. *International Journal of Inclusive Education, 23*(2), 209–228.

Strouse, G. A., Troseth, G. L., O'Doherty, K. D., & Saylor, M. M. (2018). Co-viewing supports toddlers' word learning from contingent and noncontingent video. *Journal of Experimental Child Psychology, 166*, 310–326.

Subki, A. H., Alsallum, M. S., Alnefaie, M. N., Alkahtani, A. M., Almagamsi, S. A., Alshehri, Z. S., . . . Jan, M. M. (2017). Pediatric motor stereotypies: An updated review. *Journal of Pediatric Neurology, 15*(4), 151–156.

Suh, H., Porter, J. R., Racadio, R., Sung, Y.-C., & Kientz, J. A. (2017). Baby steps text: Feasibility study of an SMS-based tool for tracking children's developmental progress. *AMIA Annual Symposium Proceedings, 2016,* 1997–2006.

Tager-Flusberg, H., & Kasari, C. (2013). Minimally verbal school-aged children with autism spectrum disorder: The neglected end of the spectrum. *Autism Research, 6*(6), 468–478.

Taguchi, K., Endo, C., Kurita, Y., & Tamura, M. (2017). The grip strength survey in infants (0–2 years old) and study of their development progress. *Japan Journal of Human Growth and Development Research, 2017*(74), 34–44.

Tahmasian, M., Khazaie, H., Golshani, S., & Avis, K. T. (2013). Clinical application of actigraphy in psychotic disorders: A systematic review. *Current Psychiatry Reports, 15*(6), 359.

Tanaka, J. W., Wolf, J. M., Klaiman, C., Koenig, K., Cockburn, J., Herlihy, L., . . . Schultz, R. T. (2010). Using computerized games to teach face recognition skills to children with autism spectrum disorder: The Let's Face It! program. *Journal of Child Psychology and Psychiatry, 51*(8), 944–952.

Tapia, E. M., Intille, S. S., Lopez, L., & Larson, K. (2006). The design of a portable kit of wireless sensors for naturalistic data collection. In K. P. Fishkin, B. Schiele, P. Nixon, & A. Quigley (Eds.), *Pervasive computing* (pp. 117–134). Berlin: Springer.

Tariq, Q., Daniels, J., Schwartz, J. N., Washington, P., Kalantarian, H., & Wall, D. P. (2018). Mobile detection of autism through machine learning on home video: A development and prospective validation study. *PLOS Medicine, 15*(11), e1002705.

Taylor, E., & Michael, K. (2016). Smart toys that are the stuff of nightmares [Editorial]. *IEEE Technology and Society Magazine, 35*(1), 8–10.

Thabtah, F. (2018). Machine learning in autistic spectrum disorder behavioral research: A review and ways forward. *Informatics for Health and Social Care, 44*(175), 1–20.

Thabtah, F. (2019). An accessible and efficient autism screening method for behavioural data and predictive analyses. *Health Informatics Journal, 25*(4), 1739–1755.

Thabtah, F., Kamalov, F., & Rajab, K. (2018). A new computational intelligence approach to detect autistic features for autism screening. *International Journal of Medical Informatics, 117,* 112–124.

Tharpe, A. M., & Ashmead, D. H. (2001). A longitudinal investigation of infant auditory sensitivity. *American Journal of Audiology, 10*(2), 104–112.

Thelen, E. (1980). Determinants of amounts of stereotyped behavior in normal human infants. *Evolution and Human Behavior, 1*(2), 141–150.

Thelen, E. (1995). Motor development: A new synthesis. *American Psychologist, 50*(2), 79–95.

Thill, S., Pop, C. A., Belpaeme, T., Ziemke, T., & Vanderborght, B. (2012). Robot-assisted therapy for autism spectrum disorders with (partially) autonomous control: Challenges and outlook. *Paladyn, 3*(4), 209–217.

Thomas, A., & Chess, S. (1968). *Temperament and behavior disorders in children.* New York: New York University Press.

Thomas, A., Chess, S., Birch, H. G., Hertzig, M. E., & Korn, S. (1963). *Behavioral individuality in early childhood.* New York: New York University Press.

Troseth, G. L., & DeLoache, J. S. (1998). The medium can obscure the message: Young children's understanding of video. *Child Development, 69*(4), 950–965.

Tröster, H., Brambring, M., & Beelmann, A. (1991). Prevalence and situational causes of stereotyped behaviors in blind infants and preschoolers. *Journal of Abnormal Child Psychology, 19*(5), 569–590.

Tryfona, C., Oatley, G., Calderon, A., & Thorne, S. (2016). M-Health solutions to support the National Health Service in the diagnosis and monitoring of autism spectrum disorders in young children. In M. Antona & C. Stephanidis (Eds.), *Universal access in human-computer interaction users and context diversity* (pp. 249–256). Cham, Switzerland: Springer International.

Turner, M. (1999). Annotation: Repetitive behaviour in autism: A review of psychological research. *Journal of Child Psychology and Psychiatry and Allied Disciplines, 40*(6), 839–849.

Turner, W. A., & Casey, L. M. (2014). Outcomes associated with virtual reality in psychological interventions: Were are we now? *Clinical Psychology Review, 34*(8), 634–644.

Turner-Brown, L. M., Lam, K. S. L., Holtzclaw, T. N., Dichter, G. S., & Bodfish, J. W. (2011). Phenomenology and measurement of circumscribed interests in autism spectrum disorders. *Autism, 15*(4), 437–456.

Valenti, S. S., & Gold, J. M. M. (1991). Social affordances and Interaction: I. Introduction. *Ecological Psychology, 3*(2), 77.

van der Meer, L., Sigafoos, J., O'Reilly, M. F., & Lancioni, G. E. (2011). Assessing preferences for AAC options in communication interventions for individuals with developmental disabilities: A review of the literature. *Research in Developmental Disabilities, 32*(5), 1422–1431.

Vereijken, B. (2010). The complexity of childhood development: Variability in perspective. *Physical Therapy, 90*(12), 1850–1859.

Vereijken, B., & Adolph, K. (1999). Transitions in the development of locomotion. In G. J. P. Savelsbergh, H. L. J. van der Maas, & P. C. L. van Geert (Eds.), *Non-linear analyses of developmental processes* (pp. 137–149). Amsterdam: Elsevier.

Vernetti, A., Senju, A., Charman, T., Johnson, M. H., & Gliga, T. (2018). Simulating interaction: Using gaze-contingent eye-tracking to measure the reward value of social signals in toddlers with and without autism. *Developmental Cognitive Neuroscience, 29*, 21–29.

Vidal, M., Turner, J., Bulling, A., & Gellersen, H. (2012). Wearable eye tracking for mental health monitoring. *Computer Communications, 35*(11), 1306–1311.

Vismara, L. A., McCormick, C. E. B., Wagner, A. L., Monlux, K., Nadhan, A., & Young, G. S. (2018). Telehealth parent training in the Early Start Denver Model: Results from a randomized controlled study. *Focus on Autism and Other Developmental Disabilities, 33*(2), 67–79.

Voos, A. C., Pelphrey, K. A., & Kaiser, M. D. (2013). Autistic traits are associated with diminished neural response to affective touch. *Social Cognitive and Affective Neuroscience, 8*(4), 378–386.

Wall, D. (2013). Autworks: A cross-disease analysis application for autism and related disorders. *AMIA Summits on Translational Science Proceedings, 2013*, 42–43.

Wall, D. P., Kosmicki, J., DeLuca, T. F., Harstad, E., & Fusaro, V. A. (2012). Use of machine learning to shorten observation-based screening and diagnosis of autism. *Translational Psychiatry, 2*(4), e100.

Wang, Q., Campbell, D. J., Macari, S. L., Chawarska, K., & Shic, F. (2018). Operationalizing atypical gaze in toddlers with autism spectrum disorders: A cohesion-based approach. *Molecular Autism, 9*, 25.

Wang, Q., Celebi, F. M., Flink, L., Greco, G., Wall, C., Prince, E., . . . Shic, F. (2015).

Interactive eye tracking for gaze strategy modification. In *Proceedings of the 14th International Conference on Interaction Design and Children* (pp. 247–250). New York: ACM.

Wang, Q., DiNicola, L., Heymann, P., Hampson, M., & Chawarska, K. (2017). Impaired value learning for faces in preschoolers with autism spectrum disorder. *Journal of the American Academy of Child and Adolescent Psychiatry, 57*(1), 33–40.

Warlaumont, A. S., Richards, J. A., Gilkerson, J., & Oller, D. K. (2014). A social feedback loop for speech development and its reduction in autism. *Psychological Science, 25*(7), 1314–1324.

Warren, S. F., Gilkerson, J., Richards, J. A., Oller, D. K., Xu, D., Yapanel, U., & Gray, S. (2009). What automated vocal analysis reveals about the vocal production and language learning environment of young children with autism. *Journal of Autism and Developmental Disorders, 40,* 555–569.

Warren, Z. E., Zheng, Z., Swanson, A. R., Bekele, E., Zhang, L., Crittendon, J. A., . . . Sarkar, N. (2013). Can robotic interaction improve joint attention skills? *Journal of Autism and Developmental Disorders, 45*(11), 3726–3734.

Wass, S., Porayska-Pomsta, K., & Johnson, M. H. (2011). Training attentional control in infancy. *Current Biology, 21*(18), 1543–1547.

Watt, N., Wetherby, A. M., Barber, A., & Morgan, L. (2008). Repetitive and stereotyped behaviors in children with autism spectrum disorders in the second year of life. *Journal of Autism and Developmental Disorders, 38*(8), 1518–1533.

Weng, M., Wall, C. A., Kim, E. S., Whitaker, L., Perlmutter, M., Wang, Q., . . . Shic, F. (2015). Linking volitional preferences for emotional information to social difficulties: A game approach using the microsoft kinect. In *2015 International Conference on Affective Computing and Intelligent Interaction (ACII)* (pp. 588–594). Xi'an, China.

Werner, E., Dawson, G., Osterling, J., & Dinno, N. (2000). Brief report: Recognition of autism spectrum disorder before one year of age: A retrospective study based on home videotapes. *Journal of Autism and Developmental Disorders, 30*(2), 157–162.

Werner, L. A. (2007). Issues in human auditory development. *Journal of Communication Disorders, 40*(4), 275–283.

Westby, C. (2018). Why children with autism are more at risk for the negative effects of screen time. *Word of Mouth, 29*(5), 9–13.

Westeyn, T. L., Abowd, G. D., Starner, T. E., Johnson, J. M., Presti, P. W., & Weaver, K. A. (2012). Monitoring children's developmental progress using augmented toys and activity recognition. *Personal Ubiquitous Computing, 16*(2), 169–191.

Whiteley, P., & Shattock, P. (2002). Biochemical aspects in autism spectrum disorders: Updating the opioid-excess theory and presenting new opportunities for biomedical intervention. *Expert Opinion on Therapeutic Targets, 6*(2), 175–183.

Whyte, E. M., Smyth, J. M., & Scherf, K. S. (2014). Designing serious game interventions for individuals with autism. *Journal of Autism and Developmental Disorders, 45*(12), 3820–3831.

Wiggs, L., & Stores, G. (2004). Sleep patterns and sleep disorders in children with autistic spectrum disorders: Insights using parent report and actigraphy. *Developmental Medicine and Child Neurology, 46*(6), 372–380.

Wilkinson, M., Shic, F., Chawarska, K., Kim, E. S., Wall, C., Barney, E., . . . Macari, S. (2018, May). *Deployment of a multimedia screening tool for asd in a diverse community setting: Feasibility and usability.* Abstract presented at the 2018 International Society for Autism Research (INSAR 2018), Rotterdam, the Netherlands.

Wilson, H. R. (1988). Development of spatiotemporal mechanisms in infant vision. *Vision Research, 28*(5), 611–628.

Wilson, K. P., Carter, M. W., Wiener, H. L., DeRamus, M. L., Bulluck, J. C., Watson, L. R., . . . Baranek, G. T. (2017). Object play in infants with autism spectrum disorder: A longitudinal retrospective video analysis. *Autism and Developmental Language Impairments, 2,* 2–12.

Wing, L., Gould, J., & Gillberg, C. (2011). Autism spectrum disorders in the DSM-V: Better or worse than the DSM-IV? *Research in Developmental Disabilities, 32*(2), 768–773.

Wolf, J. M., Tanaka, J. W., Klaiman, C., Cockburn, J., Herlihy, L., Brown, C., . . . Schultz, R. T. (2008). Specific impairment of face-processing abilities in children with autism spectrum disorder using the "Let's Face It!" skills battery. *Autism Research, 1*(6), 329–340.

Wolff, J. J., Botteron, K. N., Dager, S. R., Elison, J. T., Estes, A. M., Gu, H., . . . Piven, J. (2014). Longitudinal patterns of repetitive behavior in toddlers with autism. *Journal of Child Psychology and Psychiatry, 55*(8), 945–953.

Woynaroski, T., Oller, D. K., Keceli-Kaysili, B., Xu, D., Richards, J. A., Gilkerson, J., . . . Yoder, P. (2017). The stability and validity of automated vocal analysis in preverbal preschoolers with autism spectrum disorder. *Autism Research, 10*(3), 508–519.

Xu, D., Yapanel, U., & Gray, S. (2009). *Reliability of the LENA™ language environment analysis system in young children's natural language home environment.* Boulder, CO: LENA Foundation.

Ye, Z., Li, Y., Fathi, A., Han, Y., Rozga, A., Abowd, G. D., & Rehg, J. M. (2012). Detecting eye contact using wearable eye-tracking glasses. In *Proceedings of the 2012 ACM Conference on Ubiquitous Computing* (pp. 699–704). New York: ACM.

Ye, Z., Li, Y., Liu, Y., Bridges, C., Rozga, A., & Rehg, J. M. (2015). Detecting bids for eye contact using a wearable camera. In *2015 11th IEEE International Conference and Workshops on Automatic Face and Gesture Recognition (FG)* (Vol. 1, pp. 1–8).

Yoder, P. J., Oller, D. K., Richards, J. A., Gray, S., & Gilkerson, J. (2013). Stability and validity of an automated measure of vocal development from day-long samples in children with and without autism spectrum disorder. *Autism Research, 6*(2), 103–107.

Yuodelis, C., & Hendrickson, A. (1986). A qualitative and quantitative analysis of the human fovea during development. *Vision Research, 26*(6), 847–855.

Zaltz, Y., Ari-Even Roth, D., Karni, A., & Kishon-Rabin, L. (2018). Long-term training-induced gains of an auditory skill in school-age children as compared with adults. *Trends in Hearing, 22*(2), 1–14.

Zheng, Z., Das, S., Young, E. M., Swanson, A., Warren, Z., & Sarkar, N. (2014). Autonomous robot-mediated imitation learning for children with autism. In *2014 IEEE International Conference on Robotics and Automation (ICRA)* (pp. 2707–2712).

Zheng, Z., Fu, Q., Zhao, H., Swanson, A., Weitlauf, A., Warren, Z., & Sarkar, N. (2015). Design of a computer-assisted system for teaching attentional skills to toddlers with ASD. In M. Antona & C. Stephanidis (Eds.), *Universal access in human-computer interaction: Access to learning, health and well-being* (pp. 721–730). Cham, Switzerland: Springer International.

Zheng, Z., Zhao, H., Swanson, A. R., Weitlauf, A. S., Warren, Z. E., & Sarkar, N. (2018). Design, development, and evaluation of a noninvasive autonomous robot-mediated joint attention intervention system for young children with ASD. *IEEE Transactions on Human-Machine Systems, 48*(2), 125–135.

Zimmerman, F. J., & Christakis, D. A. (2005). Children's television viewing and cognitive outcomes: A longitudinal analysis of national data. *Archives of Pediatrics and Adolescent Medicine, 159*(7), 619–625.

Zwaigenbaum, L., Bauman, M. L., Choueiri, R., Kasari, C., Carter, A., Granpeesheh, D., . . . Natowicz, M. R. (2015). Early intervention for children with autism spectrum disorder under 3 years of age: Recommendations for practice and research. *Pediatrics, 136*(Suppl. 1), S60–S81.

Zwaigenbaum, L., Bryson, S., & Garon, N. (2013). Early identification of autism spectrum disorders. *Behavioural Brain Research, 251,* 133–146.

Zwaigenbaum, L., Bryson, S., Lord, C., Rogers, S., Carter, A., Carver, L., . . . Dobkins, K. (2009). Clinical assessment and management of toddlers with suspected autism spectrum disorder: Insights from studies of high-risk infants. *Pediatrics, 123*(5), 1383.

Zwaigenbaum, L., Bryson, S., Rogers, T., Roberts, W., Brian, J., & Szatmari, P. (2005). Behavioral manifestations of autism in the first year of life. *International Journal of Developmental Neuroscience, 23*(2–3), 143–152.

Zwaigenbaum, L., Thurm, A., Stone, W., Baranek, G., Bryson, S., Iverson, J., . . . Sigman, M. (2007). Studying the emergence of autism spectrum disorders in high-risk infants: Methodological and practical issues. *Journal of Autism and Developmental Disorders, 37*(3), 466–480.

CHAPTER 11

• • • • • • • • •

Potential Challenges of Importing Autism Spectrum Disorder Screening and Diagnostic Tools from High-Income Countries to Resource-Poor Settings

Amina Abubakar, Kavita Ruparelia, Joseph K. Gona,
Kenneth Rimba, Rachel Mapenzi, Petrus J. de Vries,
Fons J. R. van de Vijver, Andy Shih, and Charles R. Newton

Autism spectrum disorders (ASD) are neurodevelopmental disorders associated with impairments in social interaction and communication and restricted patterns of behavior, interests, and activities; these symptoms typically manifest in the first 3 years of life (American Psychiatric Association, 2013). In 2010, it was estimated that there were 52 million people with ASD worldwide (Baxter et al., 2015), and in 2012, the global prevalence of ASD was estimated at 1–2% of the population (Elsabbagh et al., 2012). However, little is known of ASD in low- and middle-income countries (Baxter et al., 2015; Elsabbagh et al., 2012; Franz, Chambers, von Isenburg, & de Vries, 2017). In a systematic review of published data, Franz and colleagues (2017) highlight the large disparity between data emanating from resource-poor settings and those from North America and Europe.

Various factors may contribute to this lack of information, including other health care priorities, lack of resources, and expertise (Abubakar, Ssewanyana, de Vries, & Newton, 2016). In this chapter, we focus on one specific factor: the lack of screening and diagnostic tools suitable for use in resource-poor settings (RPSs); Manji & Hogan, 2014; Varma & Iskandar, 2014). We describe procedures that can be employed to develop culturally appropriate measures and challenges to developing such tools. We propose a comprehensive methodological approach that can be used in the development and translation of tools to ensure a rigorous and culturally sensitive method that maintains both quality and diagnostic fidelity. The chapter does not extensively discuss challenges of diagnosis in infancy in RPSs largely because in these settings the challenges faced are similar across the different age groups. Moreover, most children receive a diagnosis and services or placement at a relatively older age compared to the average age of diagnosis in high-income settings. Another challenge is the fact that in both high-income and resource-poor settings, anecdotal evidence indicates a lack of adequate coordination between the health and educational systems, which leads to further delay in children accessing care.

Potential Challenges of Importing Tools

One may argue that there are various well-validated screening and diagnostic tools from high-income countries that can be "imported" for use in RPSs (See Campi, Lord, and Grzadzinski, Chapter 2, this volume, for a detailed discussion on screening tools.) One obvious advantage of using well-known measures such as the Autism Diagnostic Observation Schedule (ADOS; Lord et al., 2000) and Autism Diagnostic Interview–Revised (ADI-R; Rutter, Le Couteur, Lord, & Faggioli, 2005) is that these tools can help harmonize the language used to diagnose and discuss ASD (de Vries, 2016). However, as described below, imported measures may have questionable validity (Greenfield, 1997). Similar challenges have also been reported when measures developed for a majority population in a country (e.g., measures developed for white middle-class families) were being used with minority populations or those with low income or limited literacy (Kimple, Bartelt, Wysocki, & Steiner, 2014; Janvier, Coffield, Harris, Mandell, & Cidav, 2019).

To guide our discussions, we use data from qualitative studies recently conducted at the Kenyan coast (Mombasa and Kilifi) and Dar-es-Salaam, Tanzania. These studies involved a total of 81 participants. At the Kenyan coast (largely in Kilifi, a rural area), we carried out in-depth interviews with 30 parents who were part of an ongoing cohort study to validate the Kiswahili translation of the Autism Diagnostic Observation Schedule, Second Edition (ADOS-2; Lord et al., 2000) and the Social Communication Questionnaire (SCQ; Rutter, Bailey, & Lord, 2003). In Tanzania, 51 participants (parents, teachers, social workers, and clinicians), all residing in Dar-es-Salaam, an urban area, took part in in-depth interviews and focus group discussions (FGDs). The samples from Kenya and Tanzania differ in two significant ways. First, the Kenyan sample consisted mainly of rural dwellers, while the Tanzanian one is largely made up of urban dwellers. Additionally, since the Tanzanian study also sampled professionals, the Tanzanian sample had a higher socioeconomic status (SES).

The purposes of these discussions were (1) to elicit the day-to-day experiences of children in relation to tasks presented in the ADOS-2; and (2) to capture the perceptions of participants regarding the cultural appropriateness and acceptability of the ADOS-2 tasks. The ADOS-2 is used as an example for two reasons. First, it is the tool of choice for translation and adaptation into Swahili, given that it is one of the most widely used observational tools for evaluating ASD; and second, the ADOS is considered by many researchers to be the "gold-standard" observational tool in ASD diagnosis. Table 11.1 presents a sample of the tasks from the ADOS relevant to our discussions. We use these examples acknowledging that ADOS scores are not based on a single task and that there are several tasks within the measure that are familiar to children from different sociocultural contexts.

Potential Pitfalls in Importing Tools

The history of psychological/psychiatric assessment, be it cognitive, behavioral, clinical, or personality assessment, is heavily influenced by tool development in Western countries (herein used to refer mainly to North America and western Europe). Understandably, test materials and assessment approaches are largely influenced by the cultural and contextual factors

TABLE 11.1. A Sample of the Tasks from the ADOS Relevant to Our Discussions

Task	Sample items	A summary of how the task is administered
Free play	Multiple pop-up toys, board books, toy telephone, music box, jack-in-a-box, dump truck, and baby doll with eyes that open and close	Some of the toys are placed on the table while other toys are placed on the floor. The child is allowed to play with the items as he or she chooses.
Functional and symbolic play	Birthday party items, toy car, toy figures, toy cup, toy airplane, and toy flower	Items are presented to the child in a sequence closely mirroring a birthday party, and the child is encouraged to join in.
Description of a picture	U.S. map scene, feast scene, and resort scene	The child is shown a picture and is allowed to make a story out of the picture.
Demonstration task	None, or towel and soap if needed	The assessor asks the child to tell and show how to brush his or her teeth using an imaginary sink. If this task is too complex for the child to carry out, then the child can use the alternative task of washing his or her face.

within the test developer milieu (Gopaul-McNicol & Armour-Thomas, 2002). For example, in developing measures of childhood neurodevelopment, most test developers used materials that would be relevant for children in their settings, such as climbing stairs to check motor balance and using spoons and forks for adaptive behavior. Although using spoons and forks is a normal part of day-to-day culture in Western countries, in many cultures, especially in Africa, people use their hands to eat, while in others, eating with chopsticks is the norm. Psychometric instruments that use country-specific habits to elicit the behavioral patterns of interest may therefore have limited validity elsewhere because of habits unfamiliar to individuals from other cultural contexts.

Introducing tests developed in one context to a new context risks the introduction of cultural bias. Bias refers to a situation whereby interindividual or intercultural differences and variations in test performance arise from factors that are unrelated to the construct being examined (He & van de Vijver, 2012). van de Vijver and Poortinga (1997) presented a taxonomy of bias that provides the basis of our discussions. They argued that bias can come from three sources: construct, method, and item. We discuss each of these forms of bias using examples from our work.

Construct Bias

Construct bias arises when the theoretical underpinning of a measure does not fully capture the full behavioral repertoire of the construct of interest (He & van de Vijver, 2012). Construct bias may arise from various sources, such as items that are irrelevant within the new cultural context or the absence of items that would be relevant in the new cultural context. For example, the African child's ability to participate in age-appropriate household chores, such as being sent to the shops and caregiving for siblings, is taken to be an indicator of developmental levels (Gladstone et al., 2010; Kambalametore, Hartley, & Lansdown, 2000), but that may not be the case in a Western context. Additionally, cultural bias may occur if the items in the scale only partially capture the behavioral repertoire relevant to the construct being studied, implying that other aspects of the construct are not being measured (He & van de Vijver, 2012). Little research on ASD and its behavioral manifestations has been carried out in other parts of the world to allow for a full evaluation of the degree to which construct bias may exist in the current ASD screening and diagnostic tools.

Method Bias

Method bias refers to the extent to which procedures, samples, and approaches used to collect and interpret data may compromise the validity of the test results (Abubakar, 2015). Three potential procedural aspects may contribute to method bias: sample characteristics, stimuli and materials used, and administration procedures (He & van de Vijver, 2012). Sample characteristics may influence the test administration and standardization process. A good example is the literacy levels and reading habits of a sample. In Western countries, literacy levels are high. Consequently, a written procedure is the standard mode for administering questionnaires for screening for ASD such as the SCQ (Rutter et al., 2003). However, in populations with low literacy levels and lack of experience with written questionnaires, this approach is potentially problematic (D'Alonzo, 2011; Kara et al., 2014). An example of this problem was reported in Turkey, where an attempt to administer the Modified Checklist for Autism in Toddlers (M-CHAT) in a written format resulted in a high proportion of false positives (Kara et al., 2014). Given these observations, in settings such as the one we work in and other similar settings in Africa, we largely administer questionnaires that were originally developed as written questionnaires in an oral format with trained interviewers. When switching from a written to an oral procedure, the equivalence of the two modes of administration cannot be assumed. Earlier studies indicate that the way a questionnaire is administered can significantly impact the way people respond to the questions (Bowling, 2005; Li, Ford, Zhao, Tsai, & Balluz, 2012), although some have argued that the effect is relatively small (Wettergren, Mattsson, & von Essen, 2011). For instance, Bowling noted that the mode of questionnaire administration influences the response quality due to various factors, including the level of cognitive demands placed on the respondent. He observed that a charismatic and skilled interviewer may help a respondent recall more information, compared to what he or she would have done if a self-completion questionnaire was being carried out (Bowling, 2005). Another factor is the level of anonymity and privacy afforded to participants in the different forms of responding, which may have an influence on evaluation apprehension. In dealing with sensitive topics, mode of questionnaire administration may become an important confounder (D'Ancona, 2014; Hanmer, Hays, & Fryback, 2007).

Samples may also differ in their experiences and exposure even when they share the same cultural context. Thus, one would expect significant differences between rural and urban groups and between groups of low and high SES. These differences may relate to literacy levels, living standards, and exposure to modern amenities inter alia. In Africa, the impact of rural versus urban residence and SES on performance on ASD tests has yet to be studied. Research in North America indicates that ASD screening tools may perform differently when applied to disadvantaged groups in rural settings (Scarpa et al., 2013). The authors noted that the M-CHAT had an unacceptably low internal consistency score for groups with low educational level and among ethnic minority members. This observation calls into question the validity of the M-CHAT for these groups (Scarpa et al., 2013).

A number of other sample characteristics are relevant in the context of autism assessment. When using parent-report measures, their child's developmental expectations are known to be influenced by cultural background. Studies indicate that parents from different cultural contexts can differ in their developmental expectations (Durgel, van de Vijver, & Yagmurlu, 2013; Pachter & Dworkin, 1997). Durgel and colleagues (2013), in their comparison of Dutch, Turkish-Dutch, and Turkish mothers, found that Dutch mothers tended to believe that children learn certain skills and behaviors at an earlier age than did Turkish and Turkish-Dutch mothers. They also found that mothers with more education expected earlier development. These differences in expectations in achievement of milestones and what children can do may influence parental perceptions of developmental delay.

Stimulus unfamiliarity and its influence on task performance have received considerable attention in cross-cultural research. Observations in the field of cognition indicate that a significant difference in task performance among cultural groups can be explained by either stimulus or task unfamiliarity; performance on cognitive instruments tends to be higher when the test developer and test taker have the same cultural background (Malda, van de Vijver, & Temane, 2010). However, the relevance of familiarity extends beyond the cognitive domain. In measures of ASD, it is not uncommon to come across tasks and materials that are unfamiliar to children in Africa, especially those in rural settings. For instance, in the ADOS-2, a "birthday party" task is used to elicit social communication skills and to examine the functional or symbolic use of materials (Lord et al., 2000). The steps for setting up the birthday task include use of a doll as the "baby" who is having a birthday, preparing a pretend cake with play dough, inserting pretend candles, blowing out the candles, singing a "happy birthday" song, and other steps before the baby is put to sleep. The "social presses" are based on the child's ability to follow the procedures and anticipate the next moves. To be able to carry out these next moves, the child would need to be familiar with the steps taken during the birthday party. In our in-depth interviews at the Kenyan coast, we asked the parents if their children had attended any birthday parties previously. We observed that most (57%; $n = 17/30$) children in the Kenyan sample had never attended any birthday party and that most of them who had attended did not have much experience with such events. Consequently, it can be expected that they may be totally unfamiliar with this task. Earlier studies in cross-cultural assessment of cognitive skills indicate that when children's abilities are evaluated using tasks and stimulus material that are not familiar to them, they are likely to underperform. Interestingly, among parents interviewed in Dar-es-Salaam, an urban setting in Tanzania, 98% ($n = 50/51$) indicated that their children were familiar with a birthday party. This observation emphasizes the differences between rural and urban participants in their degree of exposure to Westernization, providing another example of sample bias. As one group of teachers noted in their comments regarding birthdays "[Birthday parties are] mostly held in urban areas, not so common in rural though. In Dar it is getting increasingly common and kids love it" (teachers, FGD). In fact, some of the participants suggested that even if the child had not attended a birthday party, the child would have seen it on television: "Currently, especially in urban areas they [birthday parties] are common, even if a child has never been to one they would know as they may have seen it on TV" (parent of a child with ASD, in-depth interview).

Our qualitative work indicated that pretend play was common and that we can easily identify culturally appropriate examples for use in East African settings. Common tasks included playing "classroom scenes of a teacher instructing students" and "family scenes of mother preparing meals." Materials used included many items that came from children's environments. Figure 11.1 shows some of the materials used, such as coconut copra, stones, and sand used as part of a pretend game where children are preparing a meal.

Similarly, unfamiliar materials can be problematic. For instance, the ADOS includes a task where children are required to tell and demonstrate how to brush their teeth. A set sequence is used to administer this task. The examiner will tell the children to assume that the examiner does not know how to brush their teeth and that they need to "teach" the examiner how (Lord et al., 2000). Then the examiner will indicate a toothbrush and toothpaste, a tap with cold and hot water, and a glass. The instruction is to start from the beginning and "tell me and show me how to brush my teeth." In the sample from the Kenyan coast, we observed that 93% (*n* = 28/30) of the families did not have any sink for brushing their teeth. The participating families brushed their teeth in different open-air places

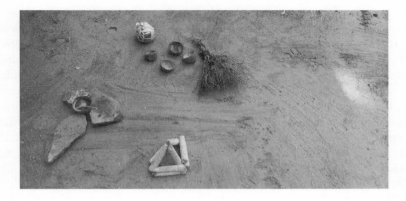

FIGURE 11.1. Some of the materials used as part of a meal preparation game.

within the compound, such as under a tree. In Dar-es-Salaam, 49% (n = 25/51) of the participants had a sink for brushing their teeth within the house. Therefore, children not familiar with the sequence may find it difficult to replicate the appropriate storyline and gestures. For example, in Kilifi where some children sometimes use stick toothbrushes cut from tree branches to clean their teeth or may brush their teeth under a tree with no sink, they will have limited options to elaborate speech and gestures. Using this task runs the risk that the "social press" for descriptive gestures (the primary purpose of the task) may not necessarily elicit the typical gestures expected in tooth brushing, thereby potentially reducing the likelihood of seeing a range of descriptive and/or other gestures.

The presence of a sink or birthday parties in the child's life may be strongly related to SES. However, other tasks may be more closely related to parental beliefs and cultural factors. For instance, the reading task may be a cultural factor. Children are expected in the ADOS to tell a story based on picture books. Many African cultures are largely oral. Therefore, children may grow up with very limited access to, or familiarity with, picture books (Holding, Abubakar, van Baar, Obiero, & van de Vijver, 2011). At the Kenyan coast, 83% (n = 25/30) of the children did not own picture books, and 93% (n = 28/30) of parents had not read stories to their children. In Dar-es-Salaam, 88% (n = 42/51) had not read to their children. As some of the parents noted, "Reading only happens at school. Not common to read in our culture, but we tell stories of the past or someone's experience and inspiration. At home it's time for house chores" [Teacher, FGD]. For children not exposed to school and even for those in school where reading to the class is not a daily task, psychological assessments that require them to read a storyline may be too unfamiliar and difficult for them.

Item Bias

A measure or a scale may be biased due to problems at item level (van de Vijver & Poortinga, 1997). Issues may arise if the item translations are not sufficiently rigorous and do not exclude ambiguous and awkward item wording (van de Vijver, & Poortinga, 1997). Even when the translation process is rigorous, challenges are likely to arise owing to lack of equivalent words or phrases in a different language. If words can be translated, care has to be taken that the translations are equivalent; that is, the items must be conceptually (psychologically) equivalent and not just literally (linguistically) equivalent (Holding, Abubakar, & Kitsao-Wekulo, 2008). For instance, in the SCQ, item 6 uses the term *rituals*, which in Swahili rituals translates to *tambiko*; the linguistic equivalence of the two words is adequate. However, the term *tambiko* is imbued with a specific cultural connotation. In the Swahili context, it is largely associated with rites and rituals carried out within the context of African traditional religious practices.

These practices sometimes carry negative connotations associated with superstition and witchcraft, among others. Therefore, using this term in a questionnaire may offend parents or influence their perceptions of causes of ASD, or even their health-seeking pattern. While *tambiko* and rituals mean the same thing literally, the conceptual meaning is totally different in this context.

A recent publication from the United States provides yet another example of the diagnostic problem that may arise during translation. The study by Kimple and colleagues (2014) observed that, unexpectedly, the Spanish version of the M-CHAT had significantly higher screening rates than the English version (23.6% vs. 11.3%). For reasons that are not entirely clear, Spanish-speaking mothers endorsed some items more than others. This led the authors to conclude that "Spanish M-CHAT questionnaires are abnormal more often than those in English even after changing to appropriate translation, despite lower prevalence of autism in Latinos. Issues with translation, interpretation, or cultural understanding of behaviors may contribute" (Kimple et al., 2014, p. 632).

Challenges Related to Resource Availability

The challenges of diagnosis go beyond those related to sociocultural factors and include resource availability. In Sub-Saharan Africa (SSA), the disease burden of both communicable and noncommunicable conditions is extremely high. This implies that health professionals are often overwhelmed by work and often lack specialized training and knowledge in areas such as ASD and other areas of child development that are yet to be considered high priority areas (Bakare & Munir, 2011; Igwe, Ahanotu, Bakare, Achor, & Igwe, 2011). The situation is no better in the education sector, where teachers have a heavy workload and lack training, particularly in areas such as ASD and other neurodevelopmental disorders (Abubakar et al., 2016). Given this lack of trained personnel, the implementation of a multidisciplinary team to carry out screening and diagnostic procedures remains a challenge. Earlier studies have indicated that part of the challenge in screening and diagnosis of ASD lies in low levels of awareness both in the general population and among health care workers. For instance, Bakare and Munir (2011) noted that "level of knowledge and awareness about autism spectrum disorder is low among the general population and health care workers in Africa. There is need for community education of the general population and continuous medical education for health care workers on issues relating to autism spectrum disorder. This would enhance early recognition and interventions and in turn improve prognosis" (p. 191). The situation is further compounded by the fact that many well-validated ASD measures are not open access (Durkin et al., 2015). Therefore, users have to pay per use and sometimes have to spend extra costs for translations and validation into local languages. This high economic burden may make it difficult for researchers in low- and middle-income countries to use these measures (Durkin et al., 2015).

Potential Solutions

Adapting Existing Tools

What should we do given the set of problems highlighted? We suggest a five-step approach that can be used to evaluate and adapt or develop measures for ASD that are contextually relevant and culturally appropriate, and possess good psychometric properties. The steps are based on various guidelines published in the field of cross-cultural psychology as well as on a four-step approach previously used in Kilifi, Kenya (Abubakar, 2008). With this approach in Kilifi, we found excellent reliability and validity of the measures we have developed (Abubakar, Holding, van Baar, Newton, & van de Vijver, 2008).

Three key factors form the core of this proposed methodology:

1. Mixed-methods approaches, where both qualitative and quantitative strategies are used during different stages of test development to ensure cultural relevancy and diagnostic fidelity.
2. Community participation, where participation not only allows for the development of culturally and contextually relevant measures, but also allows for the development of a working partnership between communities and scientists (Abubakar, van de Vijver, van Baar, Kitsao-Wekulo, & Holding, 2010).
3. Detailed documentation of the process, where the process of tool adaptation and evaluation needs to be well documented to allow for a thorough evaluation of the process and continuous improvement of scales and procedures.

In the next section we will briefly discuss each of these steps (Figure 11.2 summarizes these steps).

Step 1: Construct Clarification

The aim of this step is to clarify the range of items that are required to evaluate the construct of interest. This step ensures that both evidence-based scientific information and local perceptions and idioms for the symptoms are adequately captured early in the development of tools. A mixed-methods approach is usually recommended (Abubakar, 2015). First, a thorough review of the literature and available scales is needed to evaluate available

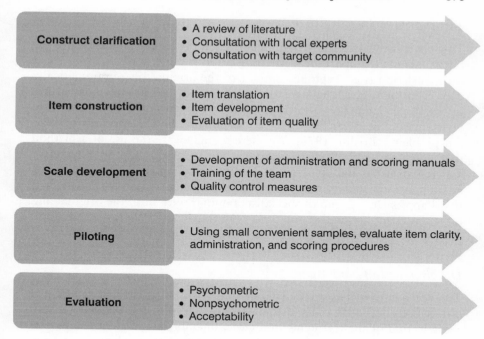

FIGURE 11.2. Five-step approach to adapting and developing measures for use across cultural contexts.

scales and their pros and cons. Moreover, this review process evaluates the extent to which the different measures have worked in other cultural contexts. Lastly, an extensive review of the existing scales highlights the three basic options in scale development: (1) choose one scale and make adaptations to it; (2) choose items from different scales and formulate a new scale; or (3) use existing theoretical frameworks to start from scratch in developing the required scales (Abubakar, 2015). The second involves consultation with local experts and communities. The aims of this consultation are to understand the local perceptions of the problem (or the attitudes, behaviors, and cognitions about a topic), identify the idioms used to describe the problem, and evaluate the extent to which existing tools and scales can be used to describe the problem.

Step 2: Item Construction

Item development can take different forms, depending on whether existing items can be translated and/or new items have to be developed.

Translation of Existing Items

This process involves transferring items from the source language into the target language. Importantly, the translation process needs to ensure that the translation is conceptually similar to the original one, grammatically correct in the target language, and easy to read, and also sounds natural in the target language. The translation–back translation approaches are widely used, but as early as 1970, it was noted to be a method with potential problems (Brislin, 1970). We therefore advocate the use of a method that combines both back translations and a "discussion by a panel of experts" or use of multiple, independent forward translations (followed by an adjudication session) to ensure high-fidelity translation. Typically, in a panel approach, a group of specialists familiar with both the original and target language, a linguist, and those who translated the measure meet and discuss the translations with an aim of harmonizing the translations.

Development of New Items

The decision to include new items should be based on the items identified during consultation with local communities. The process should document the selection of the test items in a clear, unambiguous manner. The process of developing adequate items is especially important when one is using items to be used in different linguistic and cultural contexts. Items that are short, with few if any idioms, and limited use of negations are easier to translate.

Evaluation of the Quality of the Translated and Developed Items

The purpose of this stage is to evaluate the extent to which developed and translated items meet some of the a priori set criteria such as clarity, feasibility of being administered, ease of comprehension, and conceptual clarity. Various methods exist for pretesting and piloting developed items. Methods such as cognitive interviewing (Willis, 2005) and the use of bilingual individuals can be useful in helping to investigate the degree to which the translated items are equivalent and identify faulty items early.

Step 3: Scale Development

This phase aims at ensuring that items are assembled into a proper scale. The process of scale development is important for deciding aspects such as scoring procedures and refining the administration procedures. The development of high-quality items is not sufficient; the administration procedure should also be standardized as much as possible, considering the limitations of RPSs (such as the unavailability of a quiet room to administer the test). Aspects such as the development of administration manuals and training programs are crucial to ensure quality.

Step 4: Piloting

The developed materials, including items, procedures, stimuli, and even training manuals, need to be field tested to ensure that they are performing as expected. Pilot testing, cognitive interviewing, and similar procedures may be used in an iterative manner so that initially formulated items or administration procedures are optimized in sequential steps (Malda et al., 2008).

Step 5: Evaluation

Both psychometric and nonpsychometric approaches are important in evaluating the quality of the developed scales. Key psychometric aspects to be evaluated include reliability and validity, especially clinical validity, sensitivity, and specificity. Nonpsychometric evaluation is advocated because it allows for the identification and evaluation of contextual factors, with a bearing on test scores. Among nonpsychometric approaches suggested for inclusion are observation of the person testing, feedback from participants, and observation of test-taking behavior, including time to take the test and participant reaction to test materials and procedures.

Development of Global Open-Access Measures

The first approach discussed in this chapter provides a piecemeal solution to the challenges of identification and diagnosis in low- and middle-income countries. However, there is a need for a more coordinated and collaborative approach. Piecemeal adaptation of tools tends to provide solutions to the needs of individual researchers at that specific moment but does not address the larger picture. To address some of the current concerns in the field there is a need to work toward open access tools and measures. Durkin et al. (2015) in an opinion piece noted that assessment of ASD could benefit a lot from the open-source software development movement where much gain has been made in ensuring that people from different regions of the world have access to statistical tools.

Open-access sources tools that can serve most people need to be developed in a culturally decentered or multicentered way. In this context, the tool developers will work from a global perceptive and seek to ensure that whatever tool they develop can be used across cultural contexts, and more importantly, the tool can be used by people with different levels of expertise. The development and pilot testing of such a tool would involve professionals and practitioners from different regions of the world to ensure its validity across contexts.

Conclusions

In this chapter, we highlighted some of the problems involved in importing ASD tools developed for Western countries for use in Africa. We focused on the practical steps and solutions to ensuring the validity of the imported scales. Developing adequate screening and diagnostic tools for SSA is an important step in ensuring that children receive early and adequate diagnosis, quantifying the burden of ASD in Africa, and setting up services for children and their families with ASD. The saliency of this chapter lies in its ability to provide practical solutions for those who want to develop scales for low- and middle-income countries, both for evaluating neurodevelopmental disorders and for other general health measures. Although much of the information we described refers specifically to autism, the principles underlying our approach, combining cultural sensitivity to sound practice in instrument development, can be applied more broadly in assessments made in low- and middle-income countries.

REFERENCES

Abubakar, A. (2008). *Infant–toddler development in a multiple risk environment in Kenya*. Ridderker, the Netherlands: Ridderprint.

Abubakar, A. (2015). Equivalence and transfer problems in cross-cultural research. In J. D. Wright (Ed.), *International encyclopedia of the social and behavioral sciences* (2nd ed., pp. 929–933). New York: Elsevier.

Abubakar, A., Holding, P., van Baar, A., Newton, C., & van de Vijver, F. J. (2008). Monitoring psychomotor development in a resource limited setting: An evaluation of the Kilifi Developmental Inventory. *Annals of Tropical Paediatrics: International Child Health, 28*, 217–226.

Abubakar, A., Ssewanyana, D., de Vries, P. J., & Newton, C. R. (2016). Autism spectrum disorders in sub-saharan Africa. *The Lancet Psychiatry, 3*(9), 800–802.

Abubakar, A., van de Vijver, F. J., van Baar, A., Kitsao-Wekulo, P., & Holding, P. (2010). Enhancing psychological assessment in sub-Saharan Africa through participant consultation. In A. Gari & K. Mylonas, *From Herodotus' ethnographic journeys to cross-cultural research* (pp. 169–178). Athens: Pedio Books.

American Psychiatric Association. (2013). *Diagnostic and statistical manual of mental disorders* (5th ed.). Arlington, VA: Author.

Bakare, M. O., & Munir, K. M. (2011). Autism spectrum disorders in Africa. In M. Mohammadi (Ed.), *A comprehensive book on autism spectrum disorders* (pp. 183–195). London: InTechOpen.

Baxter, A. J., Brugha, T., Erskine, H., Scheurer, R., Vos, T., & Scott, J. (2015). The epidemiology and global burden of autism spectrum disorders. *Psychological Medicine, 45,* 601–613.

Bowling, A. (2005). Mode of questionnaire administration can have serious effects on data quality. *Journal of Public Health, 27,* 281–291.

Brislin, R. W. (1970). Back-translation for cross-cultural research. *Journal of Cross-Cultural Psychology, 1,* 185–216.

D'Alonzo, K. T. (2011). Evaluation and revision of questionnaires for use among low-literacy immigrant Latinos. *Revista latino-americana de enfermagem, 19*(5), 1255–1264.

D'Ancona, M. Á. C. (2014). Measuring xenophobia: Social desirability and survey mode effects. *Migration Studies, 2*(2), 255–280.

de Vries, P. J. (2016). Thinking globally to meet local needs: Autism spectrum disorders in Africa and other low resource environments. *Current Opinion in Neurology, 29*(2), 130–136.

Durgel, E. S., van de Vijver, F. J., & Yagmurlu, B. (2013). Self-reported maternal expectations and child-rearing practices: Disentangling the associations with ethnicity, immigration, and educational background. *International Journal of Behavioral Development, 37,* 35–43.

Durkin, M. S., Elsabbagh, M., Barbaro, J., Gladstone, M., Happe, F., Hoekstra, R. A., . . . Shih, A. (2015). Autism screening and diagnosis in low resource settings: Challenges and opportunities to enhance research and services worldwide. *Autism Research, 8*(5), 473–476.

Elsabbagh, M., Divan, G., Koh, Y. J., Kim, Y. S., Kauchali, S., Marcín, C., . . . Wang, C. (2012). Global prevalence of autism and other pervasive developmental disorders. *Autism Research, 5,* 160–179.

Franz, L., Chambers, N., von Isenburg, M., & de Vries, P. J. (2017). Autism spectrum disorder in sub-Saharan Africa: A comprehensive scoping review. *Autism Research, 10*(5), 723–749.

Gladstone, M., Lancaster, G., Umar, E., Nyirenda, M., Kayira, E., van den Broek, N., & Smyth, R. (2010). Perspectives of normal child development in rural Malawi—a qualitative analysis to create a more culturally appropriate developmental assessment tool. *Child: Care, Health and Development, 36,* 346–353.

Gopaul-McNicol, S., & Armour-Thomas, E. (2002). *Assessment and culture.* New York: Academic Press.

Greenfield, P. M. (1997). You can't take it with you: Why ability assessments don't cross cultures. *American Psychologist, 52*(10), 1115–1124.

Hanmer, J., Hays, R. D., & Fryback, D. G. (2007). Mode of administration is important in U.S. national estimates of health-related quality of life. *Medical Care, 45,* 1171–1179.

He, J., & van de Vijver, F. (2012). Bias and equivalence in cross-cultural research. *Online Readings in Psychology and Culture, 2,* 8.

Holding, P., Abubakar, A., & Kitsao-Wekulo, P. (2008). A systematic approach to test and questionnaire adaptations in an African context. Paper presented at 3 MC conference. Retrieved from *http://csdiworkshop.org/v2/index.php/118-2008-3mc-conference/2008-presentations/session-9.*

Holding, P., Abubakar, A., van Baar, A., Obiero, E., & van de Vijver, F. J. R. (2011). Validation of the Infant–Toddler HOME Inventory among households in low income communities at the Kenyan Coast. In *Rendering borders obsolete* (pp. 194–206). Bremen, Germany: International Association for Cross-Cultural Psychology.

Igwe, M. N., Ahanotu, A. C., Bakare, M. O., Achor, J. U., & Igwe, C. (2011). Assessment of knowledge about childhood autism among paediatric and psychiatric nurses in Ebonyi state, Nigeria. *Child and Adolescent Psychiatry and Mental Health, 5*(1), 1.

Janvier, Y. M., Coffield, C. N., Harris, J. F., Mandell, D. S., & Cidav, Z. (2019). The developmental check-in: Development and initial testing of an autism screening tool targeting young children from underserved communities. *Autism, 23*(3), 689–698.

Kambalametore, S., Hartley, S., & Lansdown, R. (2000). An exploration of the Malawian perspective on children's everyday skills: Implications for assessment. *Disability and Rehabilitation, 22*(17), 802–807.

Kara, B., Mukaddes, N. M., Altınkaya, I., Güntepe, D., Gökçay, G., & Özmen, M. (2014). Using the Modified Checklist for Autism in Toddlers in a well-child clinic in Turkey: Adapting the screening method based on culture and setting. *Autism, 18*, 331–338.

Kimple, K. S., Bartelt, E. A., Wysocki, K. L., & Steiner, M. J. (2014). Performance of the modified checklist for autism in toddlers in Spanish-speaking patients. *Clinical Pediatrics, 53*(7), 632–638.

Li, C., Ford, E. S., Zhao, G., Tsai, J., & Balluz, L. S. (2012). A comparison of depression prevalence estimates measured by the Patient Health Questionnaire with two administration modes: Computer-assisted telephone interviewing versus computer-assisted personal interviewing. *International Journal of Public Health, 57*, 225–233.

Lord, C., Risi, S., Lambrecht, L., Cook, E. H., Jr., Leventhal, B. L., DiLavore, P. C., . . . Rutter, M. (2000). The Autism Diagnostic Observation Schedule—Generic: A standard measure of social and communication deficits associated with the spectrum of autism. *Journal of Autism and Developmental Disorders, 30*, 205–223.

Malda, M., van de Vijver, F. J. R., Srinivasan, K., Transler, C., Sukumar, P., & Rao, K. (2008). Adapting a cognitive test for a different culture: An illustration of qualitative procedures. *Psychology Science Quarterly, 50*, 451–468.

Malda, M., van de Vijver, F. J., & Temane, Q. M. (2010). Rugby versus soccer in South Africa: Content familiarity contributes to cross-cultural differences in cognitive test scores. *Intelligence, 38*, 582–595.

Manji, K., & Hogan, M. (2014). Identifying gaps in knowledge, prevalence and care of children with autism spectrum disorder in Tanzania–a qualitative review article. *Tanzania Medical Journal, 26*, 7–17.

Pachter, L. M., & Dworkin, P. H. (1997). Maternal expectations about normal child development in 4 cultural groups. *Archives of Pediatrics and Adolescent Medicine, 151*, 1144–1150.

Rutter, M., Bailey, A., & Lord, C. (2003). *The Social Communication Questionnaire: Manual.* Los Angeles: Western Psychological Services.

Rutter, M., Le Couteur, A., Lord, C., & Faggioli, R. (2005). *ADI-R: Autism Diagnostic Interview—Revised: Manual.* Florence, Italy: Organizzazioni speciali (OS).

Scarpa, A., Reyes, N. M., Patriquin, M. A., Lorenzi, J., Hassenfeldt, T. A., Desai, V. J., & Kerkering, K. W. (2013). The modified checklist for autism in toddlers: Reliability in a diverse rural American sample. *Journal of Autism and Developmental Disorders, 43*, 2269–2279.

van de Vijver, F. J., & Poortinga, Y. H. (1997). Towards an integrated analysis of bias in cross-cultural assessment. *European Journal of Psychological Assessment, 13,* 29.

Varma, A., & Iskandar, J. W. (2014). Challenges in diagnosis of autism and the struggle of using Western screening tools in different cultures psychiatrists perspective. *Indian Pediatrics, 51,* 356–357.

Wettergren, L., Mattsson, E., & von Essen, L. (2011). Mode of administration only has a small effect on data quality and self-reported health status and emotional distress among Swedish adolescents and young adults. *Journal of Clinical Nursing, 20,* 1568–1577.

Willis, G. B. (2005). *Cognitive interviewing: A tool for improving questionnaire design.* London: SAGE.

Index

Note. *f* or *t* following a page number indicates a figure or a table.

Mobile technologies, 315. *See also*
Technology
Modified Checklist for Autism in Toddlers
(M-CHAT and M-CHAT-R/F)
health care and, 279–281
overview, 48*t*, 53–55, 67
preemptive intervention and, 258
resource-poor settings (RPSs) and, 369,
373
technology and, 314–315, 316
Monitoring
of media usage, 335
technology and, 322–333, 337
Monitoring activities of others, 91
Motor activity regulation, 89
Motor skills
developmental processes and, 183–184
motor control, 254
strength and musculature and, 302–303
technology and, 303–305, 304*t*
Mullen Scales of Early Learning (MSEL)
atypical brain development in at-risk
infants, 210
early interventions and, 136, 137, 139,
258
overview, 101–102
preemptive intervention and, 258
siblings of children with ASD, 171, 183
TOBY (Therapy Outcomes by You) app
and, 124
Multimedia technologies, 316–322,
332–333. *See also* Technology
Musculature, 302–303

N

National Institute for Health and Care
Excellence (NICE), 43–44
Natural history markers, 249
Naturalistic developmental behavioral
interventions (NDBIs), 125–126
Negative Affectivity domain of
temperament, 90
Negative emotional reactivity, 175–176. *See
also* Reactivity
Negative Emotionality domain of
temperament, 91
Negative predictive value (NPV), 279

NEPSY-II, 233–234
Neurological factors. *See also* Brain
development and functioning
language development and, 102–103
neurological model of autism, 16
overview, 4
parent–child interaction and, 252
personalization of interventions and,
151
preemptive intervention and, 262
technology and, 317
Nondevelopmental approaches to
intervention, 250–251. *See also*
Interventions
Nonverbal communication. *See also*
Communication development;
Nonverbal development
adaptive functioning and, 104
alternative and augmentative
communication (AAC) systems and,
330–333
early interventions and, 120
toddlers with ASD and, 97–103
Nonverbal development. *See also*
Language development; Nonverbal
communication
attentional development and, 180
siblings of children with ASD, 183–184
toddlers with ASD and, 94–95

O

Observation, clinician. *See* Clinician
observation
Observation Scale for Autism (OSA), 48*t*,
64, 67
Observational learning
technology and, 335–336
temperament and, 91
Open-access measures, 377–378
Outcomes of siblings at risk. *See also*
Siblings
future directions and, 241–242
longer-term follow-up studies of,
228–239, 236*t*–238*t*
overview, 226–227, 239–241
preemptive intervention and, 267–268
relevance of, 227–228